T0383628

MAINTENANCE PHARMACOTHERAPIES FOR NEUROPSYCHIATRIC DISORDERS

MAINTENANCE PHARMACOTHERAPIES FOR NEUROPSYCHIATRIC DISORDERS

Stephanie S. Richards, M.D.
William S. Musser, M.D.
Samuel Gershon, M.D.

USA	Publishing Office:	BRUNNER/MAZEL *A member of the Taylor & Francis Group* 325 Chestnut Street Philadelphia, PA 19106 Tel: (215) 625-8900 Fax: (215) 625-2940
	Distribution Center:	BRUNNER/MAZEL *A member of the Taylor & Francis Group* 47 Runway Road, Suite G Levittown, PA 19057 Tel: (215) 269-0400 Fax: (215) 269-0363
UK		BRUNNER/MAZEL *A member of the Taylor & Francis Group* 1 Gunpowder Square London EC4A 3DE Tel: +44 171 583 0490 Fax: +44 171 583 0581

MAINTENANCE PHARMACOTHERAPIES FOR NEUROPSYCHIATRIC DISORDERS

1 2 3 4 5 6 7 8 9 0

Printed by Edwards Brothers, Ann Arbor, MI, 1998.

A CIP catalog record for this book is available from the British Library.
⊗ The paper in this publication meets the requirements of the ANSI Standard Z39.48-1984 (Permanence of Paper).

Library of Congress Cataloging-in-Publication Data

Richards, Stephanie.
    Maintenance pharmacotherapies for neuropsychiatric disorders/by
Stephanie Richards, William Musser, Samuel Gershon.
        p.   cm.
    Includes bibliographical references and index.
    ISBN 0–87630–894–9 (alk. paper)
    1. Mental illness—Chemotherapy—Handbooks, manuals, etc.
2. Psychopharmacology—Handbooks, manuals, etc. 3. Nervous System—
Diseases—Chemotherapy—Handbooks, manuals, etc. I. Musser,
William. II. Gershon, Samuel. III. Title.
    [DNLM: 1. Mental Disorders—drug therapy handbooks. 2. Mental
Disorders—prevention & control handbooks. 3. Nervous System
Diseases—drug therapy handbooks. 4. Nervous System Diseases—
prevention & control handbooks. WM 34 R518m 1999]
RC483.R   1999
616.89′ 18—dc21
DNLM/DLC
for Library of Congress   98–45218
                                                                                          CIP

ISBN 0-87630-894-9 (case)

CONTENTS

PREFACE

This book is designed as a reference handbook for those clinicians who treat patients with chronic neuropsychiatric disorders. In the changing health care environment, more of these patients will be the responsibility of primary care physicians and associated health professionals. We do not attempt to address acute treatment but rather focus on maintenance treatment; that is, long-term treatment beginning six months after remission of an acute episode with the goal to prevent recurrence. We have assembled guidelines and treatment recommendations based on a critical review of the existing literature on maintenance therapy for each disorder. We give guidelines on choice of medications particularly for patients with comorbid medical and psychiatric illness and patients taking other medications. We also provide guidelines for recognizing and managing adverse reactions, treating acute exacerbations, and treating nonresponders.

This book is intended not just for psychiatrists and neurologists, but also for primary care physicians (i.e., internists and family practitioners) who treat the majority of patients with mental illness. This book also will be useful for nonphysicians who care for patients with neuropsychiatric disorders including psychologists, mental health specialists, physician's assistants, and nurse practitioners.

ACKNOWLEDGMENTS

We express our special thanks to Carol Harris for preparing and typing the manuscripts. Her dedication to every detail of this project as well as her role in marshalling information from the authors ensured its high quality. We also wish to thank Benoit Mulsant, M.D., Carl Shapiro, D.O., Richard Siegel, M.D., Edward Slagle, M.D., David Tesar, M.D., and Norbert Weikers, M.D. for their assistance and critical reviews of various chapters.

MAINTENANCE
PHARMACOTHERAPIES
  FOR
NEUROPSYCHIATRIC
DISORDERS

INTRODUCTION: ROLE OF MAINTENANCE PHARMACOTHERAPY

Mental illness is a major health concern in the United States. Several groups have undertaken large epidemiological studies in the past two decades to examine the prevalence of mental illness and chemical dependency in the U.S. population. According to the Epidemiologic Catchment Area (ECA) study, 33% of the general population is affected by mental illness, 23% with a non-substance abuse mental disorder.[1] The National Comorbidity Survey (NCS) discovered a lifetime prevalence of any mental illness, including substance abuse disorders, of 48%.[2] Both studies found an almost 30% one-year prevalence rate of any mental disorder.

Despite the fact that 3 of every 10 people in the United States suffer from a major mental illness in any given year, less than one-third of them seek treatment. And of those who do seek treatment, less than half receive specialized mental health services.[3] More than half of those with diagnosed mental illness are treated exclusively by primary care physicians and receive no specialized mental health care.[4]

The pattern of service use differs among disorders. People with severe mental illness—schizophrenia and bipolar illness, for example—are more likely to seek treatment than people with less severe illness, and those with schizophrenia are more likely to receive specialty mental health services than general medical services.[3] Patients with somatization disorders are also high users of health care services, but they are more likely to use general medical services than specialty mental health services. Patients with comorbid mental illness and substance abuse disorders are also more likely to seek treatment, particularly in the specialty mental health sector, than patients with either mental illness or substance abuse alone.[3] Patients with three or more psychiatric diagnoses (with or without substance abuse) are also more likely to seek treatment and more than twice as likely to seek specialty mental health treatment than those with a single diagnosis (Figure 1–1).[2]

Patients with mental illness frequently do not seek treatment for many different reasons. Symptom clusters are often not recognized as treatable. For others, the stigma is so great as to prevent them from seeking treatment.

Even when patients do seek treatment for psychiatric symptoms, mental illness may go unrecognized by primary care physicians. Of patients who visit primary care physicians, approximately 25% have a psychiatric illness,[5]

ANNUAL PREVALENCE OF MENTAL/ADDICTIVE DISORDERS AND SERVICE

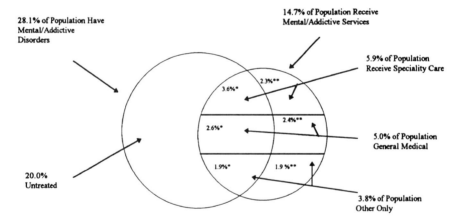

28.1% of Population Have Mental/Addictive Disorders

14.7% of Population Receive Mental/Addictive Services

5.9% of Population Receive Speciality Care

3.6%*

2.3%**

2.6%*

2.4%**

5.0% of Population General Medical

1.9%*

1.9%**

20.0% Untreated

3.8% of Population Other Only

*With Mental/Addictive Disorders in One Year - ECA
**Does not Meet Current Disorder Diagnostic Criteria (Includes Lifetime and Subthreshold Disorders)

FIG. 1–1. Annual prevalence of mental/addictive disorders and services. ECA = Epidemiologic Catchment Area. From Regier, D.A., Narrow, W.E., Rae, D.S., (1993). The de facto US mental and addictive disorders service system, Arch Gen Psychiatry, 50(2):85–94.

but only about 50% of them are recognized.[6,7] Also, in one study, only half of primary care physicians recognized depression.[8] Such physicians recognized depression more frequently than anxiety disorders and severe mental illness more frequently than mild or moderate mental illness. Despite the fact that primary care physicians recognize only about 50% of the mental illness that presents to them, almost 50% of primary and secondary diagnoses of mental disorders are made in the nonpsychiatric setting, mostly by primary care physicians (general practitioners, family practitioners, and internists).[9] Not surprisingly, those patients whose mental illness was recognized had better outcomes.[7]

Furthermore, treatment of mental illness provided by nonpsychiatric physicians may not be adequate. In a study of the treatment of depression in the primary care setting, 50% of diagnosed patients did not receive antidepressants.[10] Even when psychiatric consultation–liaison was provided to primary care physicians, only 37% of depressed patients received an adequate trial of antidepressant medications.[11]

COST OF MENTAL ILLNESS

The economic cost of mental illness to society is tremendous. The direct cost of treating mental illness constitutes 25% of the total health care expenditure and 1% of the gross national product.[12] The indirect costs, measured in lost productivity and human suffering, are even higher.

The complicated issue of pharmacoeconomics is discussed in detail in Chapter 3. The economic burden of mental illness is mentioned here briefly to underscore the tremendous cost of mental illness to our society.

ECONOMIC COST

The economic costs of mental illness can be broken down into direct costs, reflecting the cost of both psychiatric and medical treatment, and indirect costs, reflecting morbidity (decreased work productivity), mortality (lost years of productivity from premature death), and cost to family support systems. The total cost of mental illness in 1985 was estimated at $103.7 billion, with $42.5 billion attributable to direct costs.[13] This cost represents approximately 25% of the total health care expenditure for that year and includes the cost families incur by caring for their ill family member. The cost of schizophrenia in 1985 was estimated at $22.7 billion per year with $10.3 billion in direct and $12.4 billion in indirect costs.[14] Although schizophrenia affects only 1% of the general population, it accounts for 2.5% of total health care expenditure and 10% of the totally and permanently disabled.[15] The total cost of depression in 1990 was estimated at $43.7 billion, with $12.4 billion in direct costs and $31.3 billion in indirect costs.[16] This expense is comparable to the cost of coronary artery disease that has a lifetime prevalence less than half that of affective disorders.[17]

Direct costs include not only psychiatric care, but also general medical care. Mentally ill patients are disproportionately high users of general medical services.[18,19,20,21,22] Psychiatric illnesses may present with somatic symptoms that resemble medical conditions; for example, panic attacks frequently present as chest pain necessitating a two-day coronary care unit admission to rule out myocardial infarction. In a prospective study on an inpatient general medical service, 51% of patients were noted to have either psychopathology or high pain levels. These patients had a 40% longer median length of stay and a 35% greater mean hospital charge, both for more days and more procedures.[23] In the outpatient setting, patients with recent psychiatric diagnoses made more ambulatory care visits and required more medical and psychiatric admissions than those without a diagnosis.[24]

Mentally ill patients are also disproportionately high users of emergency services. Mental illness may predispose patients to high-risk behaviors that result in a higher incidence of trauma and need for emergency care. The majority of trauma patients have a history of mental illness, particularly substance abuse. Emergency rooms also provide services for overdoses and suicide attempts, panic attacks that may mimic cardiac or respiratory emergencies, somatization disorders, and somatic symptoms of depression.

HUMAN COST

In addition to the quantifiable economic cost, there is the immeasurable cost of human suffering and the decreased quality of life that affects both patients and their families.

The morbidity associated with mental illness is high. The functional disability caused by depression, for instance, affects physical, social, and role functioning. In fact, the functional disability associated with depression is comparable to, or more severe than, that associated with major chronic medical conditions including coronary artery disease, hypertension, diabetes, and arthritis.[8] Only coronary artery disease results in more disability days than depression, and only arthritis causes more chronic pain.[25] The effective treatment of depression is associated with a substantial decrease in number of disability days.[26]

Patients suffering from neuropsychiatric illness have a markedly diminished quality of life, which is much more difficult to quantify than the direct cost of health care services. They are often tormented by their symptoms, poor peer and family relationships, and low self-esteem. Their illness impairs the ability to function productively at work and the ability to maintain meaningful social relationships. Patients are often distraught and live much of their lives in solitude.

The cost of mental illness to families also is immense. Families sacrifice their own lives both financially, by investing time and money in caregiving, and emotionally, by enduring often strained and unsatisfying relationships with their ill loved ones. Family support systems often pay out of pocket for additional services for their ill family member, and they also pay a high price in lost productivity by investing time in caretaking responsibilities. This cost is estimated at $2.5 billion per year.[13] In addition, families pay a large price in their reduced quality of life and increased suffering.

NATURAL HISTORY

CHRONIC, LIFELONG ILLNESS

Neuropsychiatric disorders are largely chronic, lifelong illnesses. Early in our understanding of these disorders, particularly affective disorders, we thought that they were comprised of single episodes with little risk of recurrence. However, multiple naturalistic studies indicate otherwise. The majority of people who suffer a single episode of unipolar depression or bipolar illness go on to have recurrent illness. Many of these illnesses have a cyclical course, with recurrent acute exacerbations and a return to baseline functioning between episodes. While the morbidity might seem to be confined to discrete episodes, an episode may be so disruptive, with loss of job or separation from spouse and family, for example, that it causes permanent changes in a patient's life. Many patients then live with anticipatory dread of the next episode. Even in a cyclic disorder like bipolar illness, there is not always a complete return to baseline levels of functioning, particularly after multiple recurrent episodes over many years.

Other illnesses tend to have a more progressive course with a continuous decline in functioning. Schizophrenia, for example, is usually accompanied by progressive cognitive decline and a "downward drift" in socioeconomic status. This is related not only to the recurrent exacerbations of positive (overtly psychotic) symptomatology, but also to the negative (deficit) symptoms that result in a decline in role functioning.

In both types of illnesses, merely treating the acute exacerbations is insufficient. These are chronic disorders, frequently with interepisode sequelae, that must also be addressed and treated appropriately to effect an improvement in patients' lives.

RELAPSE RATES

The relapse and recurrence rates for many of these disorders are quite high. For example, in affective disorders (unipolar and bipolar), the relapse rate has been reported as high as 10–58% after a single episode and 18–80% after three or more episodes.[27] Rates of relapse are highest immediately after recovery[28] and increase with the number of previous episodes and with age. The relapse rate in schizophrenia is approximately 70% in the first year after a psychotic episode in unmedicated patients.[29] Relapse rates decrease 2.5–10 times with antipsychotic medications.[30]

These high rates of relapse underscore the need for effective maintenance treatment. Treating only the acute episode leaves the patient to contend with the almost inevitable future episode without any prophylaxis. Maintenance treatment decreases the risk of recurrence and thus can decrease the number of acute episodes a patient suffers, as well as the interepisode loss of functioning.

COMPLICATIONS OF MENTAL ILLNESS

Mental illness also has secondary effects on a multitude of other areas.

Patients frequently experience a significant decline in social functioning, which can lead to a lack of financial self-sufficiency and an increase in reliance upon public welfare systems. Lack of financial support may be associated with an increased rate of homelessness or living in substandard conditions. Physical illness may also be prevalent with patients' lack of access to preventive medical care and lack of health insurance.

Comorbidity of mental illness with substance abuse is remarkably high. Among individuals with any mental disorder, 29% have a comorbid alcohol or drug addictive disorder. The mentally ill have more than twice the rate of alcohol abuse disorders than the general population and greater than four times the risk of having any other drug abuse disorder.[1] Impulsivity is a symptom of many illnesses, especially substance abuse, and may contribute to criminality. Psychotic symptoms such as command auditory hallucinations, paranoia, or delusions of persecution may contribute to impulsivity and violence. There is a higher incidence of mental illness in prison populations than in the general population.[31]

COMPLICATIONS OF TREATMENT

While effective maintenance treatment for these chronic diseases can interrupt a cycle of recurrent exacerbations and possibly alter the otherwise downward course that patients might take, treatment may interfere negatively with the natural history of the illness. For example, antipsychotics may alleviate disturbing psychotic symptoms, but may leave them more aware of their functional limitations, thus contributing to depression and even to suicide. Anxiolytic agents, when initially started or abruptly discontinued, can precipitate more severe anxiety or panic than the patient had previously experienced. Although maintenance treatment may adversely effect the natural course of the illness it is meant to alleviate, the potential benefit of appropriate effective treatment far outweighs the risks.

DIAGNOSIS

The first step in initiating treatment is making the correct diagnosis.

The most appropriate and well-planned treatment strategy is misdirected if targeting the wrong illness. Therefore, careful evaluation including a detailed history with close attention to symptomatology (onset, severity and duration of symptoms), course of illness, past psychiatric history including efficacy and adequacy of past treatment trials, comorbid medical conditions, medications, family history, psychosocial stressors, social functioning, and mental status exam is necessary. Organic etiologies must be ruled out since secondary psychiatric illnesses do not respond to the same interventions as primary disorders, and therapy must be targeted to the underlying pathology: correcting hypothyroidism or removing an offending medication, for example.

Although this book is not intended to be a diagnostic manual, the section on each disorder includes diagnostic criteria and a differential diagnosis with strategies for ensuring that a correct diagnosis is made. If at any point in treatment the patient is not responding to a medication as expected, the diagnosis must be reconsidered before proceeding with the same, possibly incorrect, treatment plan.

MODES OF TREATMENT

Once a primary psychiatric disorder is recognized, a mode of treatment, or combination of treatments, must be chosen. Pharmacotherapy is based on the medical model of psychiatry and presumes a neurochemical abnormality. It is the mainstay of psychiatric treatment. Another somatic treatment is electroconvulsive therapy (ECT), also based on the medical model, that may be used as an adjunct to pharmacotherapy, usually in cases of very severe pathology or nonresponsiveness to treatment, to effect a more rapid response.

Psychotherapy may be used alone or in combination with pharmacotherapy. Psychotherapy takes many forms. Directive approaches include cognitive behavioral therapy, behavior therapy, and interpersonal psychotherapy and are often short term and time-limited. Psychodynamic or insight-oriented psychotherapies are often longer term therapies and are less directive. There is growing evidence that combinations of pharmacotherapy and psychotherapy are more effective than either alone. By intervening directly on social functioning, interpersonal relationships, and behaviors and by strengthening the physician-patient relationship resulting in increased compliance with medication regimens, psychotherapy is often an effective adjunct to medications.

This book deals with pharmacotherapy of primary neuropsychiatric disorders. Readers interested in treatment of secondary psychiatric disorders, are referred to Lishman and Stoudemire and Fogel.[32,33] For psychotherapeutic interventions, we recommend Gurman and Messer or Bongar and Beatler.[34,35]

PHASES OF TREATMENT

Treatment can be divided into three phases: (Figure 1–2) acute, continuation, and maintenance.[36] The *acute phase* involves initial treatment of the acute episode of illness with the goal of achieving remission. There is no precise time frame, but acute treatment is generally on the order of weeks to a few months.

The *continuation phase* begins when the acute episode has remitted, and the goal is to prevent relapse of the index episode. Continuation treatment is

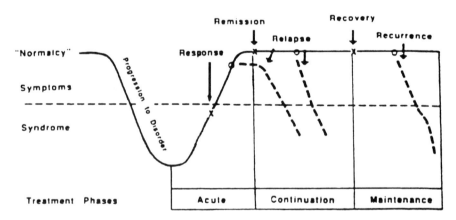

FIG. 1–2. Definitions of phases of treatment: response, remission, recovery, relapse, and recurrence of depression. From Kupfer, D.J. (1991). Long-term treatment of depression, J Clin Psychiatry, 52(5):28–34. Copyright 1991 by Physicians Postgraduate Press. Reprinted with permission.

considered by many to last 6–9 months after remission of the index episode; that is, the approximate time course of an episode if left untreated.

Maintenance treatment extends beyond the index episode into the inter-episode period. The goal is to prevent recurrence or new acute episodes of the illness. Thus, maintenance treatment is long-term prophylactic treatment against recurrence.

While much has been written about acute and continuation treatment, there is considerably less literature addressing maintenance treatment. Although it may seem obvious that long-term treatment with the same medications used to achieve remission in acute treatment should prevent recurrences, there is sparse evidence of this for many neuropsychiatric disorders. Long-term treatment carries a cost and should not be considered without clear evidence that it is advantageous. There are many disadvantages to long-term treatment including adverse effects, cost, and stigma. The risks and benefits must be weighed carefully before embarking on long-term and potentially lifelong treatment with medications that are not innocuous.

MAINTENANCE PHARMACOTHERAPY

To aid the clinician in rationally planning and following maintenance pharmacotherapy strategies, we have provided a critical review of the existing literature on maintenance pharmacotherapy for each disorder with a focus on prospective, double-blind, placebo-controlled, randomized clinical trials in which doses or levels of medications are monitored. For many disorders, this literature is small or absent.

This review is followed by a discussion of the clinically relevant issues in managing maintenance pharmacotherapy. Each chapter addresses the following points involved in planning and managing maintenance pharmacotherapy for a particular disorder or group of disorders:

- ☐ Choice of medications; mechanism of action
- ☐ Medication dosing
- ☐ Efficacy
- ☐ Predictors of response
- ☐ Adverse reactions
- ☐ Drug levels and effects on other organ systems
- ☐ Combination strategies
- ☐ Drug-drug interactions
- ☐ Treatment nonresponders
- ☐ Treatment of acute exacerbations
- ☐ Duration/discontinuation of treatment
- ☐ Compliance

- ☐ Comorbid psychiatric or medical problems
- ☐ Treatment of adolescents and the elderly
- ☐ Treatment during pregnancy and lactation

DISORDERS COVERED

This book deals with chronic neuropsychiatric disorders—those illnesses characterized by a structural or neurochemical abnormality in the brain with resultant neuropsychiatric symptomatology. We have divided these into major psychiatric disorders and primary neurological conditions with neuropsychiatric manifestations.

MAJOR PSYCHIATRIC DISORDERS

We have limited our treatment of the major neuropsychiatric disorders to the major chronic psychiatric disorders that have a clear biological component and are most prevalent and most likely to be encountered in clinical practice.

Affective disorders are a heterogeneous group including unipolar depression, bipolar (manic-depressive) disorder, and dysthymia. These disorders involve abnormalities in epinephrine, dopamine, and serotonin as well as abnormalities in the hypothalamic-pituitary-adrenal axis. While depression and mania are generally cyclic disorders with complete or almost complete return to baseline functioning between episodes, there is a high rate of recurrence, making both unipolar and bipolar illnesses chronic conditions with profound morbidity and mortality.

Schizophrenia is associated with a functional excess of dopamine, also involves norepinephrine and serotonin abnormalities, and is connected with decreased activity in the dorsolateral prefrontal cortex as well as impaired cortical connectivity. It is characterized by acute exacerbations of positive psychotic symptoms superimposed on negative deficit symptoms and is associated with a progressive decline in function and a chronic course.

Anxiety disorders (generalized anxiety disorder, panic disorder, obsessive-compulsive disorder, and post-traumatic stress disorder) involve an abnormality of catecholamine and serotonin metabolism of both cortical and subcortical structures. Anxiety disorders also are frequently chronic, lifelong illnesses that require maintenance treatment.

Several major psychiatric disorders are not covered here. Substance abuse is not dealt with as a separate disorder but is addressed as a comorbid psychiatric disorder where relevant. Unfortunately, pharmacotherapies for substance abuse are limited and there have been no long-term maintenance studies. Instead, treatment is often aimed at the comorbid psychiatric symptomatology rather than specifically at the substance being abused. There are some notable exceptions, however, including disulfiram and naltrexone for alcohol and naltrexone and methadone for opiate addictions. For a more comprehensive review of pharmacotherapy for substance abuse, we refer readers to *Pharmacological Therapies for Drug and Alcohol Addictions*.[37]

Eating disorders also frequently overlap with other major psychiatric disorders including affective disorders and anxiety disorders. These are also addressed where relevant as comorbid psychiatric disorders. For additional information on pharmacotherapy for eating disorders, see Hsu or Brownell and Fairburn.[38,39]

Personality disorders are chronic disorders requiring long-term treatment. However, there are few proven effective pharmacotherapeutic strategies and no maintenance studies have been performed.

PRIMARY NEUROLOGICAL CONDITIONS WITH NEUROPSYCHIATRIC MANIFESTATIONS

Of the neurological disorders with psychiatric manifestations, we have limited our scope to include those disorders that have a primary neurological basis. Therefore, we do not include endocrine, toxic, poison- or alcohol-related disorders. We also do not discuss delirium because this is usually not a chronic disorder.

Seizure disorders, especially complex partial seizures (temporal lobe epilepsy), are associated with an increased incidence of severe psychopathology when compared with the general population. Neuropsychiatric phenomena occur in relationship to seizure phenomena. These neuropsychiatric phenomena include psychosis, depression, personality changes, cognitive impairment, and pseudoseizures. We address the maintenance pharmacotherapy of these neuropsychiatric manifestations of seizure disorders.

Movement disorders associated with dementia and other neuropsychiatric manifestations include the extrapyramidal diseases, of which Parkinson's disease and Huntington's disease are the best understood. Our primary focus is on Parkinson's disease, which is associated with dementia, affective disorders (particularly depression), and psychosis, usually secondary to medication used to treat the movement disorder. We discuss treating these psychiatric symptoms in the context of this movement disorder.

The most common *demyelinating disorder* is multiple sclerosis (MS). Neuropsychiatric aspects of MS include affective disturbance and psychosis. We discuss the treatment of these symptoms in the context of the underlying disorder.

Dementia, frequently accompanied by neuropsychiatric syndromes, may be caused by a degenerative process (i.e., Alzheimer's disease, Pick's disease) or nondegenerative diseases (i.e., vascular disease, syphilis, and hydrocephalus). It may preferentially affect different areas of the brain. Neuropsychiatric manifestations include affective disturbance, anxiety, psychosis, personality change, sleep disturbance, and behavioral disturbance. We briefly discuss pharmacological strategies to alter the progression of Alzheimer's, but our primary focus is on psychopharmacological treatment of the neuropsychiatric symptoms that accompany dementia.

Cerebrovascular disease is associated with a wide range of neuropsychiatric manifestations depending on location and size of the lesion. Cerebrovascular disease includes atherosclerotic thrombosis, cerebral embolism, lacunae, hemorrhage, aneurysms, arteriovenous malformations, subdural and epidural hematomas, and inflammatory diseases. Neuropsychiatric manifestations are most commonly affective disorders. We deal primarily with the treatment of post-stroke depression, mania, and psychosis.

Chronic pain syndromes may occur in patients with neuropathic or non-neuropathic pain. There is considerable comorbidity between chronic pain and depressive disorders. Effective treatment usually involves a multidisciplinary approach, but we focus on the pharmacological intervention both directly for pain and for the depressive symptoms. For a more comprehensive discussion, we refer the reader to Fishbain.[41]

The neuropsychiatric deficits of *human immunodeficiency virus* (HIV) infection include those associated with primary infection of the central nervous system, those secondary to opportunistic infections or tumors systemically or within the central nervous system, and those of iatrogenic origin. The primary manifestations include cognitive decline consistent with a subcortical dementia, delirium, depression, mania, anxiety, and psychosis. Secondary and iatrogenic manifestations may overlap and are often difficult to differentiate. Opportunistic infections and tumors may have varying manifestations depending on anatomical location and size. Medications used to treat the primary infection and those to treat the opportunistic infections and tumors may cause further cognitive impairment or affective symptoms. Since the prevalence of HIV infection is increasing, this area is of growing clinical importance; treatment is rapidly changing as research efforts are concentrated in developing new treatment strategies.

Traumatic brain injury (TBI) is more common than schizophrenia, mania, panic disorder, or any neurological disease with the exception of headaches. Chronic neuropsychiatric sequelae of TBI include cognitive dysfunction, attention and concentration difficulties, affective disorders, anxiety disorders including post-traumatic stress disorder, aggression, irritability, and insomnia. Treating these disorders requires a multidisciplinary approach including psychopharmacological, behavioral, psychological, and social interventions. We address only the pharmacological treatments. Readers interested in a more comprehensive discussion of TBI are referred to *Neuropsychiatry of Traumatic Brain Injury*.[40]

DIRECTIONS FOR FUTURE RESEARCH

There are remarkably little data on the maintenance treatment of the chronic, lifelong disorders discussed in this book. While there is considerable evidence supporting the use of various pharmacological approaches in acute treatment of most neuropsychiatric disorders, there is a paucity of data on maintenance treatments. Very few research studies have been performed looking at long-term outcome with pharmacotherapy. Admittedly, these studies are time-consuming, costly, and difficult to carry out; but without them, clinicians are left to extrapolate strategies for long-term treatment from the acute treatment data. The implications for patients are long-term exposure to psychotropic agents with sometimes difficult-to-tolerate side effects and the stigma of remaining on psychiatric medication lifelong, as well as the financial cost to the patient or third-party payers. Therefore, we recommend expanding research efforts in the area of maintenance pharmacotherapy for these chronic neuropsychiatric disorders.

REFERENCES

1. Regier, D.A., Farmer, M.E., Rae, D.S., et al. (1990). Comorbidity of mental disorders with alcohol and other drug abuse: Results from the Epidemiologic Catchment Area (ECA) Study. *JAMA*, 264(19):2511–2518.
2. Kessler, R.C., McGonagle, K.A., Zhao, S., et al. (1994). Lifetime and 12-month prevalence of DSM-III-R psychiatric disorders in the United States: Results from the National Comorbidity Survey. *Arch Gen Psychiatry*, 51:8–19.
3. Regier, D.A., Narrow, W.E., Rae, D.S., et al. (1993). The de facto US mental and addictive disorders service system: Epidemiologic Catchment Area prospective 1-year prevalence rates of disorders and services. *Arch Gen Psychiatry*, 50(2):85–94.
4. Regier, D., Goldberg, I.D., Taube, C.A. (1978). The de facto mental health services system. *Arch Gen Psychiatry*, 35:685–693.
5. Barrett, J.E., Barrett, J.A., Oxman, T.E., et al. The prevalence of psychiatric disorders in a primary care practice. *Arch Gen Psychiatry*, 45(12):1100–1106.
6. Nielson, A.C., Williams, T.A. (1980). Depression in ambulatory medical patients: Prevalence by self-report questionnaire and recognition by non-psychiatric physicians. *Arch Gen Psychiatry*, 37:999–1004.
7. Ormel, J., Van Den Brink, W., Koeter, M.W., et al. (1990). Recognition, management and outcome of psychological disorders in primary care: A naturalistic follow-up study. *Psychological Med*, 20(4):909–923.
8. Wells, K.B., Stewart, A., Hays, K.D., et al. (1989). The caring and well-being of depression patients: Results from the medical outcomes study. *JAMA*, 262:914–919.

9. Schurman, R.A., Kramer, P.D., Mitchell, J.B. (1985). The hidden mental health network: Treatment of mental illness by nonpsychiatric physicians. *Arch Gen Psychiatry*, 42:89–94.
10. Hohman, A.A. (1991). Psychotropic medication prescription in U.S. ambulatory care. DICP, *Ann Pharmacother*, 25:85–89.
11. Katon, W., Schulberg, H. (1992). Epidemiology of depression in primary care. *Gen Hosp Psychiatry*, 14:237–247.
12. McGuire, T.G. (1991). Measuring the economic costs of schizophrenia. *Schizo Bull*, 17(3): 375–388.
13. Rice, D.P., Kelman, S., Miller, L.S. (1992). The economic burden of mental illness. *Hosp Comm Psychiatry*, 43(12):1227–1232.
14. Rice, D.P., Miller, L.S. (1992). The economic burden of schizophrenia. Paper presented at the Biennial Research Conference in the Economics of Mental Health, Bethesda, MD, September 21–22, 1992, pp. 1–17.
15. Rupp, A., Keith, S.J. (1993). The costs of schizophrenia: Assessing the burden. *Psychiatric Clinics N Am*, 16(2):413–423.
16. Greenberg, P.E., Stiglin, L.E., Finkelstein, S.N., et al. (1993a). The economic burden of depression in 1990. *J Clin Psychiatry*, 54(11):405–418.
17. Greenberg, P.E., Stiglin, L.E., Finkelstein, S.N., et al. (1993b). Depression: A neglected major illness. *J Clin Psychiatry*, 54(11):419–424.
18. Wallen, J., Pincus, H.A., Goldman, H.H., et al. (1987). Psychiatric consultations in short-term general hospitals. *Arch Gen Psychiatry*, 44:163–168.
19. Fulop A., Strain, J.J., Vita, J., et al. (1987). Impact of psychiatric comorbidity on length of hospital stay for medical surgical patients: A preliminary report. *Am J Psychiatry*, 144:878–882.
20. Smith, G.R., Monson, R.A., Ray, D.C. (1986). Patients with multiple unexplained symptoms: Their characteristics, functional health, and health care utilization. *Arch Int Med*, 146:69–72.
21. Katon, W., Berg, A.O., Robins, A.J., et al. (1986). Depression-medical utilization and somatization. *West J Med*, 144:564–568.
22. Thomas, R.I., Cameron, D.J., Fahs, M.C. (1988). A prospective study of delirium and prolonged hospital stay. *Arch Gen Psychiatry*, 45:937–940.
23. Levenson, J.L., Hamer, R.M., Rossiter, L.F. (1990). Relation of psychopathology in general medical inpatients to use and cost of services. *Am J Psychiatry*, 147(11):1498–1503.
24. Shapiro, S., Skinner, E.A., Kessler, L.G., et al. (1984). Utilization of mental health services: Three epidemiologic catchment sites. *Arch Gen Psychiatry*, 41:971–978.
25. Wells, K.B., Burnam, M.A. (1991). Caring for depression in America: Lessons learned from early findings of the medical outcomes study. *Psychiatric Med*, 9:503–519.
26. Von Korff, M., Ormel, J., Katon, W., et al. (1992). Disability and depression among high utilizers of health care. *Arch Gen Psychiatry*, 49:91–100.
27. Zis, A.P., Goodwin, F.K. (1979). Major affective disorder as a recurrent illness: A critical review. *Arch Gen Psychiatry*, 36:835–839.
28. Keller, M.B., Lavori, P.W., Lewis, C.E., et al. (1983). Predictors of relapse in major depressive disorder. *JAMA*, 250:3299–3304.
29. Hogarty, G.E. (1993). Prevention of relapse in chronic schizophrenic patients. *J Clin Psychiatry*, 54(3):18–23.
30. Davis, J.M. (1985). Maintenance therapy and the natural course of schizophrenia. *J Clin Psychiatry*, 11(2):18–21.
31. Snow, W.H., Briar, K.H. (1990). The convergence of the mentally disordered and the jail population. *J Offender Counseling, Serv and Rehab*, 15(1):147–162.
32. Lishman, W.A. (1987). *Organic Psychiatry: The Psychological Consequences of Cerebral Disorder*, 2nd ed. London: Blackwell Scientific Publications.
33. Stoudemire, A., Fogel, B.S. (Eds.). (1993). *Psychiatric Care of the Medical Patient*. New York: Oxford University Press.

34. Gurman, A.S., Messer, S.B. (Eds.). (1995). *Essential Psychotherapies: Theory and Practice*. New York: Guilford Press.
35. Bongar, B, Beutler, L.E. (1995). *Comprehensive Textbook of Psychotherapy: Theory and Practice*. New York: Oxford University Press.
36. Kupfer, D.J. (1991). Long-term treatment of depression. *J Clin Psychiatry*, 52(5):28–34.
37. Miller, N.S., Gold, M.S. (Eds.). (1994). *Pharmacological Therapies for Drug and Alcohol Addictions*. New York: Marcel Dekker, Inc.
38. Hsu, L.K.G. (1990). *Eating Disorders*. New York: Guilford Press.
39. Brownell, K.D., Fairburn, C.G. (Eds.). (1995). *Eating Disorders and Obesity: A Comprehensive Handbook*. New York: Guilford Press.
40. Silver, J.M., Yudofsky, S.C., Hales, R.F. (Eds.). (1994). *Neuropsychiatry of Traumatic Brain Injury*. Washington, DC: American Psychiatric Press.
41. Fishbain, D.A. (1996). Pain and Psychopathology. In Fogel, B.S., Schiffer, R.B., Rao, S.M. (Eds.), *Neuropsychiatry*. Baltimore: Williams & Wilkins.

CHAPTER

2

PHARMACOKINETICS AND PHARMACODYNAMICS OF RELEVANCE TO MAINTENANCE PHARMACOTHERAPY

Bruce G. Pollock, M.D., Ph.D.

INTRODUCTION

When medications are prescribed chronically, it is especially important that physicians be aware of pharmacokinetic and pharmacodynamic aspects if they are to navigate between loss of efficacy on one shoal and drug toxicity on the other. In particular, an understanding of rational therapeutic drug monitoring for drugs with narrow therapeutic indices, specificity of cytochrome P450 drug metabolism, and age-associated response changes is necessary for optimal treatment.

PHARMACOKINETIC PRINCIPLES

Pharmacokinetics provides a way of describing and predicting drug concentrations in plasma and various tissues over time. Typically, the

17

TABLE 2–1. FACTORS THAT CAN INFLUENCE DRUG CONCENTRATIONS IN MAINTENANCE PHARMACOTHERAPY

- □ Compliance: taking too much or to little; change in time of administration
- □ Formulation of medication: switching to generic or different brand
- □ Change in smoking, alcohol, or caffeine consumption
- □ Change in body weight or habitus
- □ Change in coadministered prescribed or over-the-counter drugs
- □ Intervening disease, especially changes in cardiac, hepatic, or renal function

phases of absorption, distribution, metabolism, and elimination provide descriptive components. Key concepts essential to the understanding of this discipline are bioavailability, volume of distribution, half-life, and clearance. The following features in Table 2–1 may affect the constancy of drug concentrations during maintenance treatments with psychotropics. Readers are encouraged to consult standard texts for more detailed definitions and derivation of pharmacokinetic formulae (e.g., Gilman et al., 1990; Evans et al., 1986; Rowland and Tozer, 1980).[1,2,3]

BIOAVAILABILITY

Bioavailability is the fraction of the dose (represented by a bioavailability factor F) of administered medication that reaches the patient's circulation. Drugs given by the intravenous route have a bioavailability of 100% and are used as a basis of comparison. For oral dosage forms, physicochemical properties, such as their formulation, degree of ionization, lipid solubility, and molecular size, affect a drug's dissolution and ability to cross biological membranes. In this regard, it is important to consider the possibility that when patients are switched between brand and generic (and indeed between generic and generic or different brand preparations) differing bioavailabilities may impact significantly on therapeutics. For example, one patient, stabilized on maintenance nortriptyline, experienced a twofold change in plasma levels when he was changed to another brand of nortriptyline.

The Drug Price Competition and Patent Term Restoration Act of 1984 resulted in greatly expedited approval of generic drugs. The U.S. Food and Drug Administration (FDA) may approve most oral, immediate-release generic products on the basis of one single-dose bioequivalency study comparing plasma concentrations in as few as 18 healthy subjects. One standard applied by the FDA is the so-called 70/70 rule. This rule as applied to phenothiazines, for example, states that the two drug products must differ by no more than 30% in the rate and extent of absorption in 70% of the test subjects. Clearly, this could permit a potentially significant degree of variation, especially clinically important for drugs with narrow therapeutic indices. In addition, since 1980 the FDA has published an annual listing "Approved Drug Products with Therapeutic Equivalence Evaluations" that categorizes under the designation "BD" documented differences in bioequivalence. In general, substitutions of differing preparations should be avoided in maintenance pharmacotherapy. If substitutions cannot be averted, the patient should be closely monitored for changes in symptomatology and side effects as well as idiosyncratic responses.

Clinicians treating patients with maintenance pharmacotherapy should also be alert to the intermittent use of over-the-counter medications that may interfere with the extent of gastrointestinal absorption such as those products with huge absorbing surfaces (e.g., Metamucil® and Maalox®) or medications with anticholinergic properties. Hepatic first-pass metabolism is another major factor in oral bioavailability. When drugs are absorbed from the upper gastrointestinal tract, they enter the portal vein and are delivered to the liver. If the drug is highly metabolized by the liver (has a high extraction ratio), then bioavailability will be markedly reduced. Compared with oral administration, intramuscular, sublingual, or transdermal preparations avoid hepatic first-pass effects and permit much smaller doses to be used. Consideration must also be given to whether taking maintenance medication with food affects bioavailability. For example, the bioavailability of sertraline, lithium, and diazepam is enhanced when they are administered with meals. Obviously, consistency in time of administration should be maintained during maintenance treatment.

VOLUME OF DISTRIBUTION

The volume of distribution is an apparent or theoretical volume that is strongly influenced by a drug's relative solubility in lipid or water and its affinity for plasma proteins. The more a drug binds to plasma proteins, the less widely it distributes. Thus, intercurrent pathophysiological states such as hypoalbuminemia during maintenance drug therapy or increases in the phase reactant protein, alpha-1-acidglycoprotein, may change the volume of distribution. The majority of psychotropics are transported in the blood bound to plasma proteins. Since only an unbound drug is pharmacologically active, acute changes in binding previously were of clinical concern. It is now recognized that a free drug is also more available for metabolism and tissue distribution. Thus, any change in the absolute concentration of a free drug would be immediately buffered and a new equilibrium established.[4]

When, however, plasma drug levels are used to monitor maintenance therapy with antidepressants or anticonvulsants, it should be appreciated that the total drug concentrations (free + bound) usually are reported. Although a change in absolute drug concentration may be caused by a change in protein binding, the new equilibrium in the proportion of bound and free drug may appear as a change in the drug's measured (total) plasma level.[5] In practice, this may be a problem if a patient who was well maintained on a monitored medication experienced a severe, intercurrent illness. The clinician in these circumstances should hesitate before changing medication doses and request free drug levels. The application of unbound drug levels in these circumstances has been found useful for lidocaine, theophylline, phenytoin, and digoxin.

Aside from changes in protein binding, it is unlikely that acute changes in volume of distribution will occur. It should be noted, however, that as patients age (Table 2–2), the proportion of adipose tissue increases from 33% in younger women to 48% in older women, and from 18–36% in men.[6] Since a drug's half-life is directly proportional to its apparent volume of distribution, the half-life of lipid soluble drugs, such as diazepam, increases as a patient ages. In contrast, the distribution of very water soluble drugs, such as lithium or digoxin, decreases with age, thus increasing the amount of drug in the blood and the risk of acute toxicity.

TABLE 2–2. AGING-ASSOCIATED PHARMACOKINETIC AND PHARMACODYNAMIC CHANGES

Physiologic Factor	Age-Related Change
Absorption	Diminished salivation may cause difficulty swallowing. Decreased gastric absorption surface, acidity, and emptying time of little clinical significance.
Distribution	Increased volume of distribution for lipid soluble drugs due to increased fat-to-muscle ratio. Lowered binding of acidic drugs due to diminished serum albumin. Increased serum alpha-1-acidglycoprotein may increase binding of basic drugs.
Cardiac output	Decreased by 30–40%, decreased hepatic and renal blood flow.
Hepatic metabolism	Little change in CYPs 2D6, and 3A4 and glucuronidation except in extreme old age and poor nutrition. CYPs 2C, and 1A may be diminished with aging.
Excretion	Decreased glomerular filtration rate and tubular secretory function may lead to increased concentrations of active metabolites.
Receptor (number and function)	Diminished CNS cholinergic and nigrostriatal dopamine functioning increases sensitivity to anticholinergics and D2 receptor antagonists.
Homeostatic mechanisms	Diminished postural control, orthostatic circulatory response, thermoregulation, and visceral muscle function increases risk of adverse consequences.

CLEARANCE AND HALF-LIFE

Clearance describes the intrinsic capacity of a patient to remove a specific drug. Expressed as a volume per unit of time, clearance does not represent how much drug is removed, but rather the theoretical volume of plasma that is completely cleared of drug. Repetitive administration of a constant dose of medication at fixed intervals leads to an accumulation in plasma concentrations until steady-state plasma levels are reached. The *concentration* at steady-state is directly proportional to the dose of medication and inversely proportional to clearance. The *rate* of drug accumulation and attainment of steady-state, however, is entirely determined by the elimination half-life. The half-life of a drug is the time necessary for its concentration to decrease by one-half after absorption and distribution are complete. Most drugs follow "first-order" kinetics: The rate of change of concentration is directly proportional to the concentration. In "zero-order" kinetics, which occur when drug metabolism is saturated, this proportionality is lost, and elimination occurs at a fixed rate. In a first-order, exponential process, it is the percentage of change during each half-life that is fixed. After five half-lives, 97% of a drug is eliminated. Thus, knowing the individual half-lives of selective serotonin reuptake inhibitors is crucial if potentially lethal interactions with monoamine oxidase inhibitors are to be avoided. At steady-state, drug elimination equals the amount ingested and the relationship of plasma to tissue concentrations remains constant at similar times on successive days. Steady-state plasma levels reflect the amount of drug available for biological action. This leads to the elaboration of dose-response data for both therapeutic and toxic effects.

Genetic and acquired (interacting medications) differences in drug metabolism cause marked differences in plasma levels among individuals given the same dose. Almost 10% of the Caucasian population lacks a functioning cytochrome P450 2D6 and is at risk of increased side effects when treated with tricyclic antidepressants[7,8] and neuroleptics.[9]

Once an individual has reached steady-state, if he or she continues to be fully compliant, the main threat to the constancy of drug concentrations comes from interacting medications. It is important that psychiatrists not only be familiar with interactions among psychotropics, but also between psychotropics and commonly prescribed and over-the-counter medications as well. Inhibition or stimulation of hepatic drug metabolizing, "microsomal" enzymes can either potentiate or negate the action of psychotropics. Recently, a structure emerged for rationalizing potential interactions occurring at the level of drug metabolism. Approximately 90% of commonly administered medications (Tables 2–3 and 2–4) are metabolized by three cytochrome P450 isozymes: CYP 2D6, 2C, and 3A.[10] Knowledge of which isozyme

text continues on page 23

TABLE 2–3. PSYCHOTROPIC OXIDATIVE METABOLISM ASSOCIATED WITH SPECIFIC P450S1

P450 2D6	P450 1A2	P450 3A3-4	P450 2C19
Desipramine	Caffeine	Alprazolam	Diazepam,
Nortriptyline	Clozapine	Midazolam	Desmethyldiazepam
Amitriptyline	Imipramine	Triazolam	Citalopram
Clomipramine ⎫ Hydroxylation	Clomipramine ⎫ Demethylation	Zolpidem	Imipramine
Imipramine ⎭	Amitriptyline ⎭	Sertraline	Clomipramine ⎫ Demethylation
Parcxetine	Fluvoxamine	Nefazodone	Amitriptyline ⎭
Maprotiline	Haloperidol	Carbamazepine	Moclobemide
Trazodone	Tacrine	Dexamethasone	Methobarbital
M-CPP (metabolite of trazodone		Imipramine ⎫ Demethylation	Hexobarbital
and nefazodone)		Amitriptyline ⎭	
Venlafaxine			
Mianserin			
Haloperidol			
Perphenazine			
Risperidone			
Thioridazine			
Coceine			

TABLE 2–4. POTENT INHIBITORS (OR INDUCERS) OF SPECIFIC P450S

P450 2D6	P450 1A2	P450 3A	P450 2C19
Chlorpromazine	Clozapine	Cimetidine	Fluoxetine
Desipramine	Fluvoxamine	Norfluoxetine	Omeprazole
Diltiazem	Theophylline	Fluvoxamine	Norethindrone
Fluoxetine,	Smoking	Sertraline	Teniposide
Norfluoxetine	(inducer)	Nefazodone	Proguanil
Fluphenazine		Ketoconazole	
Haloperidol		Erythromycin	
Labetabol		Troleoandomycin	
Lobeline		Oral contraceptives	
Paroxetine		Nifedipine	
Metadone		Alkaloids	
Perphenazine		Grapefruit juice	
Propafenone		Carbamazepine (inducer)	
Quinidine		Barbiturates (inducer)	
Sertraline,		Dexamethasone (inducer)	
Desmethylsertraline		Rifampicin (inducer)	
Thioridazine			
Vinca			

is primarily responsible for a drug's metabolism coupled with known inhibitors of that isozyme enables a predication of potential interaction. Significant change in dietary and other habits also may affect drug concentrations. Lithium levels are lowered by increased coffee consumption; grapefruit juice is a potent inhibitor of P450 3A3; smoking increases the demethylation of tricyclics through induction of P450 1A2.

PLASMA LEVELS FOR COMPLIANCE MONITORING

Altamura and Mauri[11] were the first to suggest that the longitudinal stability of quotients of amitriptyline plasma levels divided by dose may be more applicable to monitoring maintenance compliance since dosage changes may limit the usefulness of steady-state plasma levels. This approach was adopted by Frank et al.[12] in a three-year imipramine maintenance trial. Six of eight patients who had previously responded to treatment but exhibited large fluctuations in plasma level/dose values relapsed on maintenance pharmacotherapy. Patients were classified as noncompliant if two level/dose values exceeded their previously determined mean by ±2 standard deviations. An adaptation of this approach to lithium maintenance was used by Harvey and Kay.[13] They found that the standard deviation of log red blood cell lithium values was a strong predictor of relapse.

PHARMACODYNAMIC CONSIDERATIONS

DOSE-RESPONSE RELATIONSHIPS

Pharmacodynamics refers to the relationship between a drug's effect and its measurable concentration. Efficacy is defined as a drug's ability to produce a desired response while potency is the dose necessary to produce this response. Patients may differ widely in their therapeutic response to a given concentration of medication. The therapeutics of many psychotropics may not be readily discernable even if symptomatology is quantitated in a standardized fashion. Assessment is complicated by the intense subjectivity and environmental sensitivity of symptoms, such as mood and well-being, from the perspective of both patient and examiner. These difficulties are compounded by the typically long lag-times and obscure, non-linear dose-response relationships for most psychotropics.[14,15] For medications with linear dose-response relationships, the intensity of effect influences its constancy during maintenance treatment. As pointed out by Levy,[16] a drug with a steep and direct relationship of its effect to its concentration will be less "forgiving" of a missed dose than a drug with an identical half-life but a less precipitous dose-response curve. The underlying mechanisms responsible for the therapeutic effects of every psychotropic remain speculative. Much better understood are the actions of psychotropics that generate adverse effects.

TOLERANCE

Tolerance is another important pharmacodynamic concept; it reflects the dynamic nature of adaptation in the central nervous system to drug exposure over long periods of time. With benzodiazepines, for example, increasing doses are required to maintain the same degree of sedation. Conversely, no degree of tolerance to the peripheral anticholinergic side effects (i.e., increased heart rate, dry mouth, and constipation) has been found in patients treated for long periods of time with nortriptyline.[17]

AGE-ASSOCIATED CHANGES

Even in the absence of overt disease, the end organ of psychotropic action, the central nervous system, undergoes age-associated change. Recently, more definitive evidence of a less rapid antidepressant response to tricyclic antidepressants in elderly patients despite comparable pharmacotherapy has been presented.[18] More prominent are consideration of increased adverse effects in an older population secondary to the putative receptor changes, as discussed below.

As patients age, their homeostatic mechanisms (e.g., postural control, orthostatic circulatory responses, thermoregulation, visceral muscle function, higher cognitive function) are reduced. This condition may interfere with their ability to adapt to changes in the environment and may manifest as an adverse drug reaction. For instance, all psychotropics may increase the risk of falls and hip fracture in the elderly[19,20] and may increase cognitive impairment.[21]

Specific age-associated changes have been most extensively investigated for autonomic receptor-mediated effects.[22] Reductions in $\alpha 2$ (but not $\alpha 1$) adrenoceptor responsiveness may occur with age and could contribute to the increased risk of orthostatic hypotension in elderly patients. Orthostatic hypotension is the major cardiovascular concern in the elderly, and it mitigates against the use of lower potency antipsychotic drugs and tricyclic antidepressants. Tachycardia is an additional concern with the use of many psychotropics, secondary to their anticholinergic effects, and those effects not ameliorated by time.[17] Membrane-stabilizing (quinidine-like) properties of some psychotropics may delay cardiac conduction and seriously interact with either underlying pathophysiology or antiarrhythmic medication. Electrocardiogram changes have been noted most frequently for the tricyclic antidepressants and antipsychotics of the diphenylbutylpiperidine (i.e., pimozide) and piperidine (i.e., thioridazine) type. In patients with preexisting conduction disturbance, increased watchfulness is clearly needed. The risk of psychotropic-cardiovascular drug interactions is considerably amplified since many of these medications intersect both metabolically and dynamically. For example, quinidine and diltiazem not only inhibit cardiac conduction, but also P450 2D6 as well. In older patients, chronically treated with many psychotropics, the prevalence of obesity, poor nutritional status, and increased triglycerides may contribute additional cardiovascular risk factors.[23,17]

Diminished cholinergic functioning in the central nervous systems of older patients and, in particular, those suffering from Alzheimer's disease, may render them more sensitive to the central anticholinergic effects of psychotropic medication.[24] These effects can range from blurred vision and cognitive impairment to frank delirium, which may occur at therapeutic concentrations.[25,26] The increased anticholinergic effects of tertiary tricyclics and lower potency antipsychotics clearly limits their use in an older population.

Oversedation, associated with low potency neuroleptics and tertiary tricyclics because of histamine (H1) antagonism, can lead to confusion and disorientation and contribute to urinary incontinence, pneumonia, decubiti, and poor eating and aspiration. In addition to cognitive blunting, apathy, and akinesia, antipsychotics may cause depression directly.[27] Although acute neuroleptic treatment has been associated with decreased attention and vigilance in young schizophrenics, the amelioration of psychosis may improve performance on tests of sustained attention and visual-motor functions.[28]

Reductions in nigrostriatal dopamine[29] predispose the elderly to neuroleptic-induced Parkinsonism, which depends on the potency, dose, and time of antipsychotic treatment and can persist following medication discontinuation.[30]

Tardive dyskinesia constitutes a severe social handicap for patients and may impair speech, eating, breathing, and gait. Until recently the increased incidence of tardive dyskinesia in the elderly was thought to be from increased exposure to neuroleptics. A prospective study has now demonstrated that regardless of diagnosis, there is a very high onset of tardive dyskinesia in older patients taking antipsychotics for relatively brief periods of time (cumulative incidence reported as 31% after 43 weeks).[31] Four factors have been identified as increasing the risk of tardive dyskinesia in older patients: prior exposure to neuroleptics, a past history of alcohol abuse, preexisting movement disorder, and antipsychotic daily dosages greater than 3 mg of haloperidol or 150 mg chlorpromazine-equivalents. These investigators have also noted that concurrent smoking and use of anticholinergics may increase the severity of tardive dyskinesia. In addition, diabetes recently has been identified as a potent risk factor in two carefully conducted case-control studies, in which age, sex, dose, and duration of neuroleptic treatment were controlled.[32]

CONCLUSION

Nonadherence to medication regimens by patients during maintenance therapy and unanticipated drug-drug interactions through their physicians' prescriptions represent the greatest threats to the stability of drug concentrations. Periodic plasma level monitoring for psychotropics with narrow therapeutic indices (i.e., tricyclic antidepressants and lithium) is essential. As patients age, pharmacodynamic changes and concomitant illness significantly alter their responses to medication.

REFERENCES

1. Gilman, A.G., Rall, T.W., Nies, A.S., et al. (1990). *Goodman and Gilman's The Pharmacological Basis of Therapeutics.* New York: Pergamon Press.
2. Evans, W.E., Schentag, J.J., Jusko, W.J. (1986). *Applied Pharmacokinetics* (2nd ed.) Spokane, WA: Applied Therapeutics.

3. Rowland, M., Tozer, T.N. (1980). *Clinical Pharmacokinetics: Concepts and Applications.* Philadelphia: Lea & Feiger.
4. Rolan, P.E. (1994). Plasma protein binding displacement interactions—Why are they still regarded as clinically important? *Br J Clin Pharmacol*, 37:125–128.
5. Pollock, B.G., Perel, J.M. (1989). Tricyclic antidepressants: Contemporary issues for therapeutic practice. *Can J Psychiatry*, 34:609–617.
6. Greenblatt, D.J., Sellers, E.M., Shader, R.I. (1982). Drug disposition in old age. *N Engl J Med*, 306:1081–1088.
7. Tacke, U., Leinonen, E., Liisunde, P., et al. (1992). Debrisoquine hydroxylation phenotypes of patients with high versus low to normal serum antidepressant concentrations. *J Clin Psychopharmacol*, 12:262–267.
8. Bluhm, R.E., Wilkinson, G.R., Shelton, R., et al. (1993). Genetically determined drug-metabolizing activity and desipramine-associated cardiotoxicity. *Clin Pharmacol Ther*, 53:89–95.
9. Pollock, B.G., Mulsant, B.H., Sweet, R.A., et al. (1995). Prospective P450 2D6 phenotyping for neuroleptic treatment in dementia. *Psychopharmacol Bull*, 31:327–331.
10. Pollock, B.G. (1994). Recent developments in drug metabolism of relevance to psychiatrists. *Harv Rev Psychiatry*, 2:204–213.
11. Altamura, A.C., Mauri, M. (1985). Plasma concentrations, information and therapy adherence during long-term treatment with antidepressants. *Br J Clin Pharmacol*, 20:713–716.
12. Frank, E., Mallinger, A.G., Thase, M.E., et al. (1992). Relationship of pharmacologic compliance to long-term prophylaxis in recurrent depression. *Psychopharmacol Bull*, 28:231–235.
13. Harvey, N.S., Kay, R. (1991). Compliance during lithium treatment, intra-erythrocyte lithium variability, and relapse. *J Clin Pharmacol*, 11:362–367.
14. Dingemanse, J., Danhof, M., Breimer, D.D. (1988). Pharmacokinetic-pharmacodynamic modeling of CNS drug effects. *Pharmacol Ther*, 38:1–52.
15. Greenblatt, D.J., Harmatz, J.S. (1993). Kinetic-dynamic modeling in clinical psychopharmacology. *J Clin Psychopharmacol* 13:231–234.
16. Levy, G. (1993). A pharmacokinetic perspective on medicament noncompliance. *Clin Pharmacol Ther*, 54:242–244.
17. Pollock, B.G., Perel, J.M., Paradis, C.F., et al. (1994). Metabolic and physiologic consequences of nortriptyline treatment in the elderly. *Psychopharmacol Bull*, 30:145–150.
18. Reynolds, C.F., Frank, E., Kupfer, D.J., et al. (1995). *Acute and continuation treatment outcome in recurrent major depression: Comparison of elderly and mid-life patients.* Paper presented at the 34th Annual Meeting of the American College of Neuropharmacology, San Juan, PR, Dec. 12, 1995.
19. Ray, W.A., Griffin, M.R., Schaffner, W., et al. (1987). Psychotropic drug use and the risk of hip fracture. *N Engl J Med*, 316:363–369.
20. Tinetti, M.E., Speechley, M., Ginter, S.F. (1988). Risk factors for falls among elderly persons living in the community. *New Eng J Med*, 319:1701–1707.
21. Larson, E.B., Kukull, W.A., Buchner, D., et al. (1987). Adverse drug reactions associated with global cognitive impairment in elderly persons. *Ann Intern Med*, 107:169–173.
22. Pollock, B.G., Perel, J.M., Reynolds, C.F. (1990). Pharmacodynamic issues relevant to geriatric psychopharmacology. *J Geriatric Psychiatry Neurol*, 3:221–228.
23. Martinez, J.A., Velasco, J.J., Urbistondo, M.D. (1994). Effects of pharmacological therapy on anthropometric and biochemical status of male and female institutionalized psychiatric patients. *J Am Coll Nutrition*, 13:192–197.
24. McEvoy, J.P., McCue, M., Spring, B., et al. (1987). Effects of amantadine and trihexyphenidyl on memory in elderly normal volunteers. *Am J Psychiatry*, 144:573–577.
25. Schor, J.D., Levkoff, S.E., Lipsitz, L.A., et al. (1992). Risk factors for delirium in hospitalized elderly. *JAMA*, 267:827–831.

26. Feinberg, M. (1993). Therapeutic Problems of Anticholinergic Adverse Effects in Older Patients. *Drugs & Aging*, 3:335–348.

27. Harrow, M., Yonan, C.A., Sands, J.R., et al. (1994). Depression in schizophrenia: Are neuroleptics, akinesia, or anhedonia involved? *Schizophr Bull*, 20:327–338.

28. Cassens G., Inglis A.K., Appelbaum, P.S., et al. (1990). Neuroleptics: Effects on neuropsychological function in chronic schizophrenic patients. *Schizophr Bull*, 16:477–499.

29. Iyo, M., Yamasaki, T. (1993). The detection of age-related decrease of D1, D2 and serotonin 5-HT2 receptors in living human brain. *Prog Neuro Psychopharmacol Biol Psychiatry*, 17:415–421.

30. Wilson, J.A., MacLennan, W.J. (1989). Review: Drug induced Parkinsonism in elderly patients. *Age and Aging*, 18:208–210

31. Saltz, B.L., Woerner, M.G., Kane, J.M., et al. (1991). Prospective study of tardive dyskinesia incidence in the elderly. *JAMA*, 266:2402–2406.

32. Ganzini, L., Casey, D.E., Hoffman, W.F., et al. (1992). Tardive dyskinesia and diabetes mellitus. *Psychopharmacol Bull*, 28:281–286.

PHARMACOECONOMICS

Junius Gonzales, M.D. and Kevin Schulman, M.D.

INTRODUCTION

Clinicians and health policymakers have long recognized the impact of neuropsychiatric disorders on the morbidity, mortality, and quality of life of patients. More recently, efforts have been directed to extend this understanding to include an assessment of the economic impact of these disorders and to assess the economic impact of their treatments. For example, one report cited that most developed nations spend about 1% of their individual gross national product for the treatment of mental illness and that these health care costs increase at an annual rate over 10%.[1] In the United States alone, some components of treatment for neuropsychiatric disorders have increased over 75% from 1955 through 1985, whereas general health care costs did so by about 24%.

The prevalence, chronicity, and early onset of neuropsychiatric disorders have serious societal cost implications. For example, the productivity losses and high indirect costs of such disorders as schizophrenia and major depression represent, respectively, over 80% and 65% of the total costs to society of these disorders. A recent study estimated the economic burden of depressive disorders in the United States to be nearly $44 billion annually,

29

accrued through inadequate treatment that had consequences of lowered work productivity and lost wages due to disability days and suicide.[2]

Because of the escalating costs of disease and treatments and interest in fully evaluating medical technologies and clinical services, many seemingly disparate parties are involved in examining the economic parameters of these services or products. This activity has been appropriately dubbed clinical economics—an evolving discipline dedicated to the study of how different approaches to patient care and treatment influence the resources consumed in clinical medicine.[3] Clinical economics is the study of the value for money of medical technologies or services. In other words, the discipline focuses on assessing the resource use required for a new treatment and the benefit the treatment provides. The costs of a new technology are the net costs of treatment including consideration of resource offsets (those resources no longer required due to the new therapy). Clinical economics has expanded the definition of benefits of treatment from traditional clinical benefits to more expanded definitions of treatment outcomes including quality of life benefits and patient preferences for outcomes.

Within this burgeoning field of clinical economics, pharmacoeconomics is defined as that which describes, measures, analyzes, and compares the costs, or resources consumed, and outcomes including consequences of pharmaceutical products.[4] In the case of mental illness, pharmaceutical products have revolutionized the treatment of many disorders, may account for some of the abovementioned increased treatment costs, and are therefore critical to study in this way.

Due to the need to examine the value of monies spent on products or services and the usually higher premium for new pharmaceutical products, decisionmakers, at various levels and in different health care sectors, want to understand the economic impact of a product and whether it provides a reasonable value for money in relation to other treatment alternatives. These interested parties include patients, individual practitioners, hospital formulary committees, managed care executives, health insurance companies, and national health agencies, all of whom need to make decisions about choosing alternative pharmaceutical or even alternative use of resources at higher policy-making levels. While the complex and inextricable relationship between health care costs and the health needs of a population may make some people uncomfortable, its controversial nature is receding as pharmacoeconomic analyses become routine components of the assessment of new clinical products.

This chapter discusses recent developments in pharmacoeconomics, describes the major types of analyses used in pharmacoeconomics along with relevant variable domains, delineates methodological issues such as data sources, and presents relevant and exemplary pharmacoeconomic studies with particular focus on maintenance pharmacotherapy for such neuropsychiatric disorders as major depression and schizophrenia.

PHARMACOECONOMIC STUDIES: STAKEHOLDERS, APPLICATIONS, AND GUIDELINES

As mentioned, the increasing value placed on clinical economic evaluations is wide reaching, involves multiple parties, and has implications at the national health policy level, the systems health policy level (i.e., health plan, hospital), and clinical health policy level. At the national health policy level, these issues are especially relevant at the federal and state levels.[5] First, the federal Medicare program that insures the elderly and disabled provides medication benefits only for inpatient care (except for special therapies such as erythropoietin), and economic information has been incorporated in three ways: (1) the Reauthorization Act of 1992 for the Agency for Health Care Policy and Research (AHCPR), (2) a set of proposed regulations issued by the Department of Health and Human Services regarding the inclusion of new technologies or services in Medicare coverage, and (3) the use of economic analysis of therapies in AHCPR practice guidelines development.

At the state level, with federal assistance, Medicaid programs offer prescription benefits for individuals meeting inclusion criteria for this part of the program. On an experimental basis, the economic evaluation of medical therapies is being woven into the Oregon Medicaid reform program that using patient input has created condition-treatment pairs, which were ranked in terms of net benefit. In 1993 this program was approved as a Medicaid demonstration with some provisions to protect the disabled and a more extensive evaluative component examining quality of care, access, and total medical expenditures. Another state-federal endeavor provided block grants to states for services to HIV-infected persons—the Ryan White Comprehensive AIDS Resources Emergency Act of 1990—and decisions about coverage are made at the state level with consultative input from different sources such as a multidisciplinary advisory panel that may also include consumer advocacy members.

At the systems health policy level, issues such as managed care prescription plans, patient copayment, and limited plan formularies abound and affect decisionmakers at hospitals, health plans, and employment. Prepaid care plans or HMOs use pharmacoeconomic data for formulary decisions as well as to assist providers, especially physicians, in using appropriate pharmaceutical therapeutics available to the plan. Plans use their own data, which can vary in quality from one prepaid care plan to the next, to assess experience with a new agent. Hospital administrators are faced with similar issues and some hospital pharmacy committees are using detailed and targeted formulary management to examine new and/or high cost pharmaceutical products.[6]

Davey and Malek[7] describe some general conflicts that pharmacoeconomic issues pose—conflicts that may be both practical and ethical. They describe the traditional differing viewpoints between clinicians and economists on need, efficiency, and equity steeped in the ever-growing dilemma of providing health care to all in the context of limited, and perhaps, shrinking resources. At the clinical encounter level, individual patients, practitioners, and the general public are increasingly affected by pharmacoeconomic issues.

With the managed care movement providing financial risk arrangements to individual clinicians, pharmacoeconomic issues are pervasive. Pharmaceutical practice profiling is one way for health care organizations to examine the use of pharmaceutical products and attempt to influence practitioner behavior toward the use of less costly products.[8] Clinical and ethical dilemmas arise for the clinician if he or she believes the patient would benefit maximally from a more expensive medication or one that is not on the plan's formulary, resulting in out-of-pocket cost for the patient. At the individual patient level, much more work is needed in assessing preferences for care and incorporating them into the actual clinical encounter, especially given the rapidly changing health care environment in the United States. While clinicians conceptually value incorporating patient preference into decision-making, in actuality these preferences may not be attended to or elicited.

However, since out-of-pocket expenditures for new medications are high, patient advocacy groups have developed plans to work with the pharmaceutical industry to affect drug pricing for affordability. As described, the general public has been involved in large health care debates such as the Oregon project, but this involvement is still in its infancy. Important questions in this arena include:

1. Who is the public?
2. What preferences should be elicited?
3. Should preferences be aggregated and, if so, how?
4. When and at what level should preferences be included in decision-making?
5. Might preferences be unacceptable? How will rejection of preferences be handled?
6. Is consulting the public about priorities rational or ethical? [7]

While pharmacoeconomics has made the move from industry and academia into public policy, its transition has been neither smooth nor simple. The major purpose of pharmacoeconomic studies is to optimize decision-making about pharmaceutical products within limited resources.[9] Detsky (1994) outlined some general goals for these analyses: clearly defining the purpose, appropriately formatting the data, measuring outcomes and presenting data well, and understanding contractual arrangements and potential threats to the validity of the analyses.

These practical and ethical issues have surfaced in the development of pharmacoeconomic study guidelines, but it is relevant to first determine what are the primary objectives of pharmacoeconomic analyses for pharmaceutical companies. Drummond outlines four company objectives for undertaking pharmacoeconomic analyses.[10] First, analyses may assist in the early developmental phases of a product to determine whether, along with clinical efficacy, first-pass economic analyses denote a probable economic advantage to the public as well as to the company's research and development program. The second objective is to assist in product pricing. These two objectives can easily be achieved without releasing these data or publishing them in a scientific journal. Third, a company can do economic analyses to guide pricing or reimbursement strategies to meet health care standards and requirements of regulatory bodies (e.g., the Australian Pharmaceutical Benefits Scheme). Complex issues involving who did the analyses and the level of methodologic rigor have been considered, but not yet concretely placed, in guidelines. Finally, the fourth objective for economic analyses of a pharmaceutical product is for marketing that can be aimed at individual patients, practitioners, as well as decision-making bodies for formularies. Because these company objectives are potentially fraught with self-interest, companies are well aware of the need to maximize the external credibility of their economic evaluations.

In 1991, Hillman et al.[11] recommended a rudimentary code of conduct for industry-sponsored economic evaluations since the quantity and quality of potential biases were serious. Recently, four sets of guidelines have assisted in determining what the relevant concepts are in carrying out economic evaluations. These guidelines may serve several purposes that may, at one time or another, be in conflict. Major parties interested in guidelines for the provision of pharmacoeconomic data include governments, pharmaceutical industries, researchers, and health care decisionmakers. The use of guidelines has been proposed for reimbursement requirements (e.g., at the national or health care plan level), while methodological standards and ethical standards have varying levels of importance to the different groups.[10,12] For example, researchers may have more interest in the methodological standards than in reimbursement requirements or ethical standards, while industry is probably least interested in reimbursement requirements for the provision of economic data.

Nevertheless, since 1992 four sets of guidelines for pharmacoeconomic analyses have been developed and are summarized by Jacobs and colleagues.[13] The differences between these four sets—the Australian Pharmaceutical Benefits Advisor Committee, the Canadian Coordinating Office on Health Technology Assessment (CCOHTA), the Ontario Ministry of Health, and the England and Wales Department of Health—are denoted primarily by different purposes for guidelines development, different approaches to conceptual and methodological issues, and different value judgments in analytic constructs such as utility based measures. The primary aim of all guidelines, except CCOHTA's, is to assist in decision-making about the use of public monies for pharmaceuticals, whereas the Canadian guidelines reach beyond national decision-making to private drug programs and public ones at the province level. Jacobs et al.[13] describe 11 major areas that guidelines for pharmacoeconomic studies should address: study purpose, comparators, type of study, time horizon, perspective, outcome selection, method of data capture, cost items, discounting, sensitivity analyses, and analysis of global financial impact.

Interestingly, in January 1995, the Pharmaceutical Research and Manufacturers of America (PhRMA) developed and adopted a recommended, but voluntary, set of principles for the methods and conduct of pharmacoeconomic research.[14] Developed by a PhRMA Task Force, this set was "reviewed by a panel of academic experts and outside reviewers at each stage of their development." However, the process of development is not described in the article that denotes 21 general principles covering the following topics: research design, protocol/report, contents of protocol/report, costs/resources, effectiveness/benefits, data sources, and extrapolation of results to other settings.

The development of standard guidelines for design of pharmacoeconomic analyses has helped to provide recognition of the need to provide "transparency" in the planning of analyses, especially secondary analyses using literature review for data sources. It has also resulted in a call for disclosure of relationships between investigators and sponsors. However, almost concurrent with this attention to methods of economic study, the field has moved from one concerned with secondary analyses of the clinical literature to one involved in data collection within prospective clinical trials, and even to the point where clinical economics is being used to define primary endpoints for clinical trials. While guidelines are being developed to ensure the evolution of the discipline, they are not too restrictive, and the result may be they do not necessarily ensure the quality of completed studies.

Finally, the relationships between outside investigators and industry sponsors of pharmacoeconomic studies can pose numerous practical and ethical problems.[15,16] Clear issues to be specified prior to contract signing include publication rights, specification of analyses, data access and ownership, confidentiality, termination, and payment to investigators.

Clearly, the need for and interest in pharmacoeconomic studies is tremendous as evidenced by this brief description of such applications as national guidelines. However, pharmacoeconomic data must be interpreted rigorously in the specific clinical context before wide-reaching decision-making processes, especially at the policy level, can emerge. Furthermore, a clear knowledge of the current methods and constructs in pharmacoeconomics can assist in these rigorous interpretations and perhaps even in such applications as outcomes management.[17]

PHARMACOECONOMIC ANALYSES: SPECIFIC TECHNIQUES AND KEY CONSTRUCTS

The concept of efficiency, as defined by economics, underlies pharmacoeconomic analyses; that is, are resources, usually limited, being optimally used to gain the best outcome? More specifically, is the cost of a pharmaceutical product worth the therapeutic benefit of that agent? The assumption that resources are limited implies that trade-offs are mandatory and that cost is therefore defined as the consumption of a resource that could have been used for another purpose. Schulman[8] extends this concept of efficiency to clinical economics and contends that efficiency of a therapy is "the effect of a therapy as observed in actual clinical practice, outside a clinical protocol." This concept of effectiveness is in clear contrast to the efficacy of an agent that is the determined effect, usually limited, in the ideal setting of a randomized, controlled, clinical trial. The tensions between efficacy and effectiveness research are around the trade-offs between high internal validity and limited generalizability for efficacy and vice versa for effectiveness. Clearly, an examination of efficiency can be achieved through pharmacoeconomic analyses, as well as through real world randomized trials.[18]

TYPES OF PHARMACOECONOMIC ANALYSES

This section focuses on three main economic analyses: cost-identification, cost-benefit, and cost-effectiveness. Three dimensions of clinical economic analysis have been described by Bombardier and Eisenberg[19] and are represented in Figure 3–1. The first dimension along the X axis is the type of analysis listed above. Along the Y axis is the perspective that the analysis may take: that of society (most common), individual patient, payer, and health care provider. Finally, the Z axis describes the types of costs and benefits possible in an economic analysis. Most of these concepts are described in Table 3–1.

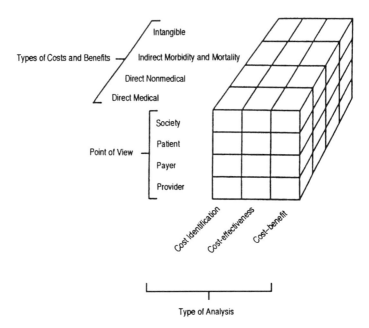

FIG. 3–1. From Bombardier, C., Eisenberg, J. (1985). Looking into the crystal ball. J Rheum, 12:201–204. Copyright 1985 by The Journal of Rheumatology. Reprinted with permission.

Cost-identification analysis is the least complex of the three main types. Its purpose is to identify the costs involved in either quantifying the economic cost of a disease or simply identifying the least expensive diagnostic or therapeutic approach to the problem; benefits are not calculated in this type of analysis.[3,4] The most obvious application of cost-identification analysis, or cost minimization, is when the two approaches are of equal efficacy or when the outcomes are presumed to be identical. The limitation to this kind of analysis is that no detailed examination of outcomes, or benefits, is possible.

Cost-benefit analysis (CBA) considers both costs and outcomes in terms of monetary units (e.g., dollars). Two primary measurements are sought: the ratio of dollars spent to dollars saved; the net saving or cost. Clearly, an intervention or medication should be used if its benefits are greater than its costs. Two general approaches to cost-benefit analysis are the net benefit approach and the cost-benefit ratio. The first simply expresses both costs and benefits in cash terms and subtracts the total cost from the total benefit. The second approach expresses a ratio in which total costs are the numerator and total benefits the denominator. The criticism of this approach is that benefits may be expressed as negative costs and costs may be expressed as negative

text continues on page 38

TABLE 3–1. GLOSSARY OF TERMS USED IN HEALTH ECONOMICS, AND
PHARMACOECONOMIC AND QUALITY-OF-LIFE ANALYSES

Term	Definition/Description
Acquisition cost	Purchase cost of a drug to an institution, agency, or person.
Analytic perspective	Viewpoint chosen for the analysis (e.g., societal, government, health care system, payer).
Average cost	Total costs of a treatment or program divided by total quantity of treatment units provided. (See also Marginal costs.)
Contingent valuation	Method for evaluation of benefit or value to individuals of therapy that uses survey methods to establish willingness to pay.
Cost/QALY gained	Measure used in cost-utility analysis to assist in comparisons among programs; expressed as monetary cost per unit of outcome.
Cost-benefit analysis (CBA)	Type of analysis that measures costs and benefits in pecuniary units and computes a net monetary gain or loss or a cost-benefit ratio.
Cost-benefit ratio	Ratio of the total monetary cost of a program divided by the benefits expressed as savings in projected expenditure.
Cost-effectiveness analysis (CEA)	Type of analysis that compares drugs or programs having a common health outcome (e.g., reduction of blood pressure, life-years saved).
Cost-effectiveness ratio	Ratio of the total cost of a program divided by the health outcome (e.g., cost per life-year gained); used in CEA to select among programs.
Cost-minimization analysis	Type of analysis that finds the least costly program among those shown or assumed to be of equal benefit.
Cost(burden)-of-illness	Study that identifies and evaluates the direct and sometimes indirect costs of a particular disease or risk factor (e.g., smoking or alcohol consumption).
Cost-utility analysis (CUA)	Type of analysis that measures benefits in utility units or quality-adjusted life-years (QALY); computes a cost per utility–measure ratio between programs.
Decision analysis	Explicit quantitative approach for prescribing decisions under conditions of uncertainty.
Decision tree	Framework for representing alternatives for use in decision analysis.
Direct medical costs	Fixed and variable costs associated directly with a health care intervention (e.g., physician salaries).
Direct nonmedical cost	Nonmedical cost associated with provision of medical services (e.g., transportation of a patient to a hospital). *(Contd.)*

TABLE 3–1. (Continued)

Term	Definition/Description
Discount rate	Rate of discount used to convert future costs and benefits into today's value; typically 2–6% per anum for costs, and 0–6% for benefits.
Effectiveness (of a drug)	Therapeutic outcome in a real world patient population (usually differs from efficacy determined in controlled clinical trials).
Formulary	List of drugs reimbursable under a health insurance plan or offered under a capitated or managed care program or preferred in a particular clinical setting.
Human capital method	Means of calculating the indirect cost of medical illness, based on the remaining lifetime economic value to society of a healthy individual of that age, measured by market earnings.
Incremental cost	Difference between the cost of a program (treatment) and the cost of the comparison program.
Indirect cost	Cost of reduced productivity resulting from illness or treatment (may be estimated by loss of wages and other means).
Intangible cost	Cost of pain and suffering occurring as a result of illness or treatment.
Marginal costs	Extra cost of one extra unit of product or service delivered (usually differs from average cost). (See also Average cost.)
Markov model	Statistical representation of recurrent events over time that can be incorporated into decision analysis.
Net benefit	Benefit (in pecuniary units) minus total cost (in pecuniary units): a basic decision criterion in CBA.
Opportunity cost	Cost of using resources for some purpose, measured as their value in their next alternative use.
Sensitivity analysis	Process through which the robustness of an economic model is assessed by examining the changes in results of the analysis when key variables are varied over a specific range.

benefits and that this kind of manipulation may be misleading. In the first approach, these kinds of changes do not affect the results of the cost benefit analysis. The limitation of the cost benefit analysis is that other variables to be included need to be expressed in monetary units, and this may be problematic when trying to assess a product's impact on additional years of life.

Cost-effectiveness analysis (CEA) has gained tremendous popularity in recent years and attempts to include not only costs, but also a wide range of benefits such as multidimensional outcomes beyond clinical symptomatology. CEA allows costs to be expressed in monetary units (dollars) and outcomes can be expressed in several ways, depending on choice of important outcome, such as years of life saved or gained, averted complications, or a combination of outcomes on a common scale. There are two approaches to CEA. The first is to determine separate cost-effectiveness ratios as costs divided by outcomes for different interventions. Consider two pharmaceutical products: A, a new medication, and B, the old standard. The second approach is to compare incremental costs and incremental benefits. The incremental cost is the cost of pharmaceutical A minus the cost of pharmaceutical B divided by incremental benefits. An example of benefits would be the number of years of life gained from pharmaceutical A minus the number of years gained from pharmaceutical B. In this kind of analysis, two possible results emerge:

1. Pharmaceutical A costs the same or more but has less impact on outcomes than B.
2. Pharmaceutical A costs less but does the same or more than pharmaceutical B.

In the first case, pharmaceutical B is said to dominate A; in the second case, pharmaceutical A is dominant. Treatments that show cost savings or equivalence with better or equal outcomes are said to be dominant and should be chosen.[8] However, treatments that cost more and are more effective should be chosen if both cost-effectiveness and incremental cost-effectiveness ratios fall within some predetermined acceptable range.

An example of combining several outcomes of interest into a common scale or unit uses both the duration and quality of life during survival and is called *quality-adjusted-life-year* (QALY).[20] One advantage of using QALYs is that a certain number of years of survival does not mean that the quality of life in each year is the same. While the use of QALYs has gained favor as an index of cost-effectiveness recently, some recommend using other units, though clear-cut empirical differences between the two methods have yet to be determined.[21]

One specific form of cost-effectiveness analysis that uses the conversion of different outcomes into a common scale is called *cost-utility analysis* (CUA). This approach uses a utility measurement approach to assign quantitative values, or utility weights, to different clinical outcomes. This utility value represents patient preferences for choosing, or avoiding, certain outcomes, and through utility analysis, these relative or comparative values can generate a utility score for a combination of seemingly intangible outcomes in which, for example, a score of 1 represents perfect health and 0 represents death.[22,23,24,25]

Finally, two types of cost-effectiveness analysis are used: marginal and incremental cost-effectiveness. Eisenberg[3] describes marginal and incremental cost-effectiveness in the following way:

> ... marginal cost-effectiveness represents the additional cost and effectiveness that can be obtained from one additional unit of service.
>
> In contrast, incremental cost-effectiveness represents the additional cost and effectiveness obtained when one option is compared with the next most intensive or next most expensive alternative...

The advantages of cost-effectiveness analysis—consideration of exchanging better outcomes for more resources and the avoidance of translating clinical or quality of life outcomes into monetary units—have made this type of pharmacoeconomic analysis most popular. It should be noted, however, that there is no one desirable cost-effectiveness ratio. Available resources may dictate the level of cost-effectiveness of a pharmaceutical product chosen for a formulary. It is critically important, however, to gather as much data as possible about the relative cost-effectiveness of multiple treatment options to guide the provider and patient in their respective decision-making processes about management.

IMPORTANT PHARMACOECONOMIC CONSTRUCTS: COSTS, PERSPECTIVES, AND SENSITIVITY COSTS

There are three major cost categories—direct, indirect, and intangible costs—that are delineated in Figure 3–1. Direct costs are made up of two types: direct medical and direct non-medical costs. Direct medical costs consist of the resources consumed by an intervention and represent expenses for medical or nonmedical products or services such as hospitalization, pharmaceuticals, diagnostic testing, equipment, and physicians' fees. Direct non-medical costs refer to costs for nonmedical services but that are clearly linked to the intervention; examples include transportation, food, clothing, and installation fees for home equipment.

The determination of direct costs is not simple and multiple issues must be included.[26] Let us examine three issues in direct costs: fixed versus variable costs, charges versus costs, and, discounting. First, one concept that applies across different cost types is whether costs are fixed—not affected by the volume of services provided—or variable—costs affected by the volume of services provided. A pharmaceutical for an illness may decrease the amount of blood work needed; but the laboratory equipment is seen as a fixed cost whereas the tubes, which depend on the volume of service, or blood tests, are classified as a variable cost. This distinction assists in clarifying the possible impact of a treatment by its ability to change resource consumption by patients.

Another issue in discussing direct costs is distinguishing between costs and charges that are not the same. Charges reflect the marketplace or regulation and may not represent the true cost, or value, of a service or pharmaceutical. Furthermore, charges often do not differentiate between fixed and variable costs and truly represent only the cost to those who pay the charges.[27]

Discounting is the technique of adjusting for costs and benefits over time. Not only does the value of money change over time (e.g., via inflation), but the issue of choosing or holding off on certain outcomes in the future always needs to be considered in a cost analysis. Thus, future values, both costs and benefits, need to be discounted and adjusted to a present value. Standard discount rates of 5 or 6% are used, particularly in developed nations. The issue of discounting is extremely complex because of conceptual and practical problems in discounting health, not just monetary, effects.[28]

The next cost category is indirect costs and these are especially significant in considering neuropsychiatric disorders. In general, indirect costs reflect the costs of morbidity and mortality that result in loss of valuable resources in the form of productivity: absenteeism or disability days, decreased earning potential because of a disability, and changes in work type due to disability. Two methods are used to calculate indirect costs: the human capital approach and the willingness to pay approach.[3] The first is the most commonly employed method and has two reputed advantages. The human capital approach quantifies morbidity as lost wages or lost livelihood and is somewhat straightforward to compute. Its second advantage is that the technique provides an evaluation of gains or losses in productivity—a unit in which governments and employers are interested. Its disadvantages are the lack of a theoretical foundation, a lower income being valued less despite being as productive via number of weekly hours worked, and the serious possibility of undervaluing certain productive individuals, such as housewives or the elderly, who do not earn classifiable wages.

The willingness to pay method has as its basic premise the notion that any outcome, whether death or disability, can be measured by the maximum amount that someone would be willing to pay to not have that outcome or program. In this way, the willingness to pay approach represents standard economic concepts and technically can incorporate all costs including intangible costs. Intangible costs are difficult to measure and are defined as pain, suffering, and grief that result from an illness, and these costs are often difficult to incorporate in pharmacoeconomic analyses. The willingness to pay method has been applied to measure intangibles by asking people how much money they would pay for a certain outcome. But issues such as posing hypothetical scenarios, baseline inequality in wealth, and beliefs about risk and certainty have an impact on this assessment method.[29]

PERSPECTIVE

Figure 3–1 denotes the various perspectives relevant to economic analysis in considering costs, benefits, and outcomes: society's, patient's, provider's, or payer's. Pharmacoeconomic analyses generally take a societal perspective and are noted as such, but conducting the analyses from more than one perspective can be useful. A simple example is choice of a medication. Consider one that is not on the managed care pharmacy formulary. A clinician may determine that a newer, more costly medication is best for the patient—to relieve symptoms and increase adherence through lower side effects (a problem with other medications the patient has tried)—but from the patient's viewpoint, monetary cost is of critical importance because he or she has to pay this out-of-pocket. Whose perspective should guide an economic analysis of this new medication? Publishing rigorous pharmacoeconomic analyses in medical journals can help keep clinicians abreast of these complex issues.

SENSITIVITY ANALYSIS

As noted in the section on costs, assumptions or estimations about costs and benefits are often made in economic analyses, and these introduce certain biases or uncertainties that limit the precision of pharmacoeconomic results. Using a group of techniques known as sensitivity analysis, evaluations of these assumptions and their impact on the results of the analyses can be performed.[30] The study results can be recalculated using different values for key study variables (e.g., cost of a medication or epidemiologic data such as survival or relapse rates) and so sensitivity analysis has the following three advantages:

☐ Demonstrating the independence or dependence of a result on particular assumptions. Establishing the minimum or maximum values of a variable that would be required to affect a recommendation to adopt or reject a program.
☐ Identifying clinical or economic uncertainties that require additional research.[4]

The first part of this chapter has been to familiarize the reader with basic terms and concepts in pharmacoeconomic analyses and those interested in more details are referred to the references. Let us now move to examples of such analyses in the maintenance pharmacotherapy treatment of high-lighted neuropsychiatric disorders.

PHARMACOECONOMIC ANALYSES OF MAINTENANCE PSYCHOPHARMACOLOGICAL TREATMENTS

The actual number of pharmacoeconomic analyses for psychopharma-cological agents used in maintenance therapy is low, considering the number of disorders and agents available. These analyses have only recently appeared in publication, over the past seven years, and the largest number of such analyses were conducted for major depressive disorder. Most studies reviewed here have been supported, in part, by pharmaceutical companies. This section focuses primarily on the published pharmacoeconomic analyses of agents for major depression and schizophrenia. The studies are described using the "study aspect" framework for pharmacoeconomic studies that Jacobs and colleagues[13] proposed in their comparative review of guidelines: study purpose, comparator, type of study, time horizon, perspective, outcome selection, method of data capture, cost items, discounting, and sensitivity analysis. Varying levels of detail are provided on different studies to illustrate key points (e.g., methodological issues).

MAJOR DEPRESSION

Major depression is a common and disabling psychiatric disorder that significantly impairs functioning and well-being, even more than many other chronic medical conditions.[31] The lifetime risk of developing major depression is nearly one in five, and point prevalence rates in the community are about 3% and about 10% in primary care settings.[32] The costs of depressive disorders, as noted, are estimated at over $44 billion.[2] Efficacious treatments, both psychopharmacologic and psychotherapeutic, exist, yet detection and treatment issues abound so that many people with this disorder go without appropriate treatment. The emergence, over the past decade, of several pharmacologic agents with better side-effect profiles, such as the selective serotonin reuptake inhibitors (SSRIs), has produced hope that the appropriateness of care for depressed people will increase. This section describes seven typical pharmacoeconomic studies and one atypical study of antidepressant pharmaceutical agents as well as discusses strengths and limitations of each.

The first pharmacoeconomic analysis of maintenance treatment for depression with imipramine was a cost-utility analysis done by Kamlet and colleagues.[33] Using a Markov state transition model and Monte Carlo simulation to examine maintenance pharmacotherapy for recurrent depression, data were taken from a clinical trial comparing imipramine, interpersonal therapy (IPT), and a combination of the two. The quality of life while depressed was quantified by using a utility value of 0.45 and derived from the literature that noted several measurement methods—health status scales (Quality of Well Being; Rand Health Status) and the time trade-off—used with different populations. Their results indicated that IPT alone did not seem to be cost-effective and that the cost-effectiveness of the other treatments, imipramine alone or with IPT, strongly depended on the quality of life, B, while clinically stable under maintenance treatment. This value B was clearly dependent on the impact of side effects of imipramine on quality of life but was not measured or approximated for this study.

Two pharmacoeconomic studies of antidepressant medications, one of sertraline and the other of citalopram (now available in the United States), were done with the same primary study purpose: to examine the cost-effectiveness of these agents for maintenance therapy in comparison to the most commonly prescribed antidepressants—tricyclics—in the United Kingdom and Germany.[34,35] The difficulty with these studies is that each of these agents is an SSRI that is better tolerated with respect to side effects versus the comparator agent.

Hatziandreu et al.[34] examined the cost utility of long-term maintenance therapy with sertraline for patients at risk of recurrent depression compared with episodic treatment with dothiepin—the most commonly prescribed tricyclic in the United Kingdom—and used a societal perspective. The treatment course with the comparator, dothiepin, is episodic and not continuous; this issue is not addressed. The dothiepin treatment course lasted for three months and the sertraline continuous treatment for two years. The study used decision analytic techniques to model events—specifically a Markov state-transition model—for the duration of patients' lives (the study time horizon); these events included remission, recurrence, or death from natural causes. The primary outcome measure was QALYs with intermediate outcomes including recurrence rates, treatment compliance, and remission rates. This analysis used utility values for different outcomes and is therefore a cost-utility analysis.

The three main categories of necessary data were probabilities for recurrence of depressive episodes, medical services utilization, and health utilities. These data were derived from the published literature, two physician panels (one of general practitioners, the other of psychiatrists), and published information on costs in the United Kingdom. Much of the data, such as medical care utilization and utilities, were derived from the physician panels. Issues about the selection of panel members and possible biases are important to consider. The conceptual validity of using utility values for *patients'* health states obtained from providers is questionable (which the authors acknowledge), especially since there are notable differences in these values by physician group. Even so, a more concrete example is a comparison of the mean utility values for treatment of a depressive episode with sertraline: 0.78 (range 0.75–0.85) and 0.66 (range 0.35–0.70) for the general practitioner and psychiatrist groups, respectively. These ranges are quite different and no notation of weighting for this effect is made. The overall mean of these values is used. Finally, this study only used direct medical costs, used two discount rates (3 and 7%), and carried out extensive sensitivity analyses. Its final result indicated that it cost 2172£ Sterling (U.S.$3,692) to save an additional QALY with maintenance sertraline treatment.

Nuijten and colleagues[35] studied the cost-effectiveness of long-term maintenance treatment with citalopram versus the three leading tricyclics in Germany. As in the previous study, decision analytic techniques, specifically Markov modeling, were used to examine one-year maintenance pharmacotherapy: continuous therapy with citalopram and episodic treatment with doxepin, amitriptyline, or trimipramine. The decision to use different treatment durations for the two different agents is not supported in the reports. The perspective taken was that of the German statutory sickness fund—a third-party payer—within Germany in 1993.

Primary outcomes or endpoints for this analysis were time without depression, direct costs, and indirect costs in the form of days lost from work. The primary sources of data for this study included published literature, the AHCPR *Practice Guidelines for the Diagnosis and Treatment of Depression in Primary Care*, clinical trials data, and expert opinion. The direct costs category included medication costs, consultation, psychotherapy, and hospitalization, while indirect costs captured only days lost from work over two months. No discounting was done given the one-year study time line. Sensitivity analyses were performed and the primary results indicated that continuous maintenance treatment with citalopram was more cost-effective than episodic treatment with the tricyclics. These results were especially sensitive to the response and relapse rates associated with citalopram and "cost-effectiveness ratios were not calculated because citalopram was both more effective and less costly than standard therapy."

The primary concerns regarding this study are the data sources, the choice of both comparator and mode of treatment (continuous versus episodic), and the lack of utility values for health states. The cost data are rudimentary, and the Markov model is fairly simple, consisting of three states: normal, depressed in outpatient care, and depressed in inpatient care. Nonetheless, these two studies can serve as examples of how basic pharmacoeconomic analyses should be set up.

The fourth pharmacoeconomic analysis compared an SSRI, paroxetine, with a tricyclic, imipramine, and was performed using decision analytic methods to compare the direct costs of treating major depression for one year.[36] Multiple sources of data—literature, clinical trials data, focus groups, and an insurance claims database—provided information on medical treatment patterns, direct medical costs, treatment failure rates, and relapse rates. This analysis was done from the perspective of a third-party payer. In contrast to the previous two studies, both medications appear to be used continuously rather than episodically. Sensitivity analyses were performed on the following variables: drug effectiveness rates, acquisition costs, and inpatient costs. If one medication was not effective or if the patient dropped out of a medication treatment, a switch to the other medication was assumed. The estimated direct medical cost per patient was slightly lower for paroxetine ($2,348) than generic imipramine ($2,448), accounted for primarily by savings in hospitalization costs. This cost analysis has several limitations: data sources, especially for costs; lack of generalizability of clinical trials data; and lack of indirect costs.

Jonsson and Bebbington[37] reported a cost-effectiveness analysis of paroxetine and imipramine and assessed the overall direct costs of depression in the United Kingdom. Using multiple sources of data—National Health Service and national survey data for costs, literature review, phase III clinical trials data, and physician and pharmacist panel data—a simulation model based on decision analytic methods was conducted. Only direct costs were examined in this study, and although it is not explicitly stated, the perspective appears to be that of society. Sensitivity analyses were conducted and the most sensitive variable was treatment failure; the relative cost-effectiveness of paroxetine compared with imipramine remained stable (e.g., average cost $824 vs. 1,024£). The differences in expected cost per patient for the two medications were negligible, and the results were for successfully treated patients. However, the authors note that even if the patient dropout rate for paroxetine was 50%, it would have a lower cost-per-successfully-treated patient compared with imipramine.

A cost-effectiveness analysis of antidepressant treatment in which the comparator medication is in the same pharmacologic class was done by Revicki and colleagues[38] who examined treating depressed women in primary care with nefazodone—a new serotonergic agent—versus imipramine or fluoxetine. Similar decision analytic methods including a Markov state-transition model were used to examine the lifetime health outcomes and costs of these three antidepressant treatments. Only direct medical costs (e.g., hospitalization costs, electroconvulsive therapy, physician services—consultation and psychotherapy—for outpatient and inpatient visits, and medication costs) were used to examine QALYs, and patient-generated utilities for 11 possible health states were used. A discount rate of 5% was used for the base study. Sensitivity analyses were conducted for discount rates, recurrence, compliance and dropout rates, and duration of the economic analysis.

Results indicated that nefazodone treatment cost $1,447 (Canadian) less per patient than imipramine while increasing the number of QALYs by 0.72; costs were only $14 less than for fluoxetine while resulting in only 0.11 increased QALYs. The cost-effectiveness ratios found nefazodone to be $17,326 per QALY gained compared with imipramine, and $7,327 per QALY gained compared with fluoxetine. This study overcame previous study limitations, but the authors recognize the problems with the utility values, data sources, and missing indirect costs and direct nonmedical costs associated with depression. The authors rightly suggest a prospective comparative study.

OTHER ECONOMIC ANALYSES OF ANTIDEPRESSANT TREATMENTS

An interesting and noteworthy economic analysis that did not focus on one medication but rather on appropriate treatment for depression was done by Sturm and Wells[39] using data from the Medical Outcomes Study (MOS). Using decision analytic methods and simulations, the study purpose was to examine the cost and health effects of changes in care of patients with depression treated in prepaid settings with shifts from specialty mental health care to the general medical specialty mental health. The three primary outcome measures in this cost-effectiveness analysis were change in serious functional limitations, annual treatment costs per patient, and costs per reduction in one functional limitation. The MOS was an extensive observational longitudinal study of five chronic conditions, including depression, in typical practice settings. Multidimensional outcome variables were examined and all data, such as utilization rates and costs, for this analysis came from this one source.

A model was developed to simulate different rates of processes of care across care sector and shifts in specialty mix. The analysis first examined the probabilities of types of treatment for severely depressed patients— receiving treatment from a specific provider, using appropriate antidepressant medication, regular use of a minor tranquilizer, receiving counseling at baseline, and being detected as depressed. These treatments, and their combinations, were then associated with functioning and cost outcomes. The analysis then examined three levels of "quality treatment" (e.g., level 1: using appropriately dosed antidepressant medication with four to five follow-up visits), and then simulating the costs per patient of providing the three levels of care (level 3 as best) by different providers and the resulting reductions in functional limitations for each respective level of care. These parameters were then placed into a cost-effectiveness ratio. Although somewhat obvious, the results showed that increasing levels of appropriate care were associated with improved functioning; the most appropriate and higher levels of care were more likely to occur in specialty mental health. Although total costs were increased with better care, the value, or cost-effectiveness, of care is higher due to the improved functioning outcomes. The models of care in the general medical sector showed less reduction in limitations, less costs per patient, but similar cost-effectiveness ratios ($790–$1,030) to care in mental health by psychiatrists ($510–$1,380) because of increased reduction in functional limitations.

Cost-effectiveness analyses provide extensive and useful information, but they do not provide "consumer" preferences for trade-offs between costs and outcomes. As described, the willingness to pay approach rarely has been used in economic evaluations of health programs.

O'Brien and colleagues[40] examined how additional reduction in medication side effects was associated with paying more for the medication. They used interviews to determine common side effects and the frequency and duration of each, and asked for ranking these side effects using category rating. The willingness to pay scenario presented the risk of seven individual side effects with graphic and numeric presentations. Respondents then proposed monetary amounts they were willing to pay to avoid side effects, and estimates were derived for multiple risk reductions. Since there are few studies examining this approach in health care, interesting issues emerge about who should be asked these questions and their experience with the scenarios proposed. More careful examination of the feasibility and implementation of this method is needed.

PHARMACOECONOMIC ANALYSES OF CLOZAPINE FOR SCHIZOPHRENIA

Clozapine, a relatively new antipsychotic with atypical structure and properties, has certain advantages for treating refractory schizophrenia. The cost of treating schizophrenia in the United States has been estimated at $30 billion a year (both direct and indirect costs),[41] so the promise of clozapine's clinical efficacy seemed to outweigh its initial increased cost at about ten times greater than the cost of standard antipsychotic medications (Table 3–2). While some severe side effects are possible (e.g., agranulocytosis) and may have contributed to clozapine's high cost in the United States (for monitoring), the cost-effectiveness of the medication is being carefully studied since its clinical benefits may produce improved functioning and reduced hospitalizations for these patients, thereby resulting in economic benefits.[42,43]

Three cost-effectiveness studies of clozapine have been reported, although there are active federally funded research endeavors that have just been

text continues on page 50

TABLE 3–2. COST ANALYSES OF MAINTENANCE ANTIDEPRESSANT AND CLOZAPINE THERAPIES

Study	Study Purpose	Comparator	Type of Study	Time Horizon	Perspective	Outcome Selection	Method of Data Capture	Cost Item	Discounting	Sensitivity Analysis
Kamlet 1992	imipramine	IPT combination none	CUA	lifetime	society	QALY	clinical trials literature	direct	yes	yes
Hatziandreu 1994	sertraline	dothiepin	CUA	lifetime	society	QALY	clinical trials literature provider panel	direct	yes	yes
Nuijten 1995	citalopam	tricyclics (3)	CEA	one year	third-party payer	costs	clinical trials literature provider panel national $ data	direct indirect	no	yes
Benkover 1995	paroxetine	imipramine	CBA	one year	third-party payer	costs	clinical trials literature insurance data focus groups	direct	no	yes
Jonsson 1994	paroxetine	imipramine	CEA	one year	society	costs	clinical trials literature provider panel national $ data	direct	yes	yes
Revicki 1995	nefazodone	imipramine fluoxetine	CUA	lifetime	society	QALY	clinical trials literature provider panel national data	direct	yes	yes
Sturm 1995	appropriate depression care	varying levels of care care sector	CEA	two years	society	QALY	Medical Outcomes Study	direct	no	yes
Revicki 1990	clozapine	standard neuroleptics	CEA	three years	third-party payer	costs	clinical trials literature varied $ sources	direct	no	no
Meltzer 1993	clozapine	standard neuroleptics	CEA	two years	society	costs	literature interviews $ per Revicki	direct	no	no
Davies 1993	clozapine	standard neuroleptics	CEA	one year lifetime	society	costs, disability	literature clinical interview national stats	direct indirect	yes	yes

completed. The first study was a retrospective analysis of patients who were treated with clozapine prior to its release, and the study perspective was that of the insurer.[44] The study examined only direct costs and compared 133 patients on clozapine and 51 comparison patients using data back to 1983; these data were scrutinized for a three-year period. Hospital and outpatient psychiatric records were used to get information on clinical issues, service use, and outcomes. Cost estimates were calculated using various sources (e.g., representative sample of participating institutions and Medicaid), but were valued in 1987 dollars. Clinical input about the average length of hospital stay for changing medications in treatment refractory schizophrenic patients was addressed by surveying nine psychiatrists—seven from research facilities and two from independent settings. The results indicated that clozapine saved direct costs particularly by decreasing inpatient costs, even with the offset of increased outpatient services.

Using the study aspect framework, several aspects cannot be assessed: type of study, discounting, and sensitivity analysis. It appears that a simulation model was used, but this is not clearly specified. Discounting is not addressed, and no sensitivity analysis results are presented. This work was criticized because it did not include the costs of the dropouts (N=46), and a re-analysis determined that savings would persist but at reduced amounts.[45]

In 1993 Meltzer and colleagues[46] reported on the cost-effectiveness of clozapine using data on 96 treatment refractory patients with the following study time frame: two years prior to beginning and the first two years after starting clozapine, 61.5% of patients (N=59) remained on the drug for two years, and complete cost data could only be obtained on 37 of the 59 and on 10 of the 37 dropouts. Sources of data were obtained from patient records, direct interview, and questionnaires. Cost data were those used by Revicki et al.[44] from a composite sampling of institutions, Medicaid carriers, and so on. The results indicated that for those patients treated with clozapine, even dropouts, $8,702 was saved annually per patient. Primary savings appeared in reduced hospitalizations even when an index hospitalization of 21 days is left in the analysis. Several study aspects are unclear. The perspective of the study is unclear, and only direct costs were used in the final cost analyses, despite the availability of quality of life data. No sensitivity analyses were conducted, and no cost-effectiveness ratios are presented; the study appears to be a cost-benefit analysis.

Finally, another 1993 study from the United Kingdom used a decision analytic model to determine the likelihood of different outcomes.[47] Sources of data included physician panels, clinical interview and records, literature review, and National Health Service statistics. A discount rate of 6% was used, and results indicated that patients on clozapine had an expected lifetime gain of nearly six years with mild or no disability compared with standard antipsychotic medication treatments. Sensitivity analyses were conducted and found that in most situations clozapine was cost-neutral or cost-effective. Results were calculated for both one-year and lifetime outcomes.

CONCLUSION

Given the recent evidence documenting the prevalence of neuropsychiatric disorders, the younger age of onset, and the efficacious treatments available, economic evaluations of treatments are tremendously important and timely. Given that recent treatment inroads have been made
in psychopharmacology, such as new antidepressants and antipsychotics,
the time is ripe for pharmacoeconomic analyses of these medications. This
chapter has summarized basic concepts of clinical economics and reviewed
the relevant research. What is clear is that pharmacoeconomic analyses for
maintenance psychotropic treatments are in an early developmental stage.
Most of the studies cited were retrospective studies, many of which lacked
critical components. Clearly, prospective clinical trials with economic analyses built in from the start are imperative.

Several methodological issues have been addressed in this review, and
it is clear that this evolving research field, like most others, would benefit
from some standardization, especially in considering similar medications
for the same disorder. For example, a basic core set of outcomes, clinical
and otherwise (e.g., quality of life), should be employed and would cer-
tainly be useful in making comparisons about the effectiveness and cost-
effectiveness of medications across different populations in different treatment settings. Similarly, costing methods in maintenance pharmacotherapy
cost analyses should be standardized and have a basic level of comprehen-
siveness.

While these methodological issues are critical to pharmacoeconomics research, the larger challenge is conducting this work in real-world settings.
Simon and colleagues put forth the challenge:

> Accurate assessment of "real world" effectiveness and cost, however, may re-
> quire modification of nearly all aspects of randomized trial design including:
> patient recruitment and selection; therapeutic approach; training and skill of
> treating clinicians; procedures for clinical management; outcome assessment;
> and, analysis.... While questions of treatment efficacy are best examined within
> the controlled environment of a typical randomized trial, cost-effectiveness
> questions involve all of the complexities of an organic health care delivery sys-
> tem. Research methods...must incorporate these complexities including het-
> erogenous patients and providers.[18]

This challenge can and should be met by furthering collaboration between
clinical and health services researchers as the fundamental question in

clinical economics—is the treatment a good value for the resources put forth—continues to loom large.

REFERENCES

1. Souetre, E. (1994). Economic evaluation in mental disorders: Community versus institutional care. *PharmacoEconomics*, 6(4):330–336.
2. Greenberg, P., Stiglin, L., Finkelstein, S., et al. (1993). The economic burden of depression in 1990. *J Clin Psychiatry*, 54:405–418.
3. Eisenberg, J.M. (1989). Clinical economics: A guide to the economic analysis of clinical practices. *JAMA*, 262(20):2879–2886.
4. Eisenberg, J.M., Schulman, K.A., Glick, H., et al. (1994). Pharmacoeconomics: Economic evaluation of pharmaceuticals. In Strom B.L. (Ed.), *Pharmacoepidemiology* (2nd ed.) (pp. 369–493). Chichester, England: John Wiley & Sons Ltd.
5. Schulman, K.A. (1993). The use of evaluation in pharmaceutical reimbursement decisions in the United States. *Canadian Collaborative Workshop on Pharmacoeconomics*, Proceedings, 19–23.
6. Cooke, J. (1994). The practical impact of pharmacoeconomics on institutional managers. *PharmacoEconomics*, 6(4):289–297.
7. Davey, P., Malek, M. (1994). The impact of pharmacoeconomics on the practitioner and the patient: A conflict of interests? *PharmacoEconomics*, 6(4):298–309.
8. Schulman, K.A. (1996). Pharmacoeconomics and clinical practice: A physician's view. In L. Bootman, *Principles of Pharmacoeconomics* (2nd ed.) (pp. 253–270). Cincinnati, OH: Harvey Whitney Books.
9. Detsky, A.S. (1994). Using cost-effectiveness analysis for formulary decision making: From theory into practice. *PharmacoEconomics*, 6(4):281–288.
10. Drummond, M.F. (1994). Issues in the conduct of economic evaluations of pharmaceutical products. *PharmacoEconomics*, 6(5):405–411.
11. Hillman, A.L., Eisenberg, J., Pauly, M. et al. (1991). Avoiding bias in the conduct and reporting of cost-effectiveness research sponsored by pharmaceutical companies. *N Engl J Med*, 324(19):1362–5.
12. Drummond, M.F. (1994). Guidelines for pharmacoeconomic studies: The ways forward. *PharmacoEconomics*, 6(6): 493–497.
13. Jacobs, P., Bachynsky, J., Baladi, J-F. (1995). A comparative review of pharmacoeconomic guidelines. *PharmacoEconomics*, 8(3):182–189.
14. Clemens, K., Townsend, R., Luscombe, F., et al. (1995). Methodological and conduct principles for pharmacoeconomic research. *PharmacoEconomics*, 8(2):169–174.
15. Schulman, K.A., Rubenstein, E.L., Glick, H.A., et al. (1995). Relationships between sponsors and investigators in pharmacoeconomic and clinical research. *PharmacoEconomics*, 7(3):206–220.
16. Schulman, K.A., Sulmasy, D.P., Roney, D. (1994). Ethics, economics, and the publication policies of major medical journals. *JAMA*, 272(2):154–156.
17. McGhan, W.F., Briesacher, B.A. (1994). Implementing pharmacoeconomic outcomes management. *PharmacoEconomics*, 6(5):412–416.
18. Simon, G., Wagner, E., Vonkorff, M. (1995). Cost-effectiveness comparisons using "real world" randomized trials: The case of new antidepressant drugs. *J Clin Epidemiol*, 48(3):363–373.
19. Bombardier, C., Eisenberg, J. (1985). Looking into the crystal ball: Can we estimate the lifetime cost of rheumatoid arthritis? *J Rheumatol*, 12:201–204.

20. Coast, J. (1993). Developing the QALY concept: Exploring the problems of data acquisition. *PharmacoEconomics*, 4(4):240–246.
21. Gafni, A., Birch, S., Mehrez, A. (1993). Economics, health and health economics: HYEs versus QALYs. *J Health Economics*, 11:325–339.
22. Froberg, D.G., Kane, R.L. (1989a). Methodology for measuring health-state preferences - I: Measurement strategies. *J Clin Epidemiol*, 42:345–354.
23. Froberg, D.G., Kane, R.L. (1989b). Methodology for measuring health-state preferences - II: Scaling methods. *J Clin Epidemiol*, 42:459–471.
24. Froberg, D.G., Kane, R.L. (1989c). Methodology for measuring health-state preferences - III: Population and context effects. *J Clin Epidemiol*, 42:585–592.
25. Froberg, D.G., Kane, R.L. (1989d). Methodology for measuring health-state preferences - IV: Progress and a research agenda. *J Clin Epidemiol*, 42:675–685.
26. Dranove, D. (1995). Measuring costs. In Sloan, F.A. (Ed.), *Valuing Health Care* (pp. 61–75). New York: Cambridge University Press.
27. Glick, H., Kington, R. (1992). Pharmacoeconomics: Principles and basic techniques of economic analysis. In Strom, B.L., Velo, G. (Eds.), *Drug Epidemiology and Post Marketing Surveillance* (pp. 115–124). New York: Plenum Press.
28. Viscusi, W.K. (1995). Discounting health effects for medical decisions. In Sloan, F.A. (Ed.), *Valuing Health Care* (pp. 125–147). New York: Cambridge University Press.
29. Pauly, M.V. (1995). Valuing health care benefits in money terms. In Sloan, F.A. (Ed.), *Valuing Health Care* (pp. 99–122). New York: Cambridge University Press.
30. Richardson, W.S., Detsky, A.S. (1995). Users' guides to the medical literature: VII. How to use a clinical decision analysis; B. What are the results and will they help me in caring for my patients? *JAMA*, 273(20):1610–1613.
31. Wells, K., Hays, R.D., Burnam, M.A., et al. (1989). The functioning and well-being of depressed patients: Results from the Medical Outcomes Study. *JAMA*, 262:914–919.
32. Agency for Health Care Policy and Research Publication Number 93-0550, *Clinical Practice Guideline, Depression in Primary Care*. Rockville, MD, April 1993.
33. Kamlet, M.S., Wade, M., Kupfer, D.J., et al. (1992). Cost-utility analysis of maintenance treatment for recurrent depression: A theoretical framework and numerical illustration. In Frank, R.G., Manning, Jr., W.G. (Eds.), *Economics and mental health* (pp. 267–291). Baltimore and London: Johns Hopkins University Press.
34. Hatziandreu, E., Brown, R.E., Revicki, D.A., et al. (1994). Cost utility of maintenance treatment of recurrent depression with sertraline versus episodic treatment with dothiepin. *PharmacoEconomics*, 5(3):249–264.
35. Nuijten, M.J., Hardens, M., Souetre, E. (1995). A Markov process analysis comparing the cost effectiveness of maintenance therapy with citalopram versus standard therapy in major depression. *PharmacoEconomics*, 8(2):159–168.
36. Bentkover, J.D., Feighner, J.P. (1995). Cost analysis of paroxetine versus imipramine in major depression. *PharmacoEconomics*, 8(3):223–232.
37. Jonsson, B., Bebbington, P.E. (1994). What price depression? The cost of depression and the cost-effectiveness of pharmacological treatment. *Br J Psychiatry*, 164:665–673.
38. Revicki, D.A., Brown, R.E., Palmer, W., et al. (1995). Modelling the cost effectiveness of antidepressant treatment in primary care. *PharmacoEconomics*, 8(6):524–540.
39. Sturm, R., Wells, K. (1995). How can care for depression become more cost-effective? *JAMA*, 273:51–58.
40. O'Brien, B.J., Novosel, S., Torrance, G., et al. (1995). Assessing the economic value of a new antidepressant: A willingness-to-pay approach. *PharmacoEconomics*, 8(1):34–35.
41. Rupp, A., Keith, S. (1993). The costs of schizophrenia. *Psychiatric Clin North Am*, 16:413–423.
42. Frankenburg, F.R. (1993). Is clozapine worth its cost? *PharmacoEconomics*, 4(5):311–314.

43. Fitton, A., Benfield, P. (1993). Clozapine, an appraisal of its pharmacoeconomic benefits in the treatment of schizophrenia. *PharmacoEconomics*, 4(2):131–156.
44. Revicki, D.A., Luce, B.R., Weschler, J.M., et al. (1990). Cost-effectiveness of clozapine for treatment-resistant schizophrenic patients. *Hosp Comm Psychiatry*, 41(8):850–854.
45. Revicki, D.A., Luce, B.R., Weschler, J.M., et al. (1991). Clozapine's cost benefits. Correspondence. *Hosp Comm Psychiatry*, 42:93–94.
46. Meltzer, H.Y., Cola, P., Way, L., et al. (1993). Cost effectiveness of clozapine in neuroleptic-resistant schizophrenia. *Am J Psychiatry*, 150(11):1630–1638.
47. Davies, L., Drummond, M. (1993). Assessment of costs and benefits of drug therapy for treatment-resistant schizophrenia in the United Kingdom. *Br J Psychiatry*, 162, 38–42.

C H A P T E R

4

DEPRESSIVE DISORDERS

INTRODUCTION

Depressive disorders include both unipolar and bipolar affective disorders. This chapter addresses the primary unipolar depressive disorders: recurrent major depressive disorder (MDD) and dysthymia, with emphasis on MDD. Bipolar disorders are discussed in Chapter 5. The secondary depressive disorders, those due to a medical condition, medications, or drugs, are mentioned briefly. The term "depression" can be used to describe an affective state, a symptom, or a syndrome. Depression is used in this chapter to refer to the syndrome including depressive episodes and the range of depressive disorders.

EPIDEMIOLOGY

PREVALENCE

Depressive disorders affect approximately 20% of the population at one time in their lives. Angst reviewed studies from the United States and Europe and found point prevalence rates for MDD varying from 1.5–6.9%, with lifetime prevalence rates varying from 4.4–19.5%.[1] The rate of dysthymia is similar; the point prevalence rates were 1–4%, with a lifetime prevalence rate of 3–20%. Two large epidemiologic studies have been conducted recently in the United States. The largest study, the Epidemiologic Catchment Area (ECA) Study, reports a relatively low prevalence of depressive disorders: a 1-month prevalence of 2.3% for major depressive episode (MDE) and a lifetime prevalence of only 5.9%.[2] The prevalence of dysthymia was 3.3% both at 1 month and over a lifetime. Results from the National Comorbidity Survey indicate a 10.3% 12-month prevalence of MDE, a 17.1% lifetime prevalence of MDE, and a 2.5% 12-month and 6.4% lifetime prevalence of dysthymia.[3] Although there is considerable variation between studies, when taken together, the lifetime prevalence of depressive disorders is accepted as about 20%.

COMORBIDITY WITH SUBSTANCE-RELATED DISORDERS

There is significant comorbidity between depressive disorders and substance-related disorders; 32% of individuals with at least one affective disorder diagnosis also suffer from some form of substance abuse or dependence.[2] Of patients with unipolar MDD, 27.2% have a comorbid diagnosis of substance abuse or dependence; 16.5% have comorbid MDD and alcohol diagnosis, while 18% have comorbid MDD and some other drug diagnosis (there is considerable overlap, with many patients having both alcohol and other drug diagnoses). Of patients with dysthymia, 31.4% suffer from substance abuse.

GENDER

The prevalence of depressive disorders is two to four times higher in females than in males across all adult ages. Hypotheses for this gender difference range from artifactual differences to real psychosocial, genetic, and endocrine differences between genders. None has been proven.

AGE

There is a bimodal peak age of onset for MDD in the late twenties and again in the fifties. There is no difference between males and females in age of onset. Patients with a later age of onset are more likely to have recurrent depressive episodes. Increasing age is associated with increased frequency of depressive episodes and decreased interepisode well time. Psychotic features are more frequent with older age.

COST

Depression places a great burden on society in both economic cost and the cost of human suffering. The total cost of depression in the United States in 1990 was $43.7 billion, with $12.4 billion in direct costs and $31.7 billion in indirect costs.[4] Much of the indirect cost reflects cost to industry of absence from work and decreased productivity. Compared with major medical illnesses with similar costs, depression is highly treatable, with response rates approaching 80%.

Unfortunately, depression is frequently underrecognized and under-treated. When depression is not recognized early in its presentation, costly and unnecessary tests may be performed in an attempt to find an organic etiology for the patient's symptoms. This not only adds to the direct cost of treatment, but also delays appropriate treatment. A study of the California Medicaid program estimated the cost of treatment failure in major depression at $1,043 per person in the first year, mostly reflected in higher hospital costs.[5] The cost of treatment failure is high, but it is a cost that might be diminished with adequate recognition, treatment, and prophylaxis.

NATURAL HISTORY

There have been many naturalistic studies of the course of depression. All indicate that it is a recurrent, lifelong, chronic illness.[6,7] Depression is a cyclic illness marked by discrete depressive episodes with interepisode return to premorbid level of functioning in most cases. In some, residual symptoms remain after an episode has resolved, resulting in subsyndromal depression, impaired interepisode functioning, and functional disability.

Recovery rates from a depressive episode are approximately 80%. In one study, 88% of patients recovered over a five-year period, with more than 50% recovering in the first six months. Only 18% of those who were still ill at one year were recovered at five years.[8] In another study, 21% of patients had not fully recovered three years after the onset of the index episode despite treatment.[9] Patients who only attain a partial remission have an increased risk of recurrent depressive episodes as well as poor interepisode functioning with chronic disability.

The average duration of a depressive episode is six months. When symptoms have decreased and are mild but persistent, the patient has achieved a partial remission. When symptoms have completely resolved, the remission is considered complete. If symptoms return to the severity of meeting criteria for a MDE within six months, it is called a relapse. If symptoms return after six months, it is a recurrence.

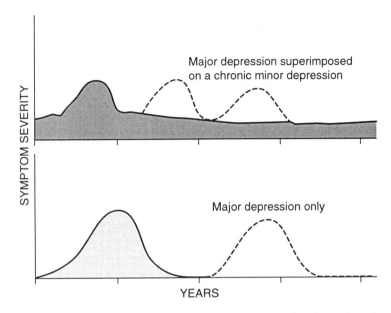

FIG. 4–1. *Symptom course in double depression and major depression alone. From Keller, M.B. (1994). Depression: A long-term illness. <u>Br J Psychiatry</u>, 165(suppl 26):9–15. Copyright 1994 by Royal College of Psychiatrists. Reprinted with permission.*

Relapse rates after remission are highest immediately after recovery and then decrease steadily. Of those patients who recovered from a depressive episode, 25% relapsed within 12 weeks and half of them relapsed within the first 4 weeks.[10] In another study, relapse rates were 15% at 6 months and 22% at 12 months.[11] The majority of those who relapse early have chronic depression: (dysthymia) punctuated by MDEs; also known as "double depression" (Figure 4–1).

For the majority of patients, depression is a recurrent illness: as many as 70–80% have multiple episodes.[1] After a first episode, 50–60% of patients go on to have a second. Of those, 70% have a third episode and 90% of those have a fourth. With an increasing number of prior episodes, the likelihood of recurrence increases and the time to relapse shortens. The duration of interepisode well time also decreases with increasing age.[11]

Predictors of relapse (Table 4–1) include greater number of previous episodes, longer duration of the index episode, increased severity of the index episode, secondary depression, history of nonaffective psychiatric disorder, bipolar illness, early age of onset, increasing age, and low family income.[1,9,11,12]

TABLE 4–1. PREDICTORS OF RELAPSE OF DEPRESSIVE EPISODE

Course	Comorbidity	Demographics	Psychosocial
Greater number of previous episodes Longer duration of index episode Increased severity of index episode	Secondary depression History of comorbid nonaffective psychiatric disorder Bipolarity Dysthymic symptoms after recovery Chronic medical condition	Early age of onset Increasing age	Low family income

The long-term impact of depression can be devastating to a person's life. In a 20-year follow-up of depressed patients, 15–20% developed a chronic course (over two years of an unremitting MDE) and 10–15% committed suicide.[13] Of patients with a chronic course, 75% recovered for at least eight weeks but only about 33% of patients sustained a six-month recovery.[14] Some patients with chronic unipolar depression spent almost a quarter of their lives in MDEs.[15] Many patients who do recover have residual symptoms that contribute to a decreased quality of life.

Patients with dysthymia, or chronic mild depression, have an increased risk of developing MDEs and recurrent episodes and also have poor interepisode recovery with functional impairment.

MORBIDITY

Recurrent depressive illness is associated with significant functional morbidity in all areas including physical, social, and role functioning. Because of the stigma of mental illness, the morbidity of depression is often misidentified and mistreated. Depression impairs the patient's ability to perform his or her usual social, academic, and work roles. The consequences of this diminished functioning may be neglected children, strained family relationships, and poor academic or job performance.

The functional disability associated with depression is comparable to or worse than that associated with eight major medical conditions: hypertension, diabetes, coronary artery disease, angina, arthritis, back disease, lung disease, and gastrointestinal disease.[16] Depression is more debilitating than diabetes, arthritis, and hypertension in physical, role, and social functioning. Only advanced coronary artery disease accounts for more disability days than depression and only arthritis causes more chronic pain (Figure 4–2).[17] The best way to prevent or minimize this disability is to recognize

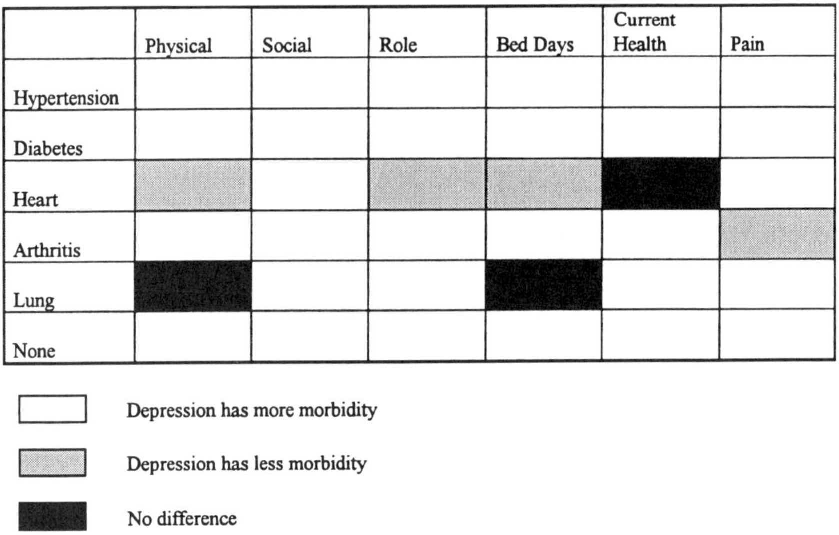

	Physical	Social	Role	Bed Days	Current Health	Pain
Hypertension						
Diabetes						
Heart	▒		▒	▒	█	
Arthritis						▒
Lung	█			█		
None						

☐ Depression has more morbidity

▒ Depression has less morbidity

█ No difference

FIG. 4–2. Comparison of the Unique Association of Depression of Chronic Medical Conditions with Daily Functioning and Well-Being. From Wells, K.B. and Burnam, M.A. (1991). Caring for depression in America. Psychiatric Med, 9(4):512. Copyright 1991 by Ryandic Publishing, Inc. Reprinted with permission.

depression early, provide appropriate treatment, and institute appropriate maintenance treatment to prevent future recurrences.

MORTALITY

Mortality in major depression is as high as 15%, with suicide the major cause of death in both short- and long-term follow-up.[18] Short-term follow-up revealed a 3% suicide rate in depression with equal rates in patients with primary, secondary, and bipolar depression.[19] Suicide accounted for about 30% of the deaths in this cohort. About 70% of people who complete suicide suffer from a depressive disorder. The suicide rate in the general population in 1988 was 12.4 per 100,000.[20] There is a bimodal age distribution with the first peak in the 30–34 year age group of 15.4 per 100,000 and a higher peak in late life at 80–84 years of 28 per 100,000. The group at highest risk for suicide is elderly white men ages 80–84 with a rate of 72.6/100,000, more than six times the age adjusted rate. Females are more likely to make suicide attempts but males are more likely to be successful, usually due to the use of more lethal means such as firearms. The ratio of completed to attempted suicide increases with increasing age among

TABLE 4–2. PREDICTORS OF SUICIDE

Affective Symptoms	Comorbidity	Past History	Demographics	Psychosocial
Hopelessness Mood cycling with an episode Loss of mood reactivity	Psychotic symptoms Substance abuse Chronic medical condition	History of previous attempts Family history of completed suicide	Increasing age Male White	Married Social isolation Negative life event

both sexes.[21] More than half of suicides are associated with alcohol or drug use and over one-quarter of addicts commit suicide.[22] Predictors of suicide among depressed patients are listed in Table 4–2.[23,24,25,26,27]

Prevention of suicide requires adequate long-term treatment of the underlying depressive disorder to prevent future episodes of depression. However, treatment is not always successful. A time of high risk for suicide is 6 to 12 months after discharge from hospital, and 40% of suicide victims visited a physician within one month of their death, but only 20% communicated suicidal ideation to their physician.[28]

Suicide is not the only cause of death in depression. Patients with depression tend to have poorer physical health and to recover more slowly from physical illness. Thus, depression increases the mortality associated with comorbid medical conditions. Patients with depression-induced psychotic symptoms are more likely to act irrationally, take greater risks, and have poor judgment, which results in higher mortality from accidents and high-risk behavior.

DIAGNOSIS

RECOGNITION

Successful treatment of depressive disorders depends first on recognition and accurate diagnosis. Unfortunately, depression often remains unrecognized and inadequately treated. Over 50% of depressed patients are treated in the primary care setting by internists and family practitioners, and only 20% are treated in the mental health sector.[29] Primary care physicians recognize depression in only 50% of their patients who suffer from depression, leaving half of their depressed patients undiagnosed and untreated.[30] Of the patients treated by primary care physicians for depression, fewer than 50% are appropriately treated with appropriate antidepressant medications and doses for an adequate length of time.[31,32]

The most important strategy for improving recognition of depression is increasing physician awareness. Primary care physicians must look actively for depression in their patients and should think of it early in the differential diagnosis, particularly in patients who complain primarily of disturbed sleep, appetite, and energy as well as multiple somatic symptoms. Certain tools may help physicians accurately recognize depression including screening questionnaires, screening interviews, self-report scales, and structured scales for depression.

SCREENING INSTRUMENTS

Screening instruments include self-report scales and structured interviews. A relatively new instrument, the PRIME-MD (Figure 4–3), has been developed as a tool for primary care physicians to quickly screen their patients for the presence of mood, anxiety, somatoform, alcohol abuse, and eating disorders.[33] It consists of a one-page patient questionnaire, followed by a structured interview conducted by the physician to follow-up on positive responses from the questionnaire. The structured interview takes an average of eight minutes to administer and has an 83% sensitivity and 88% specificity when compared with evaluations by mental health professionals.

Self-report scales such as the Beck Depression Inventory are useful tools when depression is suspected.[34] This instrument must be followed by a clarification of symptoms by the physician. Other self-report scales include the Zung Self-Rating Depression Scale (SDS), the Hopkins Symptom Checklist (SCL-90), the Inventory for Depressive Symptomatology–Self-Report (IDS-SR), and the CES-D (Figure 4–4).[35,36,37,38] These may be useful in identifying depressive symptoms but cannot be used in isolation to make a diagnosis.

DSM-IV CLASSIFICATION

The system of classification of psychiatric disorders currently employed in the United States is the *Diagnostic and Statistical Manual of Mental Disorders*, fourth edition, (DSM-IV).[39] According to this system, primary depressive disorders can be divided into major depressive disorder (MDD), dysthymic disorder, and depressive disorder not otherwise specified (NOS). Unipolar depressive disorders are differentiated from bipolar disorders by having only depressive episodes without manic, hypomanic, or mixed episodes (see Chapter 5). Secondary depressive disorders are mood disorder due to a general medical condition (GMC) and substance-induced mood disorder.

NAME: _____

INSTRUCTION: This questionnaire will help your doctor better understand problems that you may have. Your doctor may ask you more questions about some of these items. Please make sure to check a box for <u>every</u> item.

During the **PAST MONTH**, have you **OFTEN** been bothered by...	YES	NO
1. stomach pain	☐	☐
2. back pain	☐	☐
3. pain in your arms, legs, or joints (knees, hips, etc)	☐	☐
4. menstrual pain or problems	☐	☐
5. pain or problems during sexual intercourse	☐	☐
6. headaches	☐	☐
7. chest pain	☐	☐
8. dizziness	☐	☐
9. fainting spells	☐	☐
10. feeling your heart pound or race	☐	☐
11. shortness of breath	☐	☐
12. constipation, loose bowels, or diarrhea	☐	☐
13. nausea, gas, or indigestion	☐	☐
14. feeling tired or having low energy	☐	☐
15. trouble sleeping	☐	☐
16. the thought that you have a serious undiagnosed disease	☐	☐
17. your eating being out of control	☐	☐
18. little interest or pleasure in doing things	☐	☐
19. feeling down, depressed, or hopeless	☐	☐
20. "nerves" or feeling anxious or on edge	☐	☐
21. worrying about a lot of different things	☐	☐

During the **PAST MONTH**...	YES	NO
22. have you had an anxiety attack (suddenly feeling fear or panic)	☐	☐
23. have you thought you should cut down on your drinking of alcohol	☐	☐
24. has anyone complained about your drinking	☐	☐
25. have you felt guilty or upset about your drinking	☐	☐
26. was there ever a single day in which you had five or more drinks of beer, wine, or liquor	☐	☐

Overall, would you say your health is:

Excellent ☐
Very good ☐
Good ☐
Fair ☐
Poor ☐

FIG. 4–3. Patient questionnaire PRIME-MD (Primary Care Evaluation of Mental Disorders). One-page questionnaire is completed by patient before seeing the physician. PRIME-MD is registered trademark of Pfizer Inc., which also is the holder of the copyright to PRIME-MD materials. Reprinted with permission.

63

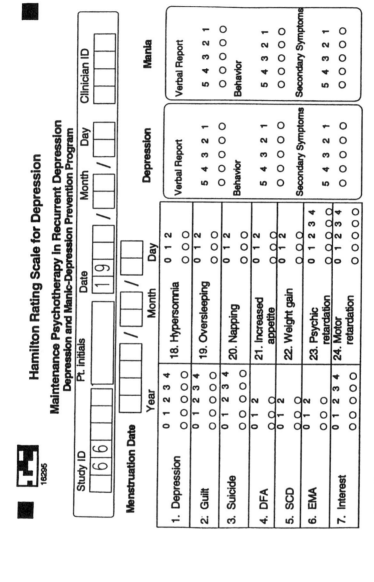

FIG. 4–4. Hamilton Rating Scale for Depression. *J Neurol Neurosurge and Psychiatry,* 23:56–61. Copyright 1960. Reprinted with permission from the BMJ Publishing Group.

64

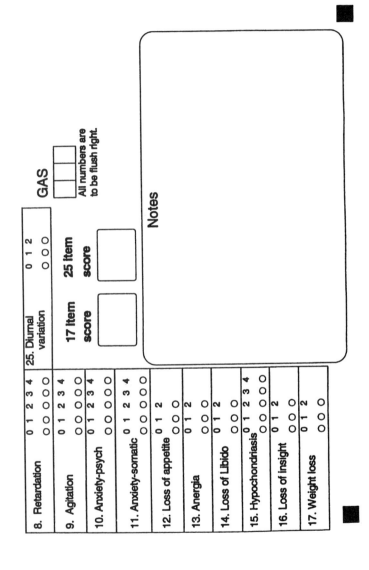

FIG. 4-4. Hamilton Rating Scale for Depression. *J Neurol Neurosurge and Psychiatry.* 23:56–61. Copyright 1960. Reprinted with permission from the BMJ Publishing Group.

MAJOR DEPRESSIVE EPISODE (MDE)

See Table 5–1 in Chapter 5. Symptoms of "masked" depression include insomnia, fatigue, and somatic complaints, particularly of the cardiovascular, gastrointestinal, genitourinary, and musculoskeletal systems. Masked depression is especially difficult to identify and treat as these patients frequently resist receiving a diagnosis of depression.

In adolescence, a MDE may be associated with substance abuse, antisocial behavior, truancy, promiscuity, rejection hypersensitivity, and decreased hygiene. In the elderly, depressive episodes may be accompanied by state-dependent cognitive deficits that resemble dementia.

MAJOR DEPRESSIVE DISORDER (MDD)

Table 4–3 presents the DSM-IV specifiers for both single episode and recurrent major depressive disorders.

COMORBIDITY WITH PSYCHIATRIC ILLNESSES

MDD may be comorbid with dysthymic disorder. Dysthymic disorder may precede MDD in 10–25% of patients. Other frequent comorbidities of MDD include substance-related disorders, panic disorder, obsessive-compulsive disorder, anorexia nervosa, bulimia nervosa, and borderline personality disorder.

COMORBIDITY WITH MEDICAL/NEUROLOGICAL ILLNESSES

MDD may be comorbid with any physical illness, particularly chronic medical conditions. At times it may be difficult to determine if the medical condition plays an etiological role in the development of the depression. In cases in which there is a comorbid neurological illness, it is often etiologically related to the depression. Depression frequently is seen with endocrine abnormalities, cardiovascular disease, gastrointestinal illnesses, malignancies, and stroke. The differentiation of primary versus comorbid medical or neurological illness may be aided by a history of symptoms coincident with the onset of the medical illness, resolution of symptoms with successful treatment of the medical condition, and atypical features of an MDE. Depression may interfere with the treatment of the medical illness and may account for a poorer outcome.

TABLE 4-3. DIAGNOSTIC CRITERIA FOR MAJOR DEPRESSIVE DISORDER

Single Episode

Presence of a single major depressive episode.

The major depressive episode is not better accounted for by schizoaffective disorder and is not superimposed on schizophrenic, schizophreniform disorder, delusional disorder, or psychotic disorder not otherwise specified.

There has never been a manic episode, a mixed episode, or a hypomanic episode. Note: This exclusion does not apply if all the maniclike or hypomaniclike episodes are substance or treatment-induced or are due to the direct physiological effects of a general medical condition.

Specify (for current or most recent episode):
Severity/psychotic/remission specifiers
Chronic
  with catatonic features
  with melancholic features
  with atypical features
  with postpartum onset

Recurrent Disorder

Presence of two or more major depressive episodes.
Note: To be considered separate episodes, there must be an interval of at least two consecutive months in which criteria are not met for a major depressive episode.

The major depressive episodes are not better accounted for by schizoaffective disorder and are not superimposed on schizophrenic, schizophreniform disorder, delusional disorder, or psychotic disorder not otherwise specified.

There has never been a manic episode, a mixed episode, or a hypomanic episode. Note: This exclusion does not apply if all the maniclike or hypomaniclike episodes are substance or treatment-induced or are due to the direct physiological effects of a general medical condition.

Specify (for current or most recent episode):
Severity/psychotic/remission specifiers
Chronic
  With catatonic features
  With melancholic features
  With atypical features
  With postpartum onset

Specify:
Longitudinal course specifiers (with and without interepisode recovery)
  With seasonal pattern

Adapted with permission from the *Diagnostic and Statistical Manual of Mental Disorders,* 4th ed. (pp. 344–345). Copyright 1994 by American Psychiatric Association.

LABORATORY FINDINGS

There are no diagnostic laboratory findings for depression although there are characteristic laboratory abnormalities that are usually state-dependent and are more common in melancholic, psychotic, or severe depressions. These include abnormalities in the sleep and waking electroencephalogram (EEG), neuroendocrine challenges including the dexamethasone suppression test (DST) and the thyrotropin-releasing hormone (TRH) test, functional and structural brain imaging, evoked potentials, and neurotransmitter metabolism. These studies cannot be used to make a diagnosis.

CULTURAL FACTORS

Mood disorders exist in all societies but are expressed through a wide array of symptoms. Cultural influences affect both the experience and expression of depressive symptoms that may contribute to the underdiagnosis or misdiagnosis of depression in different cultures. The practitioner must therefore be aware of these cultural influences when evaluating a patient. For example, in some cultures depression may be experienced primarily in somatic terms, with patients complaining chiefly of headaches, weakness, tiredness, "nerves," or imbalance. Also, Western psychiatrists may over diagnose psychosis in Asian patients.

AGE

The clinical presentation of depression changes with age. In children and adolescents, depression may present with a predominantly irritable rather than sad mood. Children are more likely to have somatic complaints and social withdrawal but are less likely to experience psychomotor retardation, hypersomnia, and delusions. Children may come to medical attention when their grades start falling, they lose interest in social activities, or they turn to illicit substances (alcohol or other drugs) in attempts to self-medicate. Depression during childhood may have important developmental consequences. Children who are depressed and drop out from activities may fall behind in social and academic achievements, which may also affect personality development and contribute to lifelong adjustment difficulties. Depression in adulthood is more likely to present with the classic features described in DSM-IV.

Depression in the elderly frequently presents with anxiety symptoms, somatic complaints, and cognitive deficits. The cognitive deficits may mimic dementia and are frequently state-dependent, resolving as the depressive episode resolves. However, patients who experience cognitive impairment of depression or "pseudodementia" are more likely to proceed to dementia in later years.

COURSE

Symptoms of an MDE usually develop over days to weeks and may be preceded by prodromal anxiety and mild depressive symptoms. A depressive episode usually lasts six months or longer with complete remission of symptoms and return to premorbid level of functioning in the majority of patients.

FAMILY HISTORY

The incidence of depression is significantly higher in first degree relatives of people with depressive disorders than in the general population.[40] There is also an association between family history of substance abuse disorders and depressive disorders. The genetic component for unipolar depression is not as strong as for bipolar depression.

DIFFERENTIAL DIAGNOSIS

The differential diagnosis for MDD includes other affective disorders, nonaffective psychiatric disorders, and a primary substance use or general medical condition causing depressive symptoms.

Periods of sadness also are a normal part of the human condition and should not be labelled MDD unless they meet full criteria of severity and duration with clinically significant distress or functional impairment.

Bereavement occurs after the loss of a loved one; enough symptoms may be present to meet criteria for MDE. However, symptoms should be attributed to bereavement unless they persist for more than two months after the loss or include marked functional impairment, morbid preoccupation with worthlessness, suicidal ideation, psychotic symptoms, or psychomotor retardation.

An MDE must be differentiated from a **mixed episode** or **manic episode with irritable mood**, which would indicate a **bipolar disorder**. If a patient develops a manic, hypomanic, or mixed episode as a result of treatment for depression with an antidepressant, it is considered a substance-induced episode and the diagnosis of MDD still holds.

Adjustment disorder with depressed mood or with **mixed anxiety and depressed mood** is a depressive episode that does not meet full criteria for an MDE precipitated by a psychosocial stressor.

Schizoaffective disorder is differentiated from MDD by the presence of at least two weeks of delusions or hallucinations in the absence of prominent mood symptoms.

Depressive symptoms associated with **schizophrenia, schizophreniform disorder, delusional disorder,** or **psychotic disorder not otherwise specified** should be considered an associated feature of the primary disorder and do not merit the diagnosis of MDD. However, if depressive symptoms meet full criteria for MDE, an additional diagnosis of depressive disorder not otherwise specified may be made.

Catatonic symptoms may be difficult to classify; that is, it may be difficult to distinguish **schizophrenia, catatonic type** from MDD with catatonic features. Previous history or family history may be helpful in making this distinction. Electroconvulsive therapy (ECT) is a useful treatment for catatonia despite the etiology.

Severe cognitive impairment or **pseudodementia** may accompany depression, especially in the elderly, and may be difficult to differentiate from dementia.

The distractibility and low frustration tolerance seen in **attention deficit hyperactivity disorder (ADHD)** may be difficult to differentiate from MDD. This is especially true in children where the mood disturbance in MDD is predominantly irritability.

Depression may be secondary to the direct physiological effects of a substance such as a drug of abuse, medication, or toxin **(substance-induced mood disorder)** or to a general medical condition **(mood disorder due to a general medical condition).**

DYSTHYMIC DISORDER

Dysthymia refers to a chronic, mild depression that does not meet the severity criteria for MDD. Dysthymia generally has an early onset and is lifelong and if punctuated by recurrent MDEs, it is called "double depression" (Table 4–4).

COMORBIDITY WITH PSYCHIATRIC ILLNESSES

Dysthymia may be comorbid with MDD, substance-related disorders, and various personality disorders including borderline, histrionic, narcissistic, avoidant, and dependent personality disorders as well as with ADHD, conduct disorder, anxiety disorders, learning disorders, and mental retardation in children.

TABLE 4–4. DIAGNOSTIC CRITERIA FOR DYSTHYMIC DISORDER

Depressed mood for most of the day, for more days than not, as indicated either by subjective account or observation by others, for at least two years. Note: In children and adolescents, mood can be irritable and duration must be at least one year.

Presence, while depressed, of two (or more) of the following:
(1) poor appetite or overeating
(2) insomnia or hypersomnia
(3) low energy or fatigue
(4) low self-esteem
(5) poor concentration or difficulty making decisions
(6) feelings of hopelessness

During the two-year period (one year for children or adolescents) of the disturbance, the person has never been without the symptoms in Criteria A and B for more than two months at a time.

No major depressive episode has been present during the first two years of the disturbance (one year for children and adolescents); i.e., the disturbance is not better accounted for by chronic major depressive disorder, or major depressive disorder, in partial remission.

Note: There may have been a previous major depressive episode provided there was a full remission (no significant signs or symptoms for two months) before development of the dysthymic disorder. In addition, after the initial two years (one year in children or adolescents) of dysthymic disorder, there may be superimposed episodes of major depressive disorder, in which case both diagnoses may be given when the criteria are met for a major depressive episode.

There has never been a manic episode, a mixed episode, or a hypomanic episode, and criteria have never been met for cyclothymic disorder.

The disturbance does not occur exclusively during the course of a chronic psychotic disorder, such as schizophrenia or delusional disorder.

The symptoms are not due to the direct physiological effects of a substance (e.g., a drug of abuse, a medication) or a general medical condition (e.g., hypothyroidism).

The symptoms cause clinically significant distress or impairment in social, occupational, or other important areas of functioning.

Specify if:
Early onset: if onset is before age 21 years
Late onset: if onset is age 21 years or older

Specify if:
With atypical features

Adapted with permission from the *Diagnostic and Statistical Manual of Mental Disorders*, 4th ed. (p. 349). Copyright 1994 by American Psychiatric Association.

COURSE

Dysthymia usually has an early and insidious onset. Early onset is associated with increased risk for developing MDD, residual interepisode symptoms and dysfunction, and recurrent MDEs with a chronic course.

DIFFERENTIAL DIAGNOSIS

MDD can be differentiated from dysthymia by the presence of at least five of the criteria for an MDE. There is an approximately 10–20% overlap between the two disorders, with recurrent MDEs superimposed on chronic dysthymia (double depression) (Figure 4–1).

Chronic psychotic disorders may be associated with persistent depressive symptoms, but dysthymia should not be diagnosed in these cases unless symptoms are present when psychotic symptoms are absent. Dysthymia is often difficult to differentiate from **personality disorders** since chronic mood symptoms may contribute to interpersonal difficulties. Primary **substance use** and **medical conditions** must also be ruled out.

DEPRESSIVE DISORDER NOT OTHERWISE SPECIFIED (NOS)

This category includes all those depressive disorders that do not meet criteria for MDD, dysthymia, or adjustment disorder.

SUBSTANCE-INDUCED MOOD DISORDER

Medications, alcohol, and illicit substances may all be associated with depressive symptoms. Depressive symptoms may be secondary to intoxication with, or withdrawal from, a drug of abuse. As substance-related disorders are frequently comorbid with depressive disorders, it is important to correlate the time course of substance use or withdrawal with depressive symptoms as well as to look for atypical features of depressive disorders that may suggest a substance-related etiology. Persistent depressive symptoms during periods of abstinence or a history of previous MDEs in the absence of substance use suggests a primary depressive disorder. Some medications may precipitate a depressive episode, and a diagnosis may be based on the temporal relationship between starting a medication and onset of symptoms. Drugs that may cause depression are listed in Table 4–5.

MOOD DISORDER DUE TO A GENERAL MEDICAL CONDITION

Depression may also be secondary to a medical or neurological illness (Table 4–6). First, the diagnosis of a medical condition must be established, then the depressive disorder must be etiologically related to this medical condition through a physiological mechanism.

TABLE 4–5. DRUGS ASSOCIATED WITH DEPRESSION*

Analgesics	Cardiac Agents
Opiates	Digitalis (Crystodigin)
	Procainamide (Pronestyl)
Antihypertensives	Propranolol (Inderal)
Guanethidine (Ismelin)	Clonidine (Catapres, Combipres)
Methyldopa (Aldomet)	
Reserpine (Serpasil)	**Sedative-Hypnotic Agents**
Hydralazine (Apresoline)	Alcohol
Propranolol (Inderal)	Chloral hydrate (Noctec)
	Benzodiazepines
Anti-infectious Agents	
Sulfonamides	**Steroids**
Clotrimazole (Lotrimin, Mycelex)	Oral contraceptives
Ethionamide (Trecator-SC)	Cortisol (Solu-Cortef)
Griseofulvin (Fulvicin)	ACTH (Acthar)
Metronidazole (Flagyl)	**Stimulants**
Anti-inflammatory Agents	Amphetamine (Benzedrine)
Phenacetin (Emprazil)	Fenfluramine (Pondimin)
Phenylbutazone (Butazolidin)	
Pentazocine (Talwin)	**Other Drugs**
Estrogen withdrawal (Premarin)	L-dopa (Carbidopa)
	Amantadine (Symmetrel)
Antineoplastic Agents	Methysergide (Sansert)
Plicamycin (Mithracin)	Acetazolamide (Diamox)
Azathioprine (Imuran)	Carbamazepine (Tegretol)
Bleomycin (Blemoxane)	Choline (Trilisate)
L-Asparaginase (Elspar)	Disulfiram (Antabuse)
	Physostigmine (Antilirium)
Antipsychotic Medications	Ethambutol (Myambutol)
	Indomethacin (Indocin)

*Association does not mean causality. Some agents (e.g., reserpine and steroids) have a clear relationship with depression, whereas many other drugs do not.
Adapted from Gelenberg, A.J., Bassuk, E.L., Schoonover, S.C. (1991). *The Practitioner's Guide to Psychoactive Drugs*, 3rd ed. (p. 74). Copyright 1991 by Plenum Publishing Corp. Reprinted with permission.

SUMMARY

Recognition and accurate diagnosis of depressive disorders are the first steps toward adequate treatment of the acute depressive episode and prophylactic treatment when appropriate. While this section has differentiated between the different depressive disorders and their associated features and provided a framework for developing diagnostic accuracy based on DSM-IV, the depressive disorders are discussed all together in the ensuing sections on acute, continuation, and maintenance treatment. Later in

TABLE 4–6. MEDICAL CONDITIONS ASSOCIATED WITH DEPRESSION

Autoimmune Systemic lupus erythematosis **Endocrine** Hypothyroidism Hyperthyroidism Cushing's syndrome Hypercalcemia Hyponatremia Diabetes mellitus **Gastrointestinal** Malabsorption Crohn's disease Irritable bowel syndrome **Infectious** Viral infections Influenza Mononucleosis Syphilis	**Malignancies** Brain tumor Pancreatic cancer Ovarian adenocarcinoma Paraneoplastic syndrome **Neurologic** Stroke Multiple sclerosis Parkinson's disease Huntington's disease Subdural hematoma Closed head injuries Seizure disorders Neurodegenerative dementias **Nutritional** Vitamin B_{12} deficiency Pellagra **Renal** Chronic renal failure

the chapter, distinctions are made about the treatment of specific depressive disorders and their particular features.

ACUTE AND CONTINUATION PHARMACOLOGICAL TREATMENT

The acute treatment of depression has been extensively studied, and treatment guidelines and recommendations have been compiled by many authors. We refer readers to the *Practice Guidelines for Major Depressive Disorder in Adults* published by the American Psychiatric Association (APA) in 1993 and a comprehensive book by Janicek et al.[41,42] There are several classes of antidepressants with many agents available in the United States that have been proven effective for acute treatment of depression.

GENERAL PRINCIPLES OF ACUTE TREATMENT

Therapeutic Alliance

Establishing and maintaining rapport with the patient during the evaluation phase and throughout treatment is crucial for an optimal outcome. In addition to creating a safe environment and actively listening, the physician should also provide psychoeducation about depression and its treatment. When patients are aware of potential adverse effects of medications and the length of time required for a therapeutic effect, they are more likely to continue with the medication for an adequate time and to report side effects that can then be addressed and ameliorated. Patients should also be informed about the need for taking antidepressant medication regularly and not just when they are feeling particularly distressed. A good relationship is crucial for maintaining compliance with the recommended treatment, especially for long-term maintenance treatment. Patients frequently stop taking antidepressant medications, as they would antibiotics or pain relievers, when they are feeling better. It is the physician's responsibility to educate patients about the need to continue medication after symptoms have resolved and patients have returned to their usual state of functioning.

INITIATING TREATMENT

Once the diagnosis of a primary major depressive episode is made, therapy should be initiated. Appropriate lab work should be obtained at baseline before initiating treatment (depending on the antidepressant). Dosing should be started low and gradually increased every few days to an appropriate initial dose to avoid severe side effects that might prompt patients to refuse to continue the trial. Antidepressants take at least two weeks to exert an effect. Some patients have an "early response" within a few days, which may be a placebo effect. Patient characteristics predictive of a placebo response, which is 20–40% in depression, are neurotic premorbid personality, fluctuating symptoms with day-to-day variation, and high mood reactivity.[42]

Once a medication trial is initiated and an appropriate dose achieved, this dose should be maintained for at least two weeks or until steady state is achieved before increasing the dose. Titration may be continued with increases approximately every two weeks until a therapeutic response is obtained or the maximum dose is achieved, or titration is limited by side effects. An adequate antidepressant trial is six to eight weeks at a therapeutic dose or level. Plasma levels should be monitored for drugs that have a relationship to clinical response (i.e., most tricyclics).

If there is only partial or no response after an adequate trial, two treatment strategies exist: switch to another agent or augment with a second agent. If switching to a different antidepressant, it is best to try first an agent from another class if possible, although a trial of another agent in the same class may be effective. Nonresponse to one antidepressant does not predict nonresponse to other antidepressants in that or other classes. Fully 50% of

TABLE 4–7. FACTORS TO CONSIDER IN CHOOSING AN
ANTIDEPRESSANT

General	Symptoms
• Efficacy	• Symptom profile
• Safety	• Suicidality
• Ease of administration	**History**
• Cost	• Personal history of response to a medication
• Patient age	• Family history of response to a medication
Side Effects	**Comorbidities**
• Tolerability	• Medical or neurological illness
• Side-effect profile	• Psychiatric illness
• Potential adverse effects	• Concomitant medications

patients respond to an initial antidepressant trial, with another 35–40%
responding to an alternative agent or augmentation. Only 10–15% of patients remain treatment nonresponsive after multiple adequate antidepressant trials.

While monotherapy is preferred, augmenting the initial antidepressant
is also an option. With augmentation, the lag time to achieving therapeutic
levels of the second agent is avoided, and there may be some benefit to a
longer trial of the initial agent.

CHOICE OF ANTIDEPRESSANT

The choice of antidepressant requires clinical judgment that should
consider drug efficacy, safety and ease of administration, tolerability,
depressive symptom profile, side-effect profile, history of response to a medication, history of a family member's response to a particular medication,
age, comorbid medical or neurological illness, comorbid psychiatric illness
(particularly substance abuse), concomitant medication, cost, and lethality (Table 4–7). This issue is discussed in greater detail in the maintenance
section.

CLASSES OF ANTIDEPRESSANTS

There are seven major classes of antidepressants currently available,
with new ones being developed and introduced regularly. These classes
are the heterocyclic antidepressants (HCAs), selective serotonin reuptake inhibitors (SSRIs), monoamine oxidase inhibitors (MAOIs), reversible

inhibitors of MAO type A (RIMAs), serotonin and norepinephrine reuptake inhibitors (SNRIs), aminoketones, and triazolopyridines. A review of efficacy for acute treatment as well as guidelines for implementation of acute treatment, including baseline studies, dosing and titration strategies, are presented briefly here (Table 4–8).

HETEROCYCLIC ANTIDEPRESSANTS

The heterocyclic antidepressants (HCAs) include the tricyclic antidepressants (TCAs) and tetracyclic antidepressants. The TCAs are the oldest class of antidepressants; the tertiary amines, imipramine (Tofranil) and amitriptyline (Elavil), are metabolized to the secondary amines desipramine (Norpramin) and nortriptyline (Pamelor), respectively. Other tertiary TCAs are trimipramine (Surmontil), doxepin (Sinequan), and clomipramine (Anafranil); another secondary TCA is protriptyline (Vivactil). Amoxapine (Asendin) is a dibenzoxazepine tricyclic antidepressant. The tetracyclic antidepressant is maprotiline (Ludiomil). Clomipramine (Anafranil), although structurally a TCA, is more selective at serotonin receptors and functionally is classified with the SSRIs.

Efficacy

Most studies report an efficacy of the HCAs around 55–80% with no significant difference between each one. Imipramine is the best studied and is effective in about 70% of patients. The other TCAs all have similar efficacy. The secondary TCAs are generally better tolerated because of weaker anticholinergic properties. Amoxapine is also equally efficacious, but because it is a demethylated metabolite of the antipsychotic loxapine, it produces significant dopamine blockade along with the associated extrapyramidal symptoms and risk of tardive dyskinesia. For this reason, it is not commonly used as an antidepressant. Combined preparations such as Triavil, which contains amitriptyline plus perphenazine, are also efficacious but should be avoided because they do not allow for optimal titration of both drugs.

Implementing Treatment

Before initiating treatment with a TCA, a medical history and physical exam should be performed, paying particular attention to the cardiac system. An electrocardiogram (EKG) is important to rule out any underlying cardiac illness particularly conduction delay, which might contraindicate use. No other baseline tests are required.

TABLE 4–8. ANTIDEPRESSANTS

Drug (Generic)	Trade Name	Half-Life (Hours)	Baseline Laboratory Studies	Initial Dose (mg)	Therapeutic Dose Range (mg)	Suggested Plasma Level (nmol/L)
Heterocyclic Antidepressants						
Imipramine	Tofranil, Tofranil PM	4–34	EKG	50	75–300	150–500
Desipramine	Norpramin	12–76	EKG	50	75–300	500–1000
Amitriptyline	Elavil	10–46	EKG	50	75–300	400–800
Nortriptyline	Pamelor	13–88	EKG	10–25	40–200	150–500
Clomipramine	Anafranil	17–28	EKG	50	75–300	300–1000
Doxepine	Sinequan	8–36	EKG	50	75–300	500–950
Protriptyline	Vivactil, Triptil	54–124	EKG	15	20–60	350–700
Trimipramine	Surmontil	7–30	EKG	25	75–300	—
Amoxipine	Asendin	8	EKG	100	100–600	—
Maprotiline	Ludiomil	27–58	EKG	25	100–225	650–950
Selective Serotonin Reuptake Inhibitors						
Fluoxetine	Prozac	24–330	None	10–20	10–80	—
Sertraline	Zoloft	24–30	None	25–50	50–200	—
Paroxetine	Paxil	3–65	None	10–20	10–50	—
Fluvoxamine	Luvox	17–22	None	50	50–300	—
Monoamine Oxidase Inhibitors						
Phenelzine	Nardil	<2	None	30–45	45–90	—
Tranylcypromine	Parnate	<2	None	20–30	30–90	—
Others						
Venlafaxine	Effexor	5–11	Blood pressure	75	75–225	—
Bupropion	Wellbutrin	10–14	None	150–200	225–450	175–350
Trazodone	Deseryl	5	None	100	200–400	—
Nefazodone	Serzone	0	None	200	300–600	—
Mirtazapine	Remeron	20–40	None	15	15–45	—

Adapted from Bezchlibnyk-Butler, K.Z., Jeffreis, J.J., Martin, B.A. (1998). *Clinical Handbook of Psychotropic Drugs*, 8th rev ed. Copyright 1998 by Hogrefe & Huber Publishers, Seattle, Toronto, Bern, Göttingen. Reprinted with permission.

[78]

Dosing

Dosing is usually started low (the equivalent of 50 mg imipramine or 25 mg nortriptyline) and given at bedtime because of their sedative effects. Lower doses (half) should be used when initiating treatment in the elderly or in patients with significant anxiety symptoms or comorbid anxiety disorder. The dose may be increased by the equivalent of 50 mg imipramine every three to five days or until side effects become troublesome. Longer intervals should be used in the elderly or anxious patient. Increased doses may be given in divided doses to minimize side effects and then may be consolidated to a bedtime dose once titration is completed. If there is no response in three to four weeks, the dose may be increased to a maximum of 300 mg imipramine or 150 mg nortriptyline if side effects allow.

SELECTIVE SEROTONIN REUPTAKE INHIBITORS (SSRIs)

There are currently five SSRIs available in the United States: fluoxetine (Prozac), sertraline (Zoloft), paroxetine (Paxil), fluvoxamine (Luvox), and citalopram. While these agents are relatively new to the antidepressant market (the first was fluoxetine released in 1987), they have rapidly become first-line agents for depression mainly because of their relatively mild side-effect profile, safety, and ease of administration. Citalopram is currently available in Europe and is now available in the United States.

Efficacy

The SSRIs all have approximately equal efficacies ranging from 60–80%. In numerous studies, most of which were conducted in the outpatient setting, they have proved to be significantly better than placebo and approximately equal to standard cyclic antidepressants.

Implementing Treatment

No laboratory studies are required before initiating treatment with an SSRI.

Dosing

Because of relative potency, half-life, and side-effect profile differences, dosing is different for each agent. Fluoxetine is usually initiated at 20 mg/day given in the morning because it has a stimulating effect in most patients. Smaller doses should be used in anxious patients or in those unable to tolerate 20 mg. Capsules of 10 mg are available, which may be opened and mixed with liquids or taken every other day for even smaller dosing. An elixir form is also available for smaller doses. A dose of 10–40 mg is usually effective in depression, although higher doses (up to 120 mg) may be required for comorbid obsessive-compulsive disorder or bulimia. Because of the long half-life, fluoxetine doses should not be increased more frequently than every four weeks. Higher doses may be given in single or divided doses.

Sertraline is initiated at 50 mg (25 mg in anxious or elderly patients) and increased by 50 mg every four to five days to a target dose of 100–200 mg/day. Because sertraline is less activating than fluoxetine, it does not need to be given in the morning. If patients find it sedating, they should take it at bedtime. Higher doses may be given in single or divided doses.

Paroxetine is started at 20 mg in a morning dose and may be increased in 10-mg increments up to a maximum of 50 mg/day. The elderly may start at 10 mg with a maximum dose of 40 mg/day.

Fluvoxamine is started at 50 mg in a bedtime dose and may be increased by 50-mg increments in a twice daily regimen to a target dose of 150–250 mg/day. Fluvoxamine may be sedating so larger doses should be given at bedtime.

MONOAMINE OXIDASE INHIBITORS (MAOIs) AND REVERSIBLE INHIBITORS OF MAO-A (RIMAs)

There are currently only two MAOIs on the market in the United States for psychiatric disorders: phenelzine (Nardil) and tranylcypromine (Parnate). These are both irreversible, nonselective inhibitors of monoamine oxidase. Phenelzine is the most rigorously studied clinically. Tranylcypromine is better tolerated and has a stimulant effect. Selegiline (l-Deprenyl), an MAOI used to treat Parkinson's disease, is an irreversible, selective MAO-B inhibitor at low doses, but at higher doses, where it may have an antidepressant effect, it becomes nonselective. There is considerable interest in reversible inhibitors of MAO-A as potentially safer antidepressants. Moclobemide among others are currently under investigation; they are in use in Europe but are not available in the United States.

Efficacy

The MAOIs have been shown to be as effective as standard tricyclics and superior to placebo. Some studies suggest that these agents may be more effective than TCAs in atypical depression and in anergic bipolar depressed patients, and they are often effective in patients who are nonresponsive to TCAs.

Implementing Treatment

There are no laboratory studies specifically required before initiating treatment with an MAOI. Patients must be educated regarding risks of interactions with certain foods and medications. Patients should also be cautioned about taking other serotonergic agents, because the combination may result in the serotonin syndrome. Other potentially lethal interactions are with meperidine (Demerol) and dextromethorphan. Drug and food interactions are discussed further in the maintenance pharmacotherapy section of this chapter.

Dosing

Phenelzine is initiated at 15 mg bid–tid and may be increased by 15 mg weekly to a target dose of 45–60 mg/day divided bid or tid. Tranylcypromine is initiated at 10 mg bid–tid and may be increased by 10 mg to a target dose of 30–40 mg/day. Although not recommended by the manufacturer, doses as high as 90 mg/day for either drug may be required.

SEROTONIN NOREPINEPHRINE REUPTAKE INHIBITORS (SNRIs)

A relatively new category of antidepressants has been termed the serotonin norepinephrine reuptake inhibitors or SNRIs. There are currently two agents in this class, venlafaxine (Effexor) and mirtazapine (Remeron), which are available for clinical use. Because these agents are relatively new, there is less clinical experience with them.

Efficacy

Efficacy is similar to TCAs and clearly better than placebo. Venlafaxine has demonstrated efficacy in both inpatient and outpatient settings. The main advantage of venlafaxine over the TCAs is a more benign side-effect profile, which is comparable to the SSRIs. It also has a wider therapeutic index than the TCAs.

Implementing Treatment

The only measurement that must be obtained prior to initiating treatment with vanlafaxine is a baseline blood pressure measurement because there is a 5–7% incidence of dose-dependent diastolic blood pressure elevation with venlafaxine.

Dosing

The usual starting dose of venlafaxine is 75 mg/day divided bid or tid with dose increases of 75 mg every few days to a target range of 150–225 mg/day with an upper dose limit of 375 mg/day. There may be a more rapid onset of action with doses >225 mg/day.[43,44,45] At lower doses, the side-effect profile is similar to the SSRIs, while at higher doses it more closely resembles that of the TCAs. Mirtazapine is initiated at 15 mg/day dosed at bedtime and may be titrated up to 45 mg.

AMINOKETONES

Another atypical class of antidepressants is the aminoketones of which bupropion (Wellbutrin) is the only representative available. It is structurally similar to amphetamine and other sympathomimetics, which accounts for its stimulantlike properties. Because its mechanism of action is different from many of the other antidepressants, bupropion often is effective in patients who have not responded to other classes of agents.

Implementing Treatment

There are no specific tests that must be performed prior to initiating treatment. Patients with a history of seizures or on anticonvulsants should be carefully monitored for seizure activity because bupropion lowers seizure threshold.

Dosing

Bupropion is usually started at 75 or 100 mg bid. If tolerated, a third dosing is added in four days to a target dose of 225–300 mg/day. The dose should not be increased by more than 100 mg in three days. The maximum single dose is 150 mg, which should be given no more frequently than every six hours. Individual doses of 100 mg may be given four hours apart. The maximum daily dose is not to exceed 450 mg because higher doses are associated with a marked increase in seizures. A slow release form is also available that is less likely to induce seizures.

TRIAZOLOPYRIDINES

This class includes trazodone (Desyrel) and the newer nefazodone (Serzone) and is chemically distinct from the other classes of antidepressants.

Efficacy

Trazodone is as effective as standard cyclic antidepressants in high doses, but adequate dosing may be limited by sedation. Several studies have demonstrated efficacy of nefazodone comparable to standard antidepressants.

Implementing Treatment

Although trazodone has been rarely associated with cardiac arrhythmias, no specific tests need to be performed before initiating treatment.

Dosing

Trazodone is initiated at 100–150 mg/day in single bedtime or divided doses with a target dose of 200–400 mg/day, but some patients may require 600 mg/day. Trazodone may be used in lower doses, 50–100 mg at bedtime, to treat insomnia induced by SSRIs, MAOIs, or bupropion. Nefazodone is usually started at 100 mg bid and increased up to 150 mg bid after one week with a range of 300–600 mg/day.

Augmentation

If a single agent is ineffective or there is only a partial response after an adequate trial (six to eight weeks) at an adequate dose or level, augmentation with a second agent may be tried. There are several options for adjunctive agents. There have been few trials of acute response to augmentation and no reported long-term maintenance studies of antidepressant augmentation.

LITHIUM

The best studied adjunctive medication is lithium, which been shown to be effective in 60% of patients who do not respond completely to a single agent. Studies of lithium augmentation of TCAs, SSRIs, and MAOIs have been reported. Onset of action is usually several days to several weeks. One study demonstrated efficacy of high-dose lithium (level 0.65–0.8 mEq/L), but not of low-dose lithium (level 0.25 mEq/L) augmentation.[46] Therefore, lithium augmentation should be to the usual target level of 0.8–1.0 mEq/L. Predictors of response to lithium are more severe depression, insomnia, and weight loss.[47]

THYROID HORMONE

Hypothyroidism has been associated with treatment refractory depression.[48] Therefore, thyroid hormone replacement as either l-triiodothyronine (T3) (25–50 mcg/day) or R-thyroxine (T4) (25–100 mcg/day) have been used as an augmentation strategy, although there are little data to support its efficacy.[47] One open study demonstrated that low normal T3 and T4 levels predicted response to thyroid hormone augmentation.[50]

PSYCHOSTIMULANTS

Augmentation of TCAs or SSRIs with psychostimulants, as well as psychostimulants alone, have also demonstrated efficacy in some studies, especially in melancholic depression or in patients with psychomotor retardation.[51] Methylphenidate 10–20 mg bid–tid has been tried and response is often seen within a few days. Patients should be monitored for insomnia, agitation, and psychosis. Psychostimulant augmentation should only be conducted by an experienced psychiatrist.

COMBINATION ANTIDEPRESSANTS

Another strategy is to augment with a second antidepressant from another class. Combinations of TCAs and SSRIs are frequently employed, but there have not been any systematic studies of this combination. Either agent may be added to the other. Due to inhibition of hepatic cytochrome P450 2D6 by both TCAs and SSRIs, the addition of a second agent further inhibits metabolism and thereby increases levels of both agents. TCA levels should be monitored as levels increase with combined therapy.

Combinations of TCAs and MAOIs occasionally have been used in refractory depression, although there are potential risks including hyperthermia, seizures, and delirium. The safest way of initiating combined treatment is to add an MAOI to an established TCA regimen or to start both simultaneously at low doses. Adding a TCA to an established MAOI regimen carries a greater risk of adverse reactions. This therapy should be initiated only by an experienced psychiatrist in a carefully monitored inpatient setting. Combination MAOI and SSRI should be avoided owing to the risk of the serotonergic syndrome.

NONPHARMACOLOGICAL SOMATIC THERAPIES

Nonpharmacological somatic therapies include phototherapy and ECT. Phototherapy has been shown to be effective for seasonal affective disorder; that is, MDD with a seasonal pattern. Light of 10,000-lux intensity is administered through a lightbox for 30–60 minutes per day, usually in the early morning, although evening or bid dosing also has demonstrated efficacy. Antidepressant effect is usually noted within the first week of treatment and may increase over several weeks.[52]

ECT is the treatment of choice for severe depression, psychotic depression, and catatonia. It is also beneficial in many patients with refractory depression. ECT typically yields a more rapid response than antidepressant medications. It is usually administered three times per week for a total of 6 to 12 treatments; initial response is usually seen after one to two weeks with recovery in two to four weeks. Efficacy is 80–90% in severe depression and 50–60% in medication-refractory depression.

CONTINUATION TREATMENT

Once the acute episode has remitted, continuation therapy should proceed with the same medication or combination of agents at the same dose that produced remission and should be maintained for another 6 to 12 months to prevent a relapse of the index episode. While continuation treatment has not been as rigorously studied as acute treatment, there is considerable evidence that continuation treatment with most antidepressants is effective in preventing relapse.

MAINTENANCE PHARMACOLOGICAL TREATMENT

The goal of maintenance therapy in depression is to prevent recurrence of depressive episodes. The efficacy of various antidepressants in preventing recurrence has been reviewed by many authors.[53,54,55,56,57,58] Several authors have also established guidelines for the long-term treatment of depression.[58,59,60,61,62,63] The purpose of this section is to provide guidelines for maintenance therapy based on data from randomized, double-blind, placebo-controlled maintenance studies.

INDICATIONS FOR MAINTENANCE TREATMENT

Longitudinal studies increasingly suggest that depressive disorders have a high probability of recurrence and chronicity and thus long-term treatment needs to be considered in the majority of patients.

Indications for maintenance pharmacotherapy are listed in Table 4–9. Patients with one or more of these risk factors should continue on maintenance antidepressant therapy.

TABLE 4–9. INDICATIONS FOR MAINTENANCE
PHARMACOTHERAPY

Depressive Episode Features
  ☐ More than three previous episodes
  ☐ Severe depressive episode
  ☐ Serious previous suicide attempts
  ☐ Neuroendocrine dysregulation
  ☐ Family history of affective disorders, especially bipolar disorder or suicide

Course
  ☐ Residual symptoms
  ☐ Seasonal pattern

Comorbidity
  ☐ Dysthymia
  ☐ Substance abuse
  ☐ Anxiety disorder
  ☐ Chronic medical condition
  ☐ Psychotic features

Demographics
  ☐ Older age of onset (>60 years)

Psychosocial
  ☐ Environmental stress
  ☐ Negative life events
  ☐ Absent social support
  ☐ High expressed emotion

DOSE OF MAINTENANCE TREATMENT

The standard of care when maintenance therapy was first introduced was to continue treatment with a smaller dose of antidepressant than was used to achieve remission. In fact, many of the earlier maintenance studies used this practice. However, several recent studies have
demonstrated superiority of full-dose over half-dose maintenance treatment. In a study of 20 patients who already had depressive recurrence
in a nonmedication cell of the Pittsburgh Maintenance Study, full-dose
imipramine (the same dose required to achieve remission) was superior
to half-dose imipramine in preventing recurrence and in significantly
increasing survival rate and survival time.[64] In a maintenance study
of phenelzine, a maintenance dose of 60 mg was better, but not significantly, than 45 mg at preventing recurrence.[65] In summary, the data point to
continuing maintenance pharmacotherapy at the same dose used to achieve remission in the acute phase, and this has become the standard of
practice.

DURATION OF MAINTENANCE TREATMENT

The longest, well-designed and carefully conducted maintenance study, known as the Pittsburgh Maintenance Study, analyzed data at three- and five-year follow-up points.[66,67] The study demonstrated a significantly lower relapse rate on medication (imipramine in this study) at both time points than placebo, providing strong support for continuing maintenance treatment for at least five years. Although there is no definitive evidence for this conclusion, the general consensus among practitioners is that patients at highest risk of relapse should continue maintenance therapy *indefinitely*.

COMBINATION WITH PSYCHOSOCIAL TREATMENT

The role of psychotherapy in the maintenance treatment of depression should not be underestimated. The combination of medication and psychotherapy, imipramine plus interpersonal therapy, has been demonstrated to be superior to medication (imipramine) alone in lengthening time to recurrence over the long term.[66] Psychotherapy may be critically important in helping patients with recurrent depressive episodes or longstanding depressive symptoms deal with the familial, social, and occupational functional impairment that may be associated with their illness. It also can enhance compliance with medication treatment.

COMPLIANCE OR ADHERENCE TO TREATMENT

Compliance with treatment, that is, taking medications as prescribed, is a particularly important issue in maintenance treatment. Perel reviewed the literature on noncompliance and found substantial evidence that almost half the patients on psychotropic medications are noncompliant.[68] For example, 70% of depressed patients on TCAs miss 25–50% of their prescribed doses. Given that antidepressant medications are superior to placebo in preventing relapse, adherence to the medication regimen is crucial. In a study of 53 depressed patients on maintenance imipramine treatment in the Pittsburgh Maintenance Study, the noncompliant patients were significantly more likely to relapse than the compliant patients, underscoring the importance of compliance in relapse prevention.[69]

Predictors of noncompliance include duration and complexity of treatment regimen, patient dissatisfaction with the treatment plan, lack of supportive follow-up, perception of invulnerability to consequences of the illness, ineffectiveness of treatment, and problems caused by the treatment. Noncompliance early in treatment predicts subsequent noncompliance.[68]

Engaging the patient's cooperation in treatment adherence is crucial and should be a high priority in treatment planning. Frank et al. outline their methodology that was very successful in engaging patients as evidenced by a <10% dropout rate over a several year protocol and >85% medication compliance as measured by level/dose ratios.[70] They advocate a combination of education, information, and active participation by the patient in the treatment process.

DRUG DISCONTINUATION

The question of how to withdraw maintenance medication has not been studied systematically. There is no clear evidence of long-term advantage to tapering medications over discontinuing them abruptly. However, there is evidence that abrupt withdrawal and even rapid taper of antidepressants, particularly the shorter half-life agents, can result in a withdrawal syndrome. Of course, there is also the high risk of recurrence. It is not known whether the rate of taper affects the risk of recurrence. There is also the risk that once a maintenance treatment is terminated, the patient may not respond again to this medication in the event of a recurrence. There is anecdotal evidence suggesting that this may occur, particularly with MAOIs.

While there are no empirically proven guidelines for discontinuing medications, current convention is to taper over several weeks to months. However, Greden suggests tapering over one year, with 25% reductions every three months.[71] For agents with longer half-lives, such as fluoxetine, doses may be reduced by switching to liquid form or reducing frequency of administration to every other day then to every third day and so on.

Discontinuation of the more anticholinergic agents (TCAs) can result in cholinergic rebound. Symptoms are likely produced by cholinergic supersensitivity and include somatic distress, gastrointestinal symptoms, disturbed sleep with vivid dreams or nightmares, psychomotor agitation, anxiety, activation, and parkinsonism.[72] MAOI withdrawal symptoms include anxiety, agitation, pressured speech, insomnia or drowsiness, hallucinations, paranoid psychosis, and delirium.[73] Some of these symptoms may mimic a relapse of depression and complicate the clinical picture.

There have also been reports of a withdrawal syndrome with the SSRIs. Reports of such symptoms include dizziness, diaphoresis, nausea, insomnia, tremor, confusion, memory difficulties, weakness, headaches, paresthesias, chest tightness, nightmares, and "electrical" sensations.[74]

ANTIDEPRESSANTS

The data supporting the efficacy of various antidepressants in long-term use for prophylaxis of depressive recurrences are limited. The number of well-designed, randomized, double-blind, placebo-controlled studies are few. This literature has been reviewed extensively by Thase, Solomon and Bauer, Kasper, Hirschfeld and Schatzberg, Montgomery, and Hirschfeld.[53,54,55,56,57,58] Following is a brief summary of this literature along with guidelines on how to use antidepressant medications in maintenance therapy presented by drug class.

HETEROCYCLIC ANTIDEPRESSANTS

EFFICACY

The largest body of data exists for the TCAs. The first group to examine the efficacy of an antidepressant in maintenance treatment for one year was Coppen et al.[75] They demonstrated that amitriptyline (average plasma level 240 ng/ml) was superior to placebo in preventing recurrence of depressive episodes in 32 patients with primary depressive illness. Glen et al. compared amitriptyline with lithium in a placebo-controlled study of 146 patients lasting three years.[76] In patients with only a single episode of depression, both amitriptyline and lithium were superior to placebo, and there was no significant difference between the two medications. Results were similar in patients with history of recurrent illness; amitriptyline and lithium demonstrated approximately equal efficacy, but there was no placebo control group. Efficacy of either medication was less in the recurrent illness group than in the single episode group, probably due to increased likelihood of recurrence in patients with a positive history of recurrent illness. Survival rates (illness free) in the recurrent group for both amitriptyline and lithium were <30%, which is much lower than in the Coppen study. This may have been due to lower blood levels of amitriptyline, with a target of 150 ng/ml compared with a mean of 240 ng/ml in the Coppen study.

A large multicenter study demonstrating maprotiline's prophylactic efficacy in unipolar depression was reported by Rouillon.[77] This study of 1,141 patients with recurrent MDD or dysthymia had a two-month open acute treatment phase with maprotiline 75–150 mg/day, no continuation phase, and follow-up for up to one year. Maprotiline 75 mg/day and 37.5 mg/day were both significantly more effective than placebo in preventing recurrence of depressive episodes in both groups.

The most thoroughly studied TCA is imipramine. In 1973, Prien et al. compared imipramine with lithium in a placebo-controlled study of 78 patients with recurrent MDD.[78] Patients were followed for an additional 20 months. Imipramine and lithium had similar efficacy, both significantly better than placebo. One limitation of this study is that the dose of imipramine was low (125 mg/day).

Two similar studies comparing imipramine, lithium, and the combination of imipramine plus lithium were conducted by Kane et al. and the NIMH Collaborative Study group.[79,80] Kane's group studied 27 patients with recurrent MDD after a six-month open continuation period during which they were on imipramine for at least the last six weeks and followed up for as long as two years. The dose of imipramine was again low at 100–150 mg/day. The groups who received lithium had fewer recurrences than the imipramine or placebo groups, and the combination of imipramine and lithium was not significantly different from lithium alone. Imipramine was not different from placebo. A similar study, the NIMH Collaborative Study, was a multicenter trial involving 150 recurrent unipolar depressed patients.[80] During the two month continuation phase, patients received imipramine (150 or 75 mg/day) and/or lithium (level 0.6–0.9 mEq/L) or placebo and were followed for up to two years. In this study, both groups receiving imipramine were significantly less likely to suffer a recurrence than those receiving either lithium or placebo. Lithium was no different from placebo. When data were analyzed separately for severity of index episode (moderate versus severe), all three active treatment groups had similar efficacy in those patients with a moderately severe index episode, but both imipramine groups were superior in patients with severe episodes. The different results obtained in these two studies are not easily explained. The Kane study was considerably smaller with only six to eight patients in each treatment cell, whereas the Prien study had at least 34 patients in each cell. Levels of imipramine and lithium were comparable. Therefore, these results suggest that imipramine is superior to lithium in preventing recurrences of depression.

The Pittsburgh Maintenance Study reported results from a three-year and a five-year follow-up.[66,60] This study employed a five cell design to compare imipramine and interpersonal therapy (IPT). One hundred twenty-eight patients were randomly assigned to imipramine plus IPT, imipramine plus medication clinic, placebo plus IPT, placebo plus medication clinic, and IPT alone. Patients were treated in the acute phase with imipramine (average 215 mg/day, level 308 ng/ml) plus IPT weekly for 12 weeks then biweekly for 8 weeks. The four months continuation phase used the same dose of imipramine and IPT before randomization into the maintenance phase. Patients receiving imipramine had significantly fewer recurrences than those receiving placebo or IPT alone. In fact, the recurrence rate on imipramine without IPT over three years was only 21%. From this cohort, 20 patients were randomized to imipramine or placebo and followed for a total of five years. There was only a 9% recurrence rate in the fourth and fifth years on imipramine compared with 67% on placebo.

Taken together, there is compelling evidence that imipramine and amitriptyline are effective in preventing recurrences of depression for up to five years after acute treatment of an index episode.

AVAILABLE AGENTS

There are many HCAs currently available. They are listed in Table 4–10. The chemical structures of these agents are shown in Figure 4–5.

MECHANISM OF ACTION

Cyclic antidepressants are thought to exert their therapeutic antidepressant effect by several mechanisms including blocking the reuptake of norepinephrine and serotonin, down-regulating beta-adrenergic receptors, and antagonizing muscarinic acetylcholine receptors.

PHARMACOKINETICS

TCAs are rapidly and completely absorbed in the gastrointestinal tract and have a high first-pass metabolism in the liver. They are metabolized in the liver by the microsomal P450 2D6 system. The tertiary tricyclics first undergo demethylation to active (secondary) metabolites, then hydroxylation, which may result in another active metabolite, and finally conjugation, which inactivates them. There may be a wide variation in metabolism depending on multiple factors including genetics, age, and concomitant drugs. The half-lives of the TCAs are listed in Table 4–8. Due to their relatively long half-lives, TCAs are usually administered in a single daily dose, and because of their sedative properties they are usually given at bedtime. TCAs are highly protein bound and are also highly lipophilic. Because they are excreted in the urine, renal disease may slow elimination and increase levels.

ADVERSE EFFECTS AND THEIR MANAGEMENT

The TCAs have a wide range of potential side effects. The side-effect profile depends on the affinity of each agent for certain receptors, particularly the muscarinic acetylcholine receptor, histamine receptor, and alpha-adrenergic receptor. Side effects are typically more pronounced at the beginning of treatment, especially if the agent is started at higher doses or rapidly titrated. Patients generally adapt to most side effects with time. The secondary TCAs are safer and better tolerated than the tertiary TCAs because they are less anticholinergic, less sedating, and less likely to cause weight gain and orthostatic hypotension.

Anticholinergic side effects are a result of antagonism at muscarinic acetylcholine receptors. These are very common, especially in the elderly, and are dose-related. They include dry mouth, dry eyes, blurred vision,

text continues on page 94

TABLE 4-10. AVERAGE COST AND AVAILABLE PREPARATIONS OF TRICYCLIC ANTIDEPRESSANTS

Compound	Trade Name	Nonparenteral Preparations	Injectable	Generic	Average Dose/Day	Average Cost/Day
Imipramine	Tofranil Tofranil PM	Tablets: 10, 25, 50 mg Injectable: 12.5 mg/ml Capsules: 75, 100, 125, 150 mg	Yes	Yes	150 mg	$2.68 (0.27)*
Desipramine	Norpramin	Tablets: 10, 25, 50, 75, 100, 150 mg	No	Yes	150 mg	$1.38 (1.09)
Amitriptyline	Elavil	Tablets: 10, 25, 50, 75, 100, 150 mg Injectable: 10 mg/ml	Yes	Yes	150 mg	$1.84 (0.27)
Nortriptyline	Pamelor	Tablets: 10, 25, 50, 75 mg Capsules: 10, 25, 50, 75 mg Solution: 10 mg/5 ml	No	Yes	75 mg	$3.22 (2.21)
Maprotilene	Ludiomil	Tablets: 25, 50, 75 mg	No	Yes	75 mg	$ 1.10 (0.69)
Clomipramine	Anafranil	Capsules: 25, 50, 75 mg	Yes	No	150 mg	$3.36 (2.66)

*Cost of generics.
From *Red Book Annual Pharmacist Reference, 1998.* Copyright 1998 by Medical Economics, Montvale, NJ. Reprinted with permission.

[92]

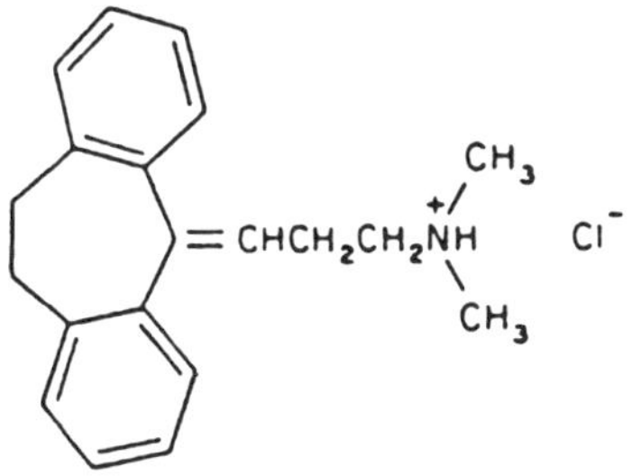

amitriptyline

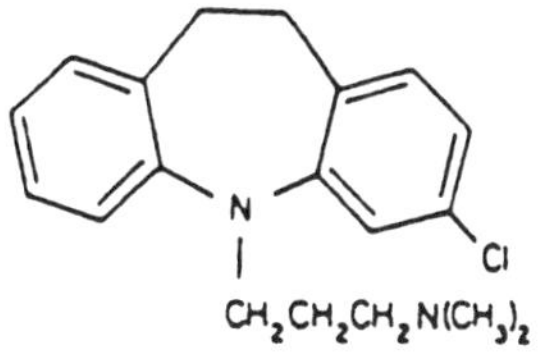

clomipramine

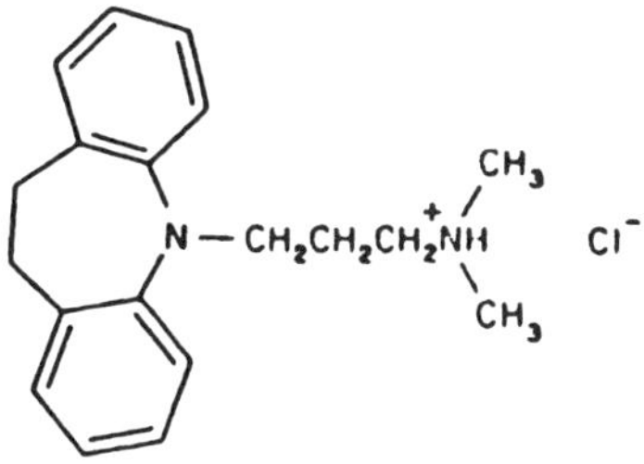

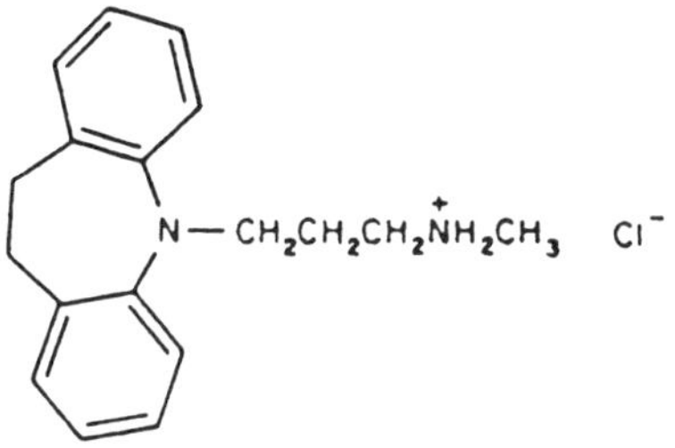

desipramine

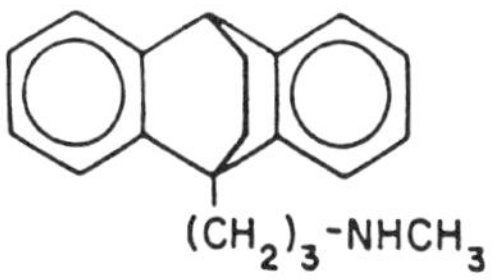

imipramine

maprotiline

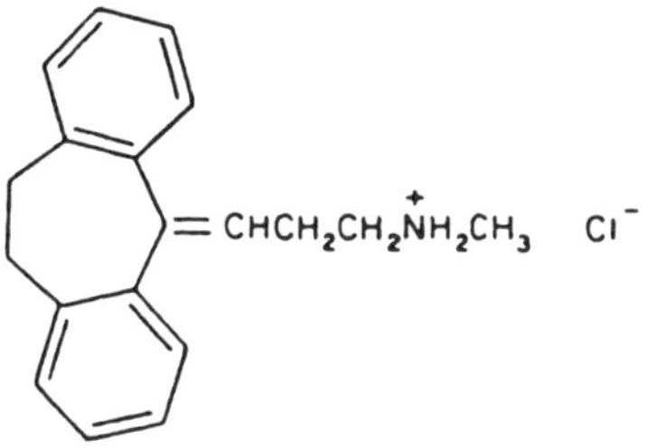

nortriptyline

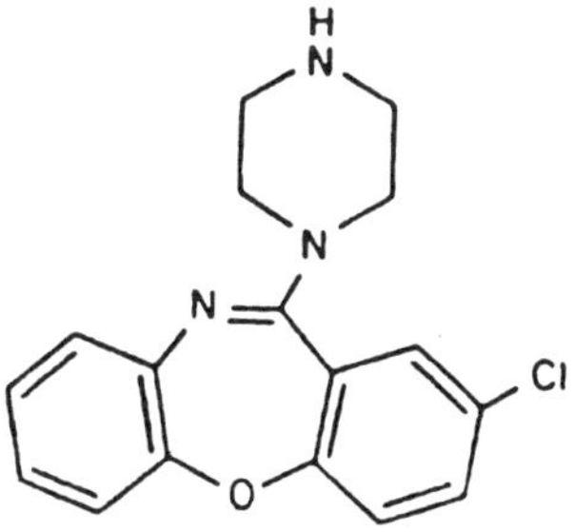

amoxapine

FIG. 4–5. Cyclic compounds (chemical structures TCAs).

tachycardia, constipation, urinary hesitancy and retention, excessive sweating, and delirium. These will each be discussed by organ system. Anticholinergic side effects may be treated with bethanechol (Urecholine) 10–50 mg three to four times per day.

Cardiovascular effects are the most worrisome. They are mediated by alpha-1-adrenergic blockade, muscarinic blockade, 5HT2 blockade, H1 receptor blockade, and quinidinelike (type 1A) antiarrhythmic activity. These effects are dose-related and carry increased risk in patients with preexisting cardiac disease.

Orthostatic hypotension, mediated by alpha-1-adrenergic blockade, is the most potentially serious of the common adverse effects of TCAs and is not dose-related; patients do not become tolerant with time. With postural change from a supine or recumbent position to a standing position, the vasculature is unable to contract sufficiently to maintain adequate blood pressure. This can cause dizziness, syncope, or falls that in the elderly may result in hip fractures. Risk factors for developing orthostatic hypotension are depression, older age, congestive heart failure, volume depletion, concomitant antihypertensive medications, impaired cardiac conduction, dysautonomias (diabetic neuropathy, Parkinson's disease, for example), and preexisting cardiac disease. Of the TCAs, nortriptyline is least likely to cause postural hypotension.[81] Management of orthostasis is simple and benign. Patients should be instructed to rise slowly from a supine position, maintain adequate fluid and salt intake, and avoid prolonged bed rest. Patients may wear supportive stockings (TEDS hose) or drink caffeinated beverages. Pharmacotherapy includes caffeine, sodium chloride 1–3 mg/day, and fludrocortisone (Florinef) 0.025–0.1 mg bid.

Tachycardia may occur with TCAs and is mediated by anticholinergic effects. It is clinically insignificant in most patients, but in patients with poorly compensated cardiac output, even a mild tachycardia may exacerbate or precipitate congestive heart failure.

TCAs are quinidinelike class 1A antiarrythmics and may cause both **conduction delay** and **arrhythmias.** At therapeutic levels, TCAs prolong PR, QRS, and QT intervals that in healthy patients are usually clinically insignificant. However, patients with preexisting first-degree atrioventricular (AV) block, second-degree block, or a bundle branch block are at increased risk of developing 2 : 1 AV block or more severe conduction defects. As with other antiarrhythmic agents, TCAs may be arrythmogenic even at therapeutic levels, but they are especially at toxic levels or in combination with other antiarrythmics.

TCAs apparently have no adverse effect on left ventricular function and therefore do not decrease cardiac output in patients with congestive heart failure. For patients with significant cardiac disease, TCAs are not first line agents and should be used only if more benign medications such as SSRIs or bupropion are ineffective. Also, TCAs should not be used in the acute recovery phase after myocardial infarction.

Monitoring for adverse cardiac effects should include pulse and orthostatic blood pressure checks at each visit. An EKG can be obtained to rule out conduction delay and arrhythmia before each dose increase in patients with cardiac disease. If TCAs must be used in patients at high risk of developing arrhythmias, Holter monitoring may be indicated. Management of heart block or arrhythmias is discontining the agent.

Constipation, another anticholinergic effect, is fairly common, especially in the elderly. In severe cases, **ileus** and **bowel obstruction** may occur and are potentially fatal. Management includes providing adequate fluids and bulk in the diet and adequate exercise. Stool softeners such as docusate sodium (Colace 100 mg bid) or bulk forming agents are helpful. Some patients may need more aggressive bowel regimens such as lactulose, laxatives, or enemas.

Gastric irritation is uncommon with the TCAs. However, some patients may experience anorexia, nausea, vomiting, or diarrhea. Some patients complain of a peculiar taste, "black tongue," or glossitis.

Dry mouth may be uncomfortable and can be treated with sugar-free candy or gum, oral lubricants (artificial saliva), pilocarpine mouthwash, or bethenechol. Decreased saliva may predispose to dental caries that can be managed by maintaining good oral hygiene and having regular dental checkups.

The TCAs may have **endocrine** effects. The dopaminergic TCAs, amoxapine and clomipramine, may cause **amenorrhea** or **galactorrhea**. Antidepressants may alter glucose regulation in patients with diabetes, usually increasing but also possibly decreasing blood glucose. They may also increase carbohydrate craving and contribute to weight gain. However, TCAs do not worsen diabetes. As do many antidepressants, TCAs may cause the **syndrome of inappropriate antidiuretic hormone (SIADH)** with hyponatremia or **idiosyncratic nephrogenic diabetes insipidus**.

TCAs may cause **blurred vision** secondary to ciliary muscle relaxation and failure of accommodation. Tolerance to this effect usually occurs within a few weeks. Treatment is with pilocarpine 0.5% eye drops. Anticholinergic effects may also produce **dry eyes** that may be treated with artificial tears. Narrow-angle glaucoma is a contraindication to TCAs as they may precipitate an acute episode. (**Narrow-angle glaucoma** can be detected by shining a light across the iris; if the light illuminates the entire iris, the patient probably does not have narrow-angle glaucoma, but if the light does not traverse all the way through the iris, the patient may have narrow-angle glaucoma.)

Hypersensitivity reactions to TCAs are rare but may present as obstructive jaundice, hepatitis, rash, urticaria, pruritus, edema, or agranulocytosis.

In addition to the desired central nervous systems effects, TCAs may also have adverse effects on the **CNS**. The TCAs, particularly the tertiary amines, are **sedating** and are best prescribed in single nighttime doses. Sedation may be minimized with caffeine or augmentation with a stimulating agent such as methylphenidate, although tolerance generally develops to sedation. Anticholinergic agents may impair recent and short-term **memory** by interfering with the encoding process. **Delirium** may occur at higher doses, especially in elderly and demented patients. Physostigmine (Antilirium) can be used to diagnose and reverse anticholinergic delirium. However, it may cause asystole, especially in patients with heart block or prolonged QRS interval on EKG. TCAs, like other antidepressants, may precipitate **mania** in patients with bipolar spectrum disorders or may increase **psychotic** symptoms. In some cases, TCAs seem to cause psychosis but they may just unmask subclinical or unrecognized preexisting psychotic symptoms.

Some patients on TCAs develop a fine **tremor** analogous to a lithium tremor that responds to benzodiazepines or beta-blockers. TCAs all decrease the seizure threshold in a dose-dependent manner. The TCAs associated with greatest risk of **seizures** are amoxapine, clomipramine, and maprotiline. Seizures are more commonly precipitated in patients with eating disorders because of lower body weight and electrolyte disturbances. **Extrapyramidal** side effects may occur with the antidopaminergic amoxapine. These include dystonias, dyskinesias, akathisia, parkinsonism, and tardive dyskinesia.

TCAs may cause **urinary hesitancy** or **urinary retention**. Urinary retention may occur acutely, especially in elderly men with enlarged prostates and this may lead to increased risk of urinary tract infections. Benign prostatic hypertrophy with urinary retention is a contraindication to TCA use.

Hyperhidrosis has been reported especially with imipramine, although it seems paradoxical given the drug's anticholinergic properties.

TCAs are also associated with **weight gain** in the majority of patients. Its etiology is unknown.

Sexual dysfunction is mediated by action at D2, 5HT2, alpha-1 adrenergic, and acetylcholine receptors. Decreased libido as well as impaired orgasm may occur in both sexes. Males may experience difficulty achieving or maintaining erections or impaired or painful ejaculation. Women may experience anorgasmia. Various management strategies have been tried, none with marked success. See the section on SSRIs for treatments.

TOXICITY

The TCAs have narrow therapeutic indices making them potentially dangerous at doses not much higher than therapeutic doses. As a result, these agents should be used with extreme caution in patients who are impulsive or at high risk for suicide. Small, nonlethal quantities should be dispensed without refillable prescriptions. Ingestion of 1 gm TCA may be toxic while 2.5 gm is frequently lethal. Therefore, a two-week supply of a TCA is generally the maximum prescribed at one time.

Symptoms of toxicity usually develop one to four hours after ingestion and include agitation, delirium, hypotension or hypertension, hypothermia, dilated sluggishly reactive pupils, hyperpyrexia, myoclonic seizures, bilateral plantar response, and cardiotoxicity including conduction defects and cardiac arrhythmias. Large overdoses may be characterized by deep coma, diminished reflexes, sluggish or nonreactive pupils, seizures, tachycardia, hypotension, hypothermia, respiratory arrest, arrhythmia, and possibly death. Cardiac effects and uncontrollable seizures are the most life-threatening complications. There is controversy regarding the association between initial TCA level and QRS interval and final outcome.[82,83] There is some evidence that a TCA level $\geq$1000 ng/ml is associated with QRS $\geq$ 0.1 seconds, which is associated with a poorer prognosis.

Management of a serious TCA overdose may be complicated. Gastric aspiration and lavage should be followed by activated charcoal every four hours and cathartics to decrease absorption and increase elimination of the drug. Forced diuresis or dialysis is ineffective. Serum TCA level, toxicology screen for other ingested drugs, and EKG should be obtained immediately. The patient should be monitored closely on a cardiac monitor and given supportive treatment including intravenous fluids and ventilatory support if needed. Seizures should be treated with diazepam. Arrhythmias may be treated with alkalinization, electrical pacing, and beta-blockers. Type 1A antiarrythmics (quinidine, procainamide, and disopyramide) should not be administered, since they will potentiate toxicity. Physostigmine (Antilirium) may be administered to counteract anticholinergic effects in serious overdose. However, risks associated with physostigmine include worsening arrhythmias, decreased respiration, and further decrease in seizure threshold, so physostigmine should not be used in respiratory or cardiovascular compromise. If there are any signs of toxicity, patients should be monitored for at least 48 hours in an intensive care unit, since recovery may be slow because of rapid and extensive tissue distribution. If there are no signs of toxicity in the first six hours after ingestion, the patient is safe and does not require further monitoring.

MONITORING

Only a few of the TCAs demonstrate a relationship between therapeutic response and serum levels. For imipramine, there is a linear relationship between combined imipramine and desipramine levels >225 ng/ml and clinical efficacy. For desipramine, there is also a linear relationship with levels >125 ng/ml. Nortriptyline levels are the best studied and demonstrate a therapeutic window with best clinical response correlated to levels between 50–150 ng/ml. Some carefully designed studies report a narrower therapeutic window of 80–120 ng/ml.[84]

Blood level monitoring may be useful in limited circumstances and should be checked in the following conditions: to monitor compliance, to rule out toxicity, to confirm adequate levels when there is no response with an adequate dose for three to four weeks, and with rapid titration. To rapidly titrate, a blood level should be checked 48 hours after a 25-mg test dose to predict the effective dose according to the formula:

$$\text{effective daily dose} = -1.65 \times (48 \text{ hour level}) + 65$$

The effective dose may then be achieved without waiting for steady-state levels with each dose increase. Pulse, orthostatic blood pressure, and serial EKGs should be monitored during titration.

Once a patient is in the maintenance phase of treatment and has demonstrated no adverse cardiac effects during the acute and continuation phases, monitoring may be less frequent. Blood levels may be checked yearly to ensure that there has been no physiologic change in metabolism and to confirm compliance. Levels should also be checked if there are changes or additions in medications that are metabolized by or inhibit the same cytochrome P450 system and therefore may alter drug metabolism and levels. Levels can also be checked if any signs or symptoms of toxicity emerge. Levels are also useful to check periodically for adherence to medication to enhance behavioral compliance. Cardiac status should be monitored by yearly electrocardiograms.

DRUG-DRUG INTERACTIONS

TCAs can interact with other medications to produce side effects or alter the effect of the TCA or the other medication. Table 4–11 presents a list of specific drug-drug interactions with TCAs. Serum levels of TCAs may also be altered by drugs that are metabolized by or inhibit metabolism of the cytochrome P450 2D6 system (Table 4–12).

Drugs that may elevate TCA levels include the SSRIs, antipsychotics, valproate, beta-blockers, calcium-channel blockers, and imidazoles. Drugs which may decrease TCA levels include carbamazepine, cholestyramine, and rifampin. TCAs may cause increased levels of carbamazepine and antipsychotics. The serotonergic syndrome may occur with SSRIs, MAOIs, and sumatriptan.

TABLE 4–11. TCAs: DRUG-DRUG INTERACTIONS

Class of Drug	Example	Interaction Effects
Antiarrhythmic	Quinidine, procainamide	Prolonged cardiac conduction
	Propafenene	Increased plasma level of desipramine reported
Anticholinergic	Antiparkinsonian agents, antihistamines, neuroleptics	Increased anticholinergic effect; may increase risk of hyperthermia, confusion, urinary retention, etc.
Anticonvulsant	Carbamazepine	Increased plasma level of carbamazepine due to inhibition of metabolism
		Decreased plasma level of tricyclic due to enzyme induction
Antidepressant	Valproate, divalproex, valproic acid	Increased plasma level of tricyclic antidepressant
Irreversible MAOI	Phenelzine, isocarboxazid, tranylcypromine	If used together, do not add cyclic antidepressants to MAOI; start cyclic antidepressant first or simultaneously with MAOI; for patients already on MAOI, discontinue MAOI 10–14 days before starting combination therapy
		Combined cyclic and MAOI therapy has additive antidepressant effects in treatment-resistant patients
SSRI	Fluoxetine, fluvoxamine, paroxetine, sertraline	Elevated tricyclic plasma level (due to release from protein binding and inhibition of oxidative metabolism); monitor plasma level and for signs of toxicity and serotonin syndrome
		Additive antidepressant effect in treatment-resistant patients
RIMA	Moclobemide	Additive antidepressant effect in treatment-resistant patients
Antihypertensive	Bethanidine, clonidine, debrisoquin, methyldopa, guanethidine, reserpine	Decreased antihypertensive effect
	Acetazolamide, thiazide, diuretics	Hypotension augmented
Beta-Blocker	Labetalol	Increased plasma level of imipramine (by 54%)
Calcium-Channel Blocker	Nifedipine	May antagonize the efficacy of antidepressant drugs
	Diltiazem, verapamil	Increased imipramine plasma level by 30% and 15%, respectively

(Contd.)

TABLE 4-11. (CONTINUED).

Class of Drug	Example	Interaction Effects
CNS Depressant	Barbiturates, hypnotics, antihistamines, alcohol, neuroleptics, benzodiazepines	Increased sedation, central nervous system depression
Cholestryramine		Decreased plasma level of antidepressant, if given together
Imidazole Compounds	Ketoconazole, fluconazole, omeprazole	Increased plasma level of antidepressant due to inhibited metabolism
L-Dopa		Increased side effects with bupropion
Lithium		Additive antidepressant effect
L-Tryptophan		Additive antidepressant effect
Narcotic	Methadone	Increased plasma level of desipramine (average increase 108%)
Neuroleptic	Chlorpromazine, haloperidol	Increased serum level of either agent
Pressor Agents	Epinephrine, norepinephrine (levarterenol), phenylephrine	Enhanced pressor response
	Isoproterenol	May increase arrhythmias
Pseudoephedrine		Report of maniclike reaction with bupropion
Rifampin		Decreased plasma level of antidepressant due to increased metabolism
Sulfonylureas	Tolbutamide	Increased hypoglycemia
Sumatriptan		Possible serotonergic reaction when combined with antidepressants with serotonergic activity (e.g., clomipramine)
Thyroid Drug	Triiodothyronine (T_3 liothyronine), L-thyroxine(T_4)	Additive antidepressant effect in treatment-resistant patients

Adapted from Bezchlibnyk-Butler, K.Z., Jeffreis, J.J., Martin, B.A. (1998). *Clinical Handbook of Psychotropic Drugs*, 8th rev ed. Copyright 1998 by Hogrefe & Huber Publishers, Seattle, Toronto, Bern, Göttingen. Reprinted with permission.

[100]

TABLE 4-12. DRUGS WITH OXIDATIVE METABOLISM ASSOCIATED WITH CYTOCHROME P450, 1A2, 2C, 2D6, AND 3A4

1A2	2C	2D6	3A4
Amitriptyline	Amitriptyline	Amitriptyline	Amitriptyline
Caffeine	Citalopram	Brofaromine	Alprazolam
Clomipramine	Clomipramine	Clomipramine	Astemizole
Clozapine	Diazepam	Codeine	Carbamazepine
Fluvoxamine	Hexobarbital	Desipramine	Clomipramine
Haloperidol	Imipramine	Dextromethorphan	Cyclosporine
Imipramine	Mephobarbital	Encainide	Dexamethasone
Phenacetin	Moclobemide	Flecainide	Dextromethorphan
Tacrine	Omeprazole	Fluoxetine	Erythromycin
Theophylline	Phenytoin	Haloperidol	Imipramine
Verapamil	Proguanil	Imipramine	Lidocaine
	Tolbutamide	Maprotiline	Midazolam
	Warfarin	Metoprolol	Nefazodone
		Mianserin	Quinidine
		Nortriptyline	Sertraline
		Paroxetine	Terfenadine
		Perphenazine	Triazolam
		Propafenone	Verapamil
		Propranolol	Vinblastine
		Remoxipride	
		Risperidone	
		Thioridazine	
		Trazodone	
		Venlafaxine	

From Nemeroff, C.B., DeVane, C.L., Pollock, B.G. (1996). Newer antidepressants and the cytochrome P450 system. *Am J Psychiatry*, 153(3): 311–320. Copyright 1996 by American Psychiatric Press. Reprinted with permission.

TCAs should not be administered with MAOIs owing to the risk of precipitating a hypertensive crisis. MAOIs should be discontinued 10–14 days before initiating treatment with a TCA. This combination has been used by experienced psychiatrists in a closely monitored inpatient setting. If used together, the TCA should be started first or simultaneously with the MAOI. TCAs given concomitantly with other type 1A antiarrythmics may be more likely to precipitate arrhythmias.

DRUG-DISEASE INTERACTIONS

TCAs must be used with caution in patients with **cardiac disease,** particularly those with **conduction defects** or **recent myocardial infarctions.** If a patient has a myocardial infarction while on TCA maintenance treatment, the drug should be discontinued and not restarted until after the acute recovery phase. Frequent EKG monitoring and possible Holter monitoring should be conducted in these patients. However, the preferred alternative is to try another class of antidepressant (such as SSRIs or bupropion).

TCAs should be used cautiously in patients with **respiratory disease**, since the medication can dry up bronchial secretions and exacerbate breathing difficulties. TCAs decrease the seizure threshold and should be used cautiously in patients with preexisting **seizure and eating disorders**. Maprotiline is not recommended at all because of the increased risk of seizures at doses over 200 mg, limiting dosing in the therapeutic range.

TCAs may precipitate mania in patients with **bipolar** disorder. Many clinicians use TCAs in bipolar patients in combination with a mood stabilizer such as lithium, valproate, or carbamazepine. Some argue, however, that TCAs should not be used at all in bipolar depression because they may induce mixed states, cycle acceleration, or rapid cycling, which is more treatment refractory.[85,86]

SELECTIVE SEROTONIN REUPTAKE INHIBITORS (SSRIs)

EFFICACY

There is limited data supporting the efficacy of the SSRIs for prophylaxis against recurrent unipolar depression. The first randomized, double-blind, placebo-controlled study of an SSRI was reported in 1988.[87] It compared fluoxetine 40 mg with placebo in 220 patients with recurrent MDD. In a one-year follow-up, fluoxetine was significantly better than placebo with a recurrence rate of only 26% on fluoxetine compared with 57% on placebo.

In a maintenance study of sertraline in 295 patients with single episode or recurrent MDD, sertraline was significantly superior to placebo in preventing recurrences in a 10-month follow-up period.[88] This study had several flaws including no clear criteria for response in the acute phase, no continuation phase, use of a low dose of sertraline (mean weekly dose 69–82 mg/day), and a >50% dropout rate. Nevertheless, survival rates for sertraline were significantly better than placebo.

A well-designed maintenance study of paroxetine was reported by Montgomery and Dunbar.[89] This was a randomized, double-blind, placebo-controlled study of paroxetine 20–30 mg/day in 135 patients with recurrent MDD with a one-year follow-up. Patients were treated openly with paroxetine 30 or 40 mg, which was decreased by 10 mg for the maintenance phase.

Recurrence rates were analyzed separately for the first four months (continuation period) and after four months (8-month maintenance phase). There were significantly fewer recurrences on paroxetine than placebo (recurrence 14% compared with 30%, $p < .05$).

Despite the limited number and quality of many of the studies, there is some evidence for efficacy of the SSRIs in preventing recurrent depressive episodes.

AVAILABLE AGENTS

There currently are four SSRIs available: fluoxetine, sertraline, paroxetine, citalopram, and fluvoxamine (Table 4–13). The chemical structures of these agents are shown in Figure 4–6.

MECHANISM OF ACTION

SSRIs are thought to exert their therapeutic effect by inhibiting reuptake of serotonin at the presynaptic neuron increasing the concentration of serotonin in the synaptic cleft. This causes down-regulation of serotonin receptors on the pre- and post-synaptic neurons. While all these agents selectively block serotonin uptake and appear to be equally effective, they have different affinities for serotonin as well as for other neurotransmitters. Paroxetine is the most potent at serotonin receptors, while fluoxetine is the least.

PHARMACOKINETICS

The SSRIs are almost completely absorbed in the gastrointestinal tract and undergo extensive first-pass metabolism in the liver. The SSRIs are metabolized in the liver by the cytochrome P450 2D6 microsomal system and are potent inhibitors of this system to varying degrees (Table 4–14).[90] Fluvoxamine is metabolized primarily by cytochrome P450 1A2 and is also a potent inhibitor of this isozyme.

Fluoxetine has the longest half-life of four to six days and is metabolized to norfluoxetine, an active metabolite with a half-life of 4–16 days. Sertraline is metabolized to its active metabolite norsertraline that has a half-life of 62–104 hours. Paroxetine, with a half-life of 24 hours, and fluvoxamine, with a half-life of 15 hours, have no active metabolites. All the SSRIs and their metabolites are excreted in the urine. Because of their long half-lives, the SSRIs (except fluvoxamine) may be given in a single daily dose, usually in the morning. Fluvoxamine is dosed twice daily. Since it may cause sedation,

text continues on page 107

TABLE 4–13. AVERAGE COST AND AVAILABLE PREPARATIONS OF ANTIDEPRESSANTS

Compound	Trade Name	Nonparenteral Preparations	Injectable	Generic	Average Dose/Day	Average Cost/Day
Trazodone	Desyrel	Tablets: 50, 100, 150 mg	No	Yes	300 mg	$7.11 (1.35)*
Bupropion	Wellbutrin	Tablets: 75, 100 mg	No	No	225 mg	$1.80
Fluoxetine	Prozac	Capsules: 10, 20 mg Solution: 20 mg/5 ml	No	No	20 mg	$2.25
Sertraline	Zoloft	Tablets: 50, 100 mg	No	No	100 mg	$2.15
Paroxetine	Paxil	Tablets: 10, 20, 30, 40 mg	No	No	20 mg	$1.98
Fluvoxamine	Luvox	Tablets: 50, 100 mg	No	No	150 mg	$4.03

*Cost of generics.
From Red Book Annual Pharmacist Reference, 1996. Copyright 1996 by Medical Economics, Montvale, NJ. Reprinted with permission.

[104]

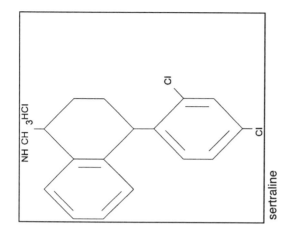

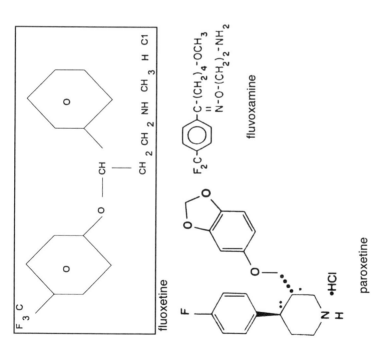

FIG. 4–6. Chemical structures of SSRIs.

TABLE 4–14. SSRIs: RELATIVE AFFINITIES FOR NEUROTRANSMITTER RECEPTORS

SSRI	Half-Life (Hours)	Half-Life of Active Metabolites	Protein Binding (%)	P450 Metabolism	5HT2 Potency	P450 2D6 Inhibition	P450 3A4 Inhibition	P450 1A2 Inhibition	P450 2C9 Inhibition
Fluoxetine	96–144	96–384	94	2D6	+++	+++	++	+	++
Sertraline	26	62–104	98	2D6	++++	++	++	+	+
Paroxetine	24	None	95	2D6	++++	++++	+	+	+
Fluvoxamine	15	None		1A2	+++	+	++	+++	++/+++

[106]

a larger dose may be administered at bedtime. Because of the long half-life of fluoxetine and its active metabolite, steady-state is not reached until approximately four weeks.

The SSRIs are highly protein-bound and displace other highly protein-bound agents such as warfarin and digoxin.

ADVERSE EFFECTS AND THEIR MANAGEMENT

The side-effect profile of the SSRIs is milder than that of the TCAs, and in general these agents are better tolerated. The adverse effects come from serotonin agonism. Most side effects are more pronounced in the beginning of treatment and abate over time.

The most frequent adverse effects involve the CNS and include headache and dizziness, insomnia or somnolence, anxiety, and restlessness and are easily managed. **Headache** often begins several hours after the dose is taken, is relieved by acetaminophen or NSAIDs, and usually resolves within several days. If patients become **somnolent**, the dose can be given in a single bedtime dose. **Insomnia** is best treated by changing the time of dosage or adding trazodone or a benzodiazepine at bedtime. **Activation, anxiety, and restlessness** may be relieved by a reduction in dose followed by slower titration. Patients with prominent anxiety symptoms as part of their depression should begin with half the usual starting dose and titrate at smaller increments and less frequently. Fluoxetine is most commonly associated with activation; paroxetine may be the least likely to cause anxiety. SSRIs, like other antidepressants, may precipitate **mania** or hypomania in patients with a prediliction to bipolar illness.

Tremor and **akathisia** are the most common neurological side effects; **bruxism, myoclonus, parasthesias, akathisia, dystonias** and **dyskinesias, tinnitus,** and **parkinsonism** are less common. The SSRIs may increase extrapyramidal side effects when given in combination with antipsychotics. Tremor may improve with dose reduction, beta-blockers, or benzodiazepines. Extrapyramidal side effects may improve with typical antiparkinsonian agents such as benztropine. Increased sweating may occur secondary to effects on the autonomic nervous system.

Gastrointestinal side effects are a direct result of serotonin inhibition. **Nausea** and **vomiting** are common and are usually transient and dose-related. Symptoms may be relieved by taking the medication with food or antacids. **Diarrhea** and **constipation** are both common and may be relieved by dietary changes or pharmacotherapy with stool softeners for constipation or loperamide (Imodium) for diarrhea.

The SSRIs frequently cause **anorexia**, which may be more pronounced in those who are overweight. Fluoxetine in particular may be abused by some eating disorder patients. Anorexia may be an intolerable side effect in some patients, especially the frail elderly who are significantly underweight initially, either as a result of other medical problems or their depression, and patients with HIV infection or who are otherwise malnourished. Weight gain is also a possible side effect but is much less common than anorexia.

The **cardiovascular** effects of the SSRIs are less common and less severe than those associated with the TCAs. Rarely, however, they may cause coronary vasoconstriction that can worsen or precipitate angina. Sinus node slowing has been reported with fluoxetine, as have tachycardia, palpitations, and atrial fibrillation. Care should be exercised in giving these drugs to patients with cardiac conduction abnormalities and poor ventricular dysfunction.

Sexual side effects are fairly common with the SSRIs and result from a combination of serotonin, dopamine, norepinephrine, and acetylcholine effects. They include decreased libido, impotence, and ejaculatory disturbances in men and anorgasmia in women. Various management strategies have been tried, none with overwhelming success.[91] Noninvasive measures include decreasing the dose, waiting for possible accommodation, or switching to a different antidepressant. Invasive measures involve adding medications. These are dosed initially only several hours before sexual activity but may be increased to daily dosing if necessary. Yohimbine (Yocon, Yohimex) is a presynaptic alpha2-blocker. It may be dosed at 5.4–16.2 mg two to four hours before sexual activity or 5.4 mg tid. Potential side effects include anxiety, insomnia, urinary frequency, diaphoresis, and fatigue. It should not be used in combination with MAOIs due to increased risk of hypertensive crisis. Cyproheptadine (Periactin) is antiserotonergic. It is dosed at 4–12 mg in the evening and may cause sedation or increased psychiatric symptoms. Bethanechol (Urecholine) is cholinergic and may cause diarrhea, cramps, and diaphoresis. Dosing is 10–40 mg before sexual activity or 30–100 mg divided daily dose. Amantadine (Symmetrel) is a dopamine agonist and can be given 100–200 mg daily. Buspirone (Buspar) is a 5HT1A agonist and can be given 5 mg two to three times daily. Other possible approaches include adding bupropion (Wellbutrin) 75–100 mg in the morning, trazodone, carbidopa-levodopa (Sinemet), or methylphenidate. Drug holidays for one to two days per week coincident with planned sexual activity also have been reported to decrease sexual side effects without worsening affective symptoms.[92]

SSRIs, as well as many other psychotropic medications, may induce **SIADH** with hyponatremia. If it cannot be adequately managed medically, it is treated by fluid restriction and stopping the medication.

Allergic reactions to the SSRIs are rare but the following have been reported: jaundice, hepatitis, rash, urticaria, psoriasis, pruritus, edema, swollen joints, lymphadenopathy, blood dyscrasia, serum sickness, petechiae, purpura, and bleeding disorders.

TOXICITY

The SSRIs have not been associated with dose-related toxicity. Patients have taken acute ingestions of up to 10 times the usual dose without adverse effects. Symptoms occurring with these ingestions include nausea, vomiting, tremor, myoclonus, and irritability. No specific treatment is necessary. Because of the safety of SSRIs in overdose, these medications may be used in patients with a high risk of suicide, impulsivity, or substance abuse.

There has been some controversy over whether fluoxetine and other SSRIs are associated with increased impulsivity, aggression, and suicide based largely upon a few studies.[93,94] Unfortunately, this controversy has been exaggerated in the lay press. Other studies, however, have reported that the rate of suicide in patients treated with SSRIs is no higher than in those treated with other antidepressants.[95,96,97]

MONITORING

There is no evidence for a dose-response relationship for the SSRIs. Therapeutic monitoring is not indicated as the dose response curve is flat. As the SSRIs are not known to have any toxic effects on organ systems, no medical tests need to be monitored.

DRUG-DRUG INTERACTIONS

The SSRIs are metabolized by the cytochrome P450 system and are also potent inhibitors of it. Their use can result in increased levels of other drugs that are metabolized by the P450 system, including tricyclic antidepressants, other cyclic antidepressants, and some antipsychotics. Potentially serious interactions involve fluvoxamine coadministered with terfenadine (Seldane) or astemizole (Hismanal), both of which may result in cardiac conduction abnormalities (i.e., heart block and fatal ventricular arrythmias) and must be avoided (Table 4–15).

The SSRIs are highly protein bound and may displace other protein-bound medications, increasing their free plasma levels. Examples include digoxin and coumadin. When adding an SSRI to a regimen that includes digoxin, digoxin levels should be monitored, and an increase in unbound drug may be anticipated by decreasing the digoxin dose when adding the SSRI.

text continues on page 112

TABLE 4–15. SSRIs: DRUG–DRUG INTERACTIONS

Class of Drug	Example	Interaction Effects
Antiarrhythmic	Propafenone, flecainide	Increased plasma level of antiarrhythmic due to inhibited metabolism
Anticonvulsant	Carbamazepine	Increased plasma level of carbamazepine due to inhibition of metabolism with fluoxetine and fluvoxamine; increased nausea with fluvoxamine; decreased plasma level of SSRIs
	Phenytoin	Increased plasma level of phenytoin with fluoxetine, fluvoxamine, and paroxetine due to decreased metabolism
	Valproate, valproic acid, divalproex	Increased plasma level of valproate (up to 50%) with fluoxetine. Valproate may increase plasma level of fluoxetine
Anticoagulant	Warfarin	65% increase in plasma level of warfarin with fluvoxamine and paroxetine; increased bleeding
Antidepressant		
Cyclic	Amitriptyline, desipramine, bupropion	Elevated plasma level of cyclic antidepressant from release from protein binding and inhibition of oxidative metabolism; monitor plasma level and for signs of toxicity
Irreversible MAOI	Phenelzine, tranylcypromine, isocarboxazid	Additive antidepressant effect in treatment-resistant patients Hypermetabolic syndrome (serotonergic syndrome) reported with combined use. Suggest waiting 5 weeks when switching from fluoxetine to MAOI and vice versa. Increased plasma level of tranylcypromine (by 15%) reported with paroxetine
RIMA	Moclobenide	Combined therapy may have additive antidepressant effect in treatment-resistant patients; use caution
Antipyrine		Increased metabolism and decreased half-life of antipyrine with sertraline
Anxiolytic	Buspirone	May potentiate antiobsessional effects
Benzodiazepine	Alprazolam, Diazepam	Increased plasma level of alprazolam (by 25%) and diazepam with fluoxetine due to inhibited metabolism
Cimetidine		Inhibited metabolism and increased plasma level of sertraline (by 25%) and paroxetine (by 50%)
CNS Depressant	Alcohol, antihistamines, chloral hydrate	Potentiation of effects; low risk Increased sedation and side effects with fluoxetine due to inhibited metabolism

(Contd.)

[110]

TABLE 4–15. (CONTINUED)

Class of Drug	Example	Interaction Effects
Cyproheptadine		Report of reversal of effect of fluoxetine
Lithium		Increased serotonergic effects; caution with fluoxetine; increased lithium level with neurotoxicity and seizures reported
		Increased tremor and nausea reported with sertraline and paroxetine; decreased lithium level and increased clearance of lithium
		Additive antidepressant effect in treatment-resistant patients
L-Tryptophan		May result in central and peripheral toxicity, hypermetabolic syndrome (serotonin syndrome) with agitation, aggressiveness, chills, palpitations, nausea, and diarrhea
Metoprolol		Increased side effects, lethargy, and bradycardia with fluoxetine due to decreased metabolism
Narcotic	Pentazocine	Report of excitatory toxicity (serotonergic) with fluoxetine
	Dextronethoptan	Visual hallucinations reported with fluoxetine
Neuroleptic	Chlorpromazine, haloperidol	Increased serum level of neuroleptic; may worsen extrapyramidal effects, akathisia
		Additive effect in treatment of obsessive–compulsive disorder
Procyclidine		Increased plasma level of procyclidine with paroxetine
Propranolol		Fivefold increase in propranolol level reported with fluvoxamine
Theophylline		Increased plasma level of theophylline with fluvoxamine due to decreased metabolism
Thyroid Drug	Triiodothyronine (T_3 liothyronine)	Antidepressant effect potentiated
Sulfonylurea	Tolbutamide	Increased hypoglycemia; increased plasma level of tolbutamide due to reduced clearance (up to 16%) with sertraline
Sumatriptan		Increased serotonergic effects

Adapted from Bezchlibnyk-Butler, K.Z., Jeffreis, J.J., Martin, B.A. (1998). *Clinical Handbook of Psychotropic Drugs*, 8th rev ed. Copyright 1988 by Hogrefe & Huber Publishers, Seattle, Toronto, Bern, Göttingen. Reprinted with permission.

[111]

Prothrombin time must be monitored carefully when an SSRI is added to warfarin. A dose decrease while initiating or increasing an SSRI may anticipate this change and prevent complications. Fluvoxamine is the least protein bound of the SSRIs.

The "serotonin syndrome" may occur when the combination of SSRIs and other serotonergic agents causes excessive serotonergic activity.[98] This results in a hypermetabolic state characterized by nausea, diarrhea, hyperpyrexia, chills, diaphoresis, palpitations, agitation, restlessness, myoclonus, hyperreflexia, tremor, excitation, and delirium. Treatment consists of discontinuation of the serotonergic agents and supportive measures. In severe cases, serotonin antagonists such as methysergide, cyproheptadine, or propranolol may be used. This syndrome usually resolves spontaneously within 24 hours, although delirium has been reported to last up to four days.

SSRIs should never be coadministered with MAOIs. MAOIs should not be started until two weeks after discontinuation of an SSRI, five weeks for fluoxetine because of its long half-life. Other serotonergic agents that may precipitate this reaction include lithium, l-tryptophan, and sumatriptan. These agents should be used with caution with SSRIs.

DRUG-DISEASE INTERACTIONS

SSRIs may precipitate mania in patients with **bipolar disorder**. Many clinicians use SSRIs in bipolar patients in combination with a mood stabilizer such as lithium, valproate, or carbamazepine. However, some argue that SSRIs should not be used at all in bipolar depression because they may induce mixed states or rapid cycling, which is more treatment refractory.[86]

Hepatic disease may slow metabolism, and **renal disease** may slow elimination of the SSRIs, thus decreasing clearance and increasing accumulation of the drug and its active metabolites. In these conditions, lower doses should be used. SSRIs may alter glycemic control in patients with **diabetes**. Insulin and oral hypoglycemic doses may need to be adjusted.

MONOAMINE OXIDASE INHIBITORS

EFFICACY

There are two maintenance treatment studies of the MAOI phenelzine. Georgotas compared phenelzine and nortriptyline with placebo and found phenelzine significantly better than placebo in preventing recurrence

TABLE 4–16. AVAILABLE PREPARATIONS AND COST OF MAOIs

Compound	Trade Name	Nonparenteral Preparations	Injectable	Generic	Average Dose/Day	Average Cost/Day
phenelzine	Nardil	Tablets: 15 mg	No	No	45 mg	$ 1.32
tranylcypromine	Parnate	Tablets: 10 mg	No	No	30 mg	$ 1.06

Cost of generics.
From *Red Book Annual Pharmacist Reference, 1996*. Copyright 1996 by Medical Economics, Montvale, NJ. Reprinted with permission.

of unipolar depression.[99] Robinson performed a dose-response study comparing phenelzine 60 mg with phenelzine 45 mg in a placebo-controlled, two-year study of 47 patients.[100] Both doses were significantly superior to placebo, but the two doses did not differ significantly from each other (Table 4–16).

AVAILABLE AGENTS

There are two types of MAOIs, the irreversible agents that include phenelzine, tranylcypromine, and isocarboxazid and the reversible inhibitors of MAO-A (RIMAs) represented by moclobemide and brofaromine, neither of which is currently available in the United States. (Table 4–16 and Figure 4–7)

MECHANISM OF ACTION

MAOIs inhibit monoamine oxidase type-A and type-B enzymes that degrade catecholamines located in the cytoplasm of the presynaptic terminals, thus increasing the amount of norepinephrine, epinephrine, dopamine, and serotonin in the nerve terminal. MAO-A preferentially degrades norepinephrine and serotonin, while MAO-B preferentially degrades dopamine, phenylethanolamine, and benzylamine. RIMAs are selective for MAO-A, targeting norepinephrine and serotonin metabolism but not affecting dopamine. They only inhibit MAO-A at lower doses but become nonselective at higher doses (>400 mg moclobemide). While both monoamine oxidase types are present in the central nervous system, MAO-A is also located in the GI tract and liver, where it catabolizes exogenous amines from ingested food. MAOIs also inhibit these peripheral enzymes that may cause an accumulation of endogenous amines and result in a hyperadrenergic/hypertensive crisis. Because the RIMAs are reversible, they pose less risk for these systemic effects.

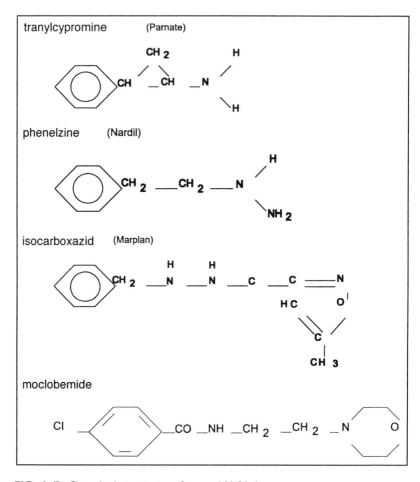

FIG. 4–7. Chemical structures of some MAOI drugs.

PHARMACOKINETICS

MAOIs are rapidly absorbed in the gastrointestinal tract and undergo hepatic metabolism with a high first-pass effect and renal excretion. Peak levels are usually achieved approximately one to two hours after dose and correlate with peak in cardiovascular side effects (orthostatic hypotension and tachycardia). The irreversible MAOIs impair their own metabolism with chronic administration resulting in nonlinear kinetics; therefore, the dose may need to be increased to maintain efficacy. The half-lives of the MAOIs are short thus requiring bid dosing. Doses are best given in the morning and midafternoon to avoid evening excitation and insomnia. Protein binding is low. Maximal MAO inhibition occurs after several days with re-peated dosing. Inhibition usually lasts approximately one to two weeks, but only 24 hours for RIMAs. Tranylcypromine inhibition reverses quicker than phenelzine because tranylcypromine reversibly binds MAO. The onset of therapeutic action may be quicker with moclobemide.

ADVERSE EFFECTS AND THEIR MANAGEMENT

The MAOIs are generally well tolerated. The most life-threatening po-tential complication from MAOIs is hypertensive crisis, which may be precipitated by certain foods or medications (see below). However, if patients can follow the restrictions, they often tolerate the MAOIs very well.

The most common limiting side effect is **postural hypotension** that may result in dizziness and falls as well as **lethargy**. Blood pressure, supine and standing, should be monitored at each visit, especially during dose titration. Orthostasis may be treated with dose reduction, since this effect is dose-related. However, it frequently occurs even at low doses. Other strategies include rising slowly from either a sitting or recumbent position, returning to a supine position when dizzy, adequate fluid and salt intake, support hose, salt tablets, or fludrocortisone. In the rare event of unremitting hypotension, intravenous fluids may be necessary; *pressor support must be avoided*, as it may precipitate a hypertensive crisis.

MAOIs have no direct **cardiac** effects and do not alter cardiac conduction or cardiac rhythm. They therefore may be a good alternative to TCAs in patients with underlying cardiac disease.

Hypertensive crisis is the most severe adverse reaction and results from the interaction of MAOIs with tyramine or other vasoactive amine-contain-ing foods or sympathomimetic drugs. Fortunately, it is rare, but it may be life-threatening. The mechanism underlying this effect is as follows: the patient ingests an exogenous pressor, such as tyramine in various prepared or processed foods, or a sympathomimetic agent; since it cannot be degraded due to inhibition of MAOI-A in the gut, liver, and blood vessels, it enters the systemic circulation causing release of catecholamine stores, resulting in hypertension. Occasionally, patients have had spontaneous hypertensive crises shortly after a dose of an MAOI.

Warning signs include a sudden severe headache, flushing, diaphoresis, palpitations, retro-orbital pain, nausea, vomiting, photophobia, and mydri-asis. These signs may herald extreme hypertension with subsequent risk of intracerebral hemorrhage or myocardial infarction. Patients should be in-structed to call their physician and to go to the emergency room immediately if any of these warning signs occur. Treatment of MAOI-associated hyperten-sive crisis is with alpha-adrenergic blockers such as phentolamine, chlorpro-mazine, or calcium channel blockers (nifedipine). Some physicians prescribe nifedipine or chlorpromazine as needed for sudden onset of headache so that patients may take an antidote immediately before arriving in the emergency room.

Hypertensive crises may be precipitated by ingesting tyramine-rich foods or sympathomimetic agents. Prior to initiating treatment, patients should be educated about food and medication restrictions and should understand and agree to these restrictions (Table 4–17).

Hypermetabolic crisis or the **serotonergic syndrome** is another medical crisis that is associated with MAOIs. It results from a hyperserotonergic state and may occur when MAOIs are used in combination with other serotonergic agents such as the SSRIs, clomipramine, meperidine (Demerol), dextromethorphan, or tryptophan. The serotonergic syndrome is characterized by profound hyperthermia, neuromuscular irritability, altered consciousness, seizures, and possibly death. Treatment is supportive. Dantrolene or cyproheptadine may be used as an antidote.

As do many of the other antidepressants, MAOIs may cause **sexual dysfunction**, most commonly decreased libido, impaired erection, delayed ejaculation, and anorgasmia. These are more frequent with phenelzine than with tranylcypromine. See the previous SSRI section for antidotes.

Fluid balance may be impaired by the MAOIs, and bipedal edema is a common side effect. If clinically significant, treatment with a thiazide or loop diuretic may be indicated, or the agent should be discontinued.

MAOIs are associated with **weight gain** through several mechanisms including increased appetite and food intake as well as fluid retention. Patients should be assisted with dietary control. Weight gain occurs more frequently with phenelzine than with tranylcypromine. In fact, weight loss may occur with tranylcypromine as a result of its amphetaminelike properties.

CNS side effects may be distressing to patients. **Agitation, anxiety**, and **restlessness** may occur, especially with tranylcypromine because of its amphetamine-like properties. Patients may complain of restless nocturnal sleep with afternoon somnolence that is not easily treated. **Insomnia** may be treated with trazodone at bedtime or change the time of dose. Euphoria and even **mania** may occur, particularly in patients with a bipolar spectrum disorder. **Confusional states** may also occur.

Nocturnal myoclonus may contribute to sleep disturbance and responds to dividing doses or giving the last dose in the afternoon. Clonazepam at bedtime often helps. **Paresthesias** may occur and are sometimes secondary to pyridoxine (vitamin B_6) deficiency, which may be caused by MAOIs. Paresthesias may respond to parenteral pyridoxine supplementation (50–150 mg/day). Headache, dizziness, and weakness may also occur.

MAOIs may cause hepatocellular damage that may lead to cirrhosis. **Hepatotoxicity** is more common with phenelzine and isocarboxazid than with

text continues on page 118

TABLE 4–17. DIETARY RESTRICTIONS NECESSARY FOR MAOI THERAPY

Dietary Guidelines	Tyramine* (mg/30 g)	Comments and Examples
Not Permitted		
Cheese, aged, overripe, or spoiled	1.0–65.0	For example, blue, cheddar, Gruyere
Smoked, pickled, or unfresh fish	0–99.0	For example, caviar, anchovies, herring
Fermented dry sausage	3.0–45	For example, pepperoni, salami, summer sausage
Semi-dry	~2.6	For example, bologna
Beer		
Imported or import-style ale	0.05–0.4	12 oz American-style beer contains
American style	0.05–0.1	about 1 mg tyramine
Red wine, sherry, liqueurs	0.05–0.4	Especially Chianti (0.76 mg/30 ml)
Beef or chicken liver	0–0.3	May be acceptable if very fresh
Meat extracts	2.9–9.1	Bovril, Marmite, some dry soup bases
Yeast extracts and supplements	2.0–68.0	Regular bakery products are permitted
Sauerkraut	0.6–2.9	Testing done on German products
Unfresh or overripe protein-rich foods	Varies	For example, leftover meats and expired dairy products
Broad beans (e.g., fava beans)	NA	Contains dopa rather than tyramine
Green banana or banana peel	0.2–2.0	Peel also contains dopamine
Permitted in Limited Amounts		
Processed American cheeses	0–1.5 0–0.7	Up to 1.5 mg tyramine in a single slice (1 oz) of American cheese
Avocado		Higher levels in overripe fruit and guacamole
Bananas, fresh	0–0.2	Avoid overripe fruit and peel
Soy sauce and variants	~0.05	Safe unless used in very large amounts
Peanuts and other nuts	?	No documentation of tyramine content
Raspberries, fresh or in jams	~0.3–2.9	Safe in very small servings
White wine and distilled spirits	?	No documentation of tyramine content
Chocolate	NA	Contains phenylethylamine
Not Restricted		
Yogurt, sour cream, cream cheese, cottage cheese	0–0.3	Avoid homemade or homemade styles and consume very fresh products
Fresh fish and meats	ND	Do not allow spoilage
Fresh fruits (except raspberries)	ND	
Figs and raisins	ND	Canned figs may contain tyramine*
Most dried soups and bouillon	ND	

*Figures based on 1-oz (30 g or 30 ml) portions. Up to 6 mg tyramine may be ingested safely while taking therapeutic doses of MAOIs.
ND = no detectable amount of tyramine; NA = not applicable, contains other pressor agents.

tranylcypromine. It typically begins one to six months after initiation of treatment and is heralded by anorexia, malaise, and insidious jaundice. Bilirubin and transaminases may be 8–100 times normal. The drug should be discontinued at the earliest sign of hepatotoxicity. Recovery is usually complete, although markedly elevated bilirubin may predict a poorer outcome with chronic liver disease. Severe hepatotoxicity is more frequent with phenelzine than tranylcypromine.

Gastrointestinal side effects are not common with MAOIs, although patients may report constipation, anorexia, or dyspepsia. **Hypersensitivity** reactions are rare. Skin rashes and photosensitivity are the most likely. **Anticholinergic** side effects can occur with the MAOIs but are usually less frequent and less severe than with the TCAs. Patients may report dry mouth and urinary retention.

TOXICITY

MAOIs are dangerous in overdose. The effects may be slow to develop, over 12–24 hours, so patients need prolonged monitoring after a significant overdose. Doses of 375–1500 mg phenelzine and 170–650 mg tranylcypromine have proved fatal. Symptoms may include hyperpyrexia, autonomic excitation, neuromuscular irritability and rigidity, tachycardia, tachypnea, and metabolic acidosis. Seizures may occur. Rhabdomyolysis may occur as a result of muscular excitement and may lead to renal failure. The late phase may be marked by cardiovascular collapse, arrhythmias, or asystole.

Treatment should include gastric lavage, activated charcoal, magnesium citrate, and acidification to decrease absorption and speed up elimination.[101] Hemodialysis is effective in removing MAOIs. Seizures and agitation may be treated with short acting benzodiazepines. Muscular irritability has been treated successfully with IV dantrolene sodium.[102] Hypertension may be treated with IV phentolamine; ventricular arrhythmias may be treated with lidocaine. Bretylium should be avoided due to its adrenergic effects.

WITHDRAWAL

Abrupt MAOI withdrawal may precipitate a withdrawal syndrome characterized by agitation, irritability, lability, aggressivity, pressured speech, insomnia or drowsiness, hallucinations, paranoid delusions, disorientation, muscle weakness, hyperreflexia, myoclonus, ataxia, choreoathetosis, and catatonia.[103] These symptoms may begin one to four days after withdrawal. A slow (over one to two weeks) taper is recommended when discontinuing an MAOI.

MAO inhibition persists for one to two weeks after withdrawal of the MAOI. Therefore, dietary and medication restrictions should continue for at least 10 days after discontinuation of tranylcypromine and 14 days after discontinuation of phenelzine. If switching to another antidepressant, a two-week wash-out period is recommended.

MONITORING

Plasma levels have not been well studied, but platelet MAO inhibition has been correlated with clinical response. Blood pressure, supine and standing, should be monitored at each visit while initiating and titrating an MAOI. Once a patient is on maintenance treatment with an MAOI, less frequent blood pressure monitoring is required unless a patient has signs or symptoms of orthostasis or hypertensive crisis.

DRUG-DRUG INTERACTIONS

As mentioned, sympathomimetic amines should be avoided, because they may precipitate a hypertensive crisis (Table 4–18). Sympathomimetic amines include amphetamine, methylphenidate, ephedrine, pseudoephedrine, phenylpropanolamine, dopamine, and tyramine. The direct-acting epinephrine, norepinephrine, isoproterenol, and methoxamine are safe. Many over-the-counter drugs contain sympathomimetics and should be avoided, including most cold remedies, nasal decongestants, antihistamines, cough medicines, allergy medicines, narcotic painkillers, appetite suppressants, and antiasthma drugs.

Serotonergic agents can interact with MAOIs to precipitate the serotonergic syndrome. These include TCAs, SSRIs, other MAOIs, lithium, l-tryptophan, and sumatriptan. Combination MAOI-TCA therapy may be used with caution by physicians who have experience with this combination. The TCA should be started first or concurrently with the MAOI. If an MAOI has been started first and a TCA is to be added, discontinue the MAOI for 10–14 days and then start the two concurrently at low doses. TCAs should not be added to an existing MAOI regimen because of increased risk of hypertensive crisis. The combination potentiates some of the adverse effects, particularly weight gain, hypotension, and anticholinergic effects.

DRUG-DISEASE INTERACTIONS

Patients with **hypertension** or **cardiovascular disease** that might predispose to a myocardial infarction should not be prescribed MAOIs.

TABLE 4–18. MEDICATIONS THAT ARE CONTRAINDICATED WITH MAOI THERAPY

Degree of Caution	Medication	Comments and Examples
Common Agents Absolutely Contraindicated	Sympathomimetic Amines	Rx—amphetamine and epinephrine analogs
		OTC—ephedrine, pseudoephedrine, phenylephrine, and phenylethylamine
	Dextromethorphan	OTC—present in Dristan, Comtrex, and many others; acts via serotonin reuptake blockade
	SSRIs	Rx—fluoxetine, sertraline, paroxetine, fluvoxamine; may produce serotonin syndrome
	Hypoglycemic agents	Rx—potentiates hypoglycemia
	L-dopa, methyldopa	Rx—enhances pressor effect. Dopa present in some food
	Reserpine, tetrabenazine	Rx—similar to serotonin syndrome
	Tryptophan	Rx—serotonin precursor
Anesthetic Agents to Be Avoided	Narcotic analgesics	Reserved to meperidine and other 5HT blockers but may also prolong action of morphine and barbiturates
	Ketamine	Theoretical risk of cardiovascular toxicity
	Suxamethonium	May prolong or increase neuromuscular blockade
	Local anesthetics	Avoid epinephrine, norepinephrine, cocaine, and analogues
Agents Causing Adverse Reactions in Rare Cases	Amantadine	Acts as a dopamine agonist; may produce hypertension
	Chloral hydrate	Hypertension reported, mechanism unknown
	Droperidol	Hypotension reported
	Fenfluramine	Delirium reported, mechanism unknown
	Guanethidine	May produce hypertension
Agents to Be Used with Caution	Tricyclic antidepressants	See guidelines in text
	Anticholinergics	Potentiation reported in humans, hyperthermia in animals
	Benzodiazepines	Reports of edema, probably safe
	Caffeine	Hypertension and agitation with excessive intake

*Rx = prescription drug, OTC = available without prescription.

[120]

Patients with **cerebral aneurysms, arteriovenous malformations,** history of **hemorrhagic strokes,** or any other condition predisposing to intracerebral hemorrhage with hypertension should not be prescribed MAOIs. Patients with **asthma** or other conditions that might need to be treated on an emergency basis with vasopressors or sympathomimetics should not be treated with MAOIs.

Pheochromocytoma causes high levels of endogenous sympathomimetic amines and is a relative contraindication to MAOI therapy. **Hepatic disease** may impair tyramine clearance and increase the risk of hypertensive crisis. Patients with **impending surgical procedures** requiring anesthesia should not be prescribed MAOIs. MAOIs should not be given concurrently with **ECT** because of the interaction with anesthetic agents.

SEROTONIN NOREPINEPHRINE REUPTAKE INHIBITOR (SNRI)

This new class of antidepressants is like a combination of a TCA and SSRI in a single agent with a relatively benign side-effect profile. Venlafaxine (Effexor) and mirtazapine (Remeron) are the two representatives of this class currently available (Table 4–19 and Figure 4–8).

EFFICACY

There are no reported randomized, double-blind, placebo-controlled studies of venlafaxine in the maintenance treatment of depression available yet.

MECHANISM OF ACTION

Venlafaxine is thought to exert its therapeutic effect by inhibiting reuptake of both serotonin and norepinephrine. There is speculation that this combination produces more rapid down-regulation of beta-adrenergic receptors, which is responsible for the therapeutic effect and possibly more rapid onset of action than the other antidepressants. Mirtazapine also inhibits serotonin and norepinephrine reuptake, but it is also an alpha-2-adrenergic and 5-HT2A and 5-HT3 receptor agonist.

PHARMACOKINETICS

Venlafaxine is metabolized in the liver by cytochrome P450 2D6 and 3A3/4. It is a weak inhibitor of P450 2D6, ten times less so than

text continues on page 123

TABLE 4–19. AVAILABLE PREPARATIONS AND COSTS FOR OTHER ANTIDEPRESSANTS

Compound	Trade Name	Nonparenteral Preparations	Injectable	Generic	Average Dose/Day	Average Cost/Day
Venlafaxine	Effexor	Tablets: 25, 37.5, 50, 75, 100 mg	No	No	225 mg	$2.20
Mirtzapine	Remeron	Tablets: 15, 30 mg	No	No	15–45 mg	$2.20
Trazodone	Desyrel	Tablets: 50, 100, 150 mg	No	Yes	300 mg	$7.11 (1.35)*
Nefazodone	Serzone	Tablets: 100, 150, 200, 250 mg	No	No	400 mg	$1.00
Bupropion	Wellbutrin	Tablets: 75, 100 mg	No	No	225 mg	$1.80

*Cost of generics.
From Red Book Annual Pharmacist Reference, 1996. Copyright 1996 by Medical Economics, Montvale, NJ. Reprinted with permission.

[122]

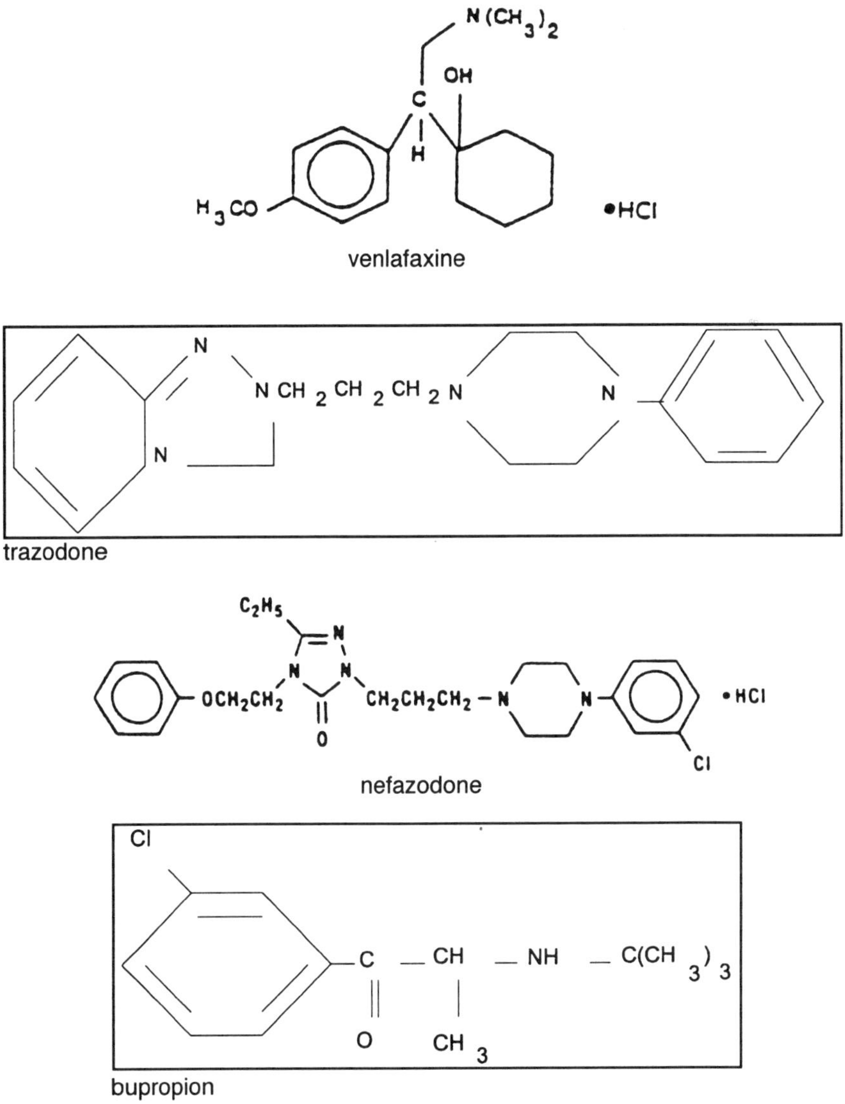

venlafaxine

trazodone

nefazodone

bupropion

FIG. 4–8. Chemical structures of other antidepressants.

sertraline. The half-life of venlafaxine is 5 hours and the half-life of the active metabolite o-desmethylvenlafaxine is 11 hours, requiring two to three daily dosings. Venlafaxine has low protein binding (25–30%) that is significantly less than the other antidepressants.

Mirtazapine is metabolized in the liver by cytochrome P450 2D6, 1A2 and 3A4 but does not significantly inhibit any of these systems. The half-life is

20–40 hours. There are active metabolites that are present in very low levels. Protein binding is 85%.

ADVERSE EFFECTS AND THEIR MANAGEMENT

The side-effect profile is more similar to that of the SSRIs than that of the TCAs, and both agents are generally well tolerated by patients. Common side effects of venlafaxine include **anxiety, agitation, insomnia, sedation, dizziness, sweating,** and **constipation.** Nausea and vomiting are common dose-limiting adverse effects in the beginning of treatment and may be ameliorated by dosing with food or adding cisapride (Propulcid), a 5-HT3 blocker, until tolerance develops.[104] Venlafaxine at higher doses may cause a persistent **elevation in diastolic blood pressure** in about 6% of patients, which is a dose-related phenomenon. For this reason, baseline blood pressure measurements should be obtained and blood pressure should be monitored throughout initiation and titration at each visit. It also causes a clinically insignificant increase in heart rate.

The most common side effects of mirtazapine are **somnolence, increased appetite, weight gain, dizziness,** and **constipation.** Due to sedation, mirtazapine is dosed at bedtime. There have been reports of agranulocytosis, but this is very rare.

Sexual side effects of delayed ejaculation and anorgasmia are reportedly more rare with either venlafaxine or mirtazapine than with the SSRIs. There is no indication of cardiac effects with either venlafaxine or mirtazapine.

MONITORING

While initiating therapy with venlafaxine, blood pressure should be checked at baseline and at each visit due to the risk of increased diastolic blood pressure. There are no other necessary medical tests. There is no need for therapeutic blood level monitoring, since there is no correlation between level and therapeutic efficacy.

DRUG-DRUG INTERACTIONS

The SNRIs should not be given with an MAOI or within 14 days of discontinuing an MAOI. Drugs that inhibit P450 2D6 may interfere with venlafaxine and mirtazapine metabolism, decreasing levels of the active metabolite.

DRUG-DISEASE INTERACTIONS

Patients with hepatic or renal disease have an increased elimination half-life so lower doses should be used.

Aminoketones

The aminoketones are structurally very different from the other classes of antidepressants. Bupropion is the only agent of this type currently available (see Figure 4–8 and Table 4–19).

EFFICACY

There have been no adequate randomized, double-blind, placebo-controlled studies reported for bupropion in the maintenance treatment of depression.

MECHANISM OF ACTION

Bupropion, unlike the other antidepressants, probably works primarily through a dopaminergic mechanism and has weak effects on serotonin and noradrenergic neurotransmission. At high doses, however, it produces down-regulation of beta-noradrenergic receptors. It is structurally related to amphetamine and has some stimulantlike effects. It does not have any anticholinergic or antihistaminic effects.

PHARMACOKINETICS

Bupropion is rapidly absorbed from the gut with peak levels achieved in two hours. It is metabolized by the liver but not through the P450 system and induces its own metabolism. Half-life is 14 hours, and active metabolites with longer half-lives than the parent compound are present, but their potency and toxicity have not been well characterized. Protein binding is about 80%.

ADVERSE EFFECTS AND THEIR MANAGEMENT

Bupropion is well tolerated by most patients, including those who are unable to tolerate the TCAs or SSRIs. Serious side effects are few, and it can be used safely in many populations for which TCAs and SSRIs are contraindicated. It is nonsedating, has few anticholinergic effects, and does not induce weight gain.

Bupropion may be activating in some patients due to its stimulantlike properties. Patients may complain of **agitation, restlessness, insomnia,** and **anxiety.** These symptoms may be relieved by benzodiazepines or trazodone at bedtime. Bupropion is associated with some anticholinergic symptoms including dry mouth, dry eyes, blurred vision, and sweating. Bupropion may also cause **psychotic** symptoms in some patients or mania in patients with bipolar spectrum disorders. Bupropion is associated with elevated blood pressure, tremor, nausea, and constipation. Because of the dopaminergic effects, bupropion may cause **menstrual irregularities.** Bupropion may cause **gait disturbance, akinesia** and **bradykinesia.** It is not associated with weight gain but may produce weight loss. Bupropion is among the least likely to cause sexual dysfunction.

Bupropion is also associated with a higher incidence of **seizures:** about 0.4%, which is four times higher than the other antidepressants. This is a dose-related effect, and for this reason, no single dose should exceed 150 mg; doses should be administered at least six hours apart, and total daily dose should not exceed 450 mg. Seizures usually occur within the first six weeks of treatment and at peak blood levels. A new sustained-release preparation may be associated with a lower incidence of seizures.

MONITORING

There is no need for therapeutic blood level monitoring, because there is no correlation between level and therapeutic efficacy. However, patients should be monitored for seizure activity. Blood pressure should also be monitored.

DRUG-DRUG INTERACTIONS

There are few drug interactions with bupropion as it is not metabolized by the hepatic cytochrome system and is not highly protein bound. It may be used safely with other drugs.

DRUG-DISEASE INTERACTIONS

Because of the increased incidence of seizures with bupropion, it should be used cautiously in patients with known **seizure disorders.** Patients should be warned about the possibility of increased seizure activity, and anticonvulsant medications may need to be increased. Bupropion should not be used in patients with **eating disorders,** because the incidence of bupropion-induced seizures is higher in this population.

TRIAZOLOPYRIDINES

There are currently two representatives of this group on the market, trazodone and nefazodone. This group is chemically unrelated to any of the other classes of antidepressants (see Table 4–19 and Figure 4–8).

EFFICACY

There are no adequate randomized, double-blind, placebo-controlled studies of the efficacy of either trazodone or nefazodone in maintenance treatment in depression. Trazodone is used frequently in combination with SSRIs or MAOIs to alleviate the agitation and insomnia associated with these medications.

MECHANISM OF ACTION

Trazodone and nefazodone both inhibit serotonin reuptake, block 5-HT2A receptors, and down-regulate noradrenergic receptors. Trazodone acts as a serotonomimetic agent, probably through its metabolite m-chlorophenylpiperazine (m-CPP), which is a post-synaptic serotonin agonist and potentiates 5-HT1A transmission. Nefazodone exhibits less alpha1-adrenergic antagonism than trazodone. Neither exhibits anticholinergic effects.

PHARMACOKINETICS

Both agents are rapidly absorbed following oral administration. They are metabolized in the liver and excreted mainly in the urine. Trazodone has an active metabolite, m-CPP. Nefazodone has three active metabolites: hydroxynefazodone, triazole dione, and m-CPP. Half-lives are short: 3 to 9 hours for trazodone and m-CPP, approximately 3 to 4 hours for nefazodone and its hydroxy metabolite, but 18–33 hours for triazole dione. At least twice daily dosing is required for both agents. Protein binding is very high (>99% for nefazodone).

Trazodone is metabolized by P450 2D6. Nefazodone does not appear to inhibit P450 2D6 or to be affected by inhibition of this enzyme. Nefazodone is metabolized by P450 3A3/4 and is also a potent inhibitor of this system.

ADVERSE EFFECTS AND THEIR MANAGEMENT

Common side effects of trazodone are **sedation, orthostatic hypotension, cognitive slowing, nausea**, and **vomiting**. Trazodone has been associated with **cardiac arrhythmias** in patients with preexisting ventricular arrhythmias.

Penile or clitoral priapism may occur with trazodone, usually in the beginning of therapy. Male patients should be cautioned that if they have an abnormally prolonged erection they should stop the trazodone and go to the emergency room for treatment. In this event, trazodone should be discontinued and never restarted. Comparable symptoms may also occur in female patients. Some clinicians have noted that trazodone may be useful in treating impotence. To date, there are no published reports of priapism with nefazodone.

The most common side effects of nefazodone are **headache, dry mouth**, and **nausea. Somnolence, dizziness, light-headedness, constipation**, and **asthenia** also have been reported. Nefazodone is less likely to cause sedation or orthostasis than trazodone and therefore may be better tolerated.

These agents are less likely to cause anxiety, agitation, or sexual dysfunction than the SSRIs. This class of antidepressants is relatively safe in overdose.

MONITORING

Orthostatic blood pressures should be checked, particularly with trazodone if patients are symptomatic. Otherwise there are no other tests that should be monitored. Therapeutic monitoring is not necessary, because there is no correlation between blood levels and therapeutic response.

DRUG-DRUG INTERACTIONS

Nefazodone inhibits P450 3A3/4, increasing levels of drugs metabolized by this system including alprazolam (Xanax) and triazolam (Halcion), leading to a 200–400% increase in levels of these benzodiazepines. Caution should be taken with these agents and lower doses should be used. Terfenadine and astemizole are also metabolized by this system and high levels may result in cardiac toxicity. These agents should not be used with nefazodone.

DRUG-DISEASE INTERACTIONS

Trazodone should not be used in patients with cardiac disease, due to the low but appreciable risk of cardiac arrhythmias.

CHOICE OF ANTIDEPRESSANT

The choice of antidepressant for acute and maintenance treatment requires consideration of many factors. Many have already been discussed: drug efficacy, both for acute alleviation of symptoms as well as long-term prophylaxis against recurrence; ease of administration (single daily versus multiple daily dosing); safety; need for baseline physical assessments and ongoing periodic monitoring; tolerability and side-effect profile; cost, and lethality. If a patient has responded to a particular medication in the past, chances are he or she will respond to the same medication again. Likewise, if a patient's family member with a similar disorder has responded to a particular agent, it is likely that the patient may as well.

Other factors that merit consideration are depressive symptom profile and depressive subtype, because some symptoms may respond preferentially to a particular agent or class of antidepressants. In addition, comorbid psychiatric illness (particularly substance abuse) and comorbid medical and neurological illness deserve close attention.

DEPRESSIVE SUBTYPE

Melancholic depression with neurovegetative symptoms (profound disturbance of sleep and appetite and psychomotor retardation), anhedonia, lack of mood reactivity, diurnal variation in symptoms, and excessive guilt is a severe form of depression and responds better to TCAs than to SSRIs. There have been few studies specifically designed to examine the efficacy of the newer antidepressants in melancholic depressed patients, although larger studies indicate that these agents are more efficacious in the subgroup of less severely depressed patients and less efficacious in more severely depressed patients. Venlafaxine and nefazodone have demonstrated efficacy in hospitalized patients.

Atypical depression, which is marked by reverse neurovegetative signs (increased sleep, increased appetite, and psychomotor activation) and is common in **seasonal affective disorder** (SAD) and bipolar depressions, responds preferentially to the SSRIs and MAOIs.

Anxious depression, marked by psychomotor agitation, restlessness, excessive worry, generalized anxiety, or panic attacks responds well to MAOIs, TCAs, and SSRIs. The MAOIs are efficacious in panic disorder and social phobia and may be the best choice for patients with comorbid anxiety symptoms if patients can follow the dietary restrictions. The TCAs are also effective treatments for anxiety disorders that may benefit from these sedating drugs.

Benzodiazepines may be used in the short term to treat anxiety until the antidepressant begins exerting its effect; a long-acting agent such as clonazepam (Klonopin) may be used on a once daily (bedtime) or twice daily schedule for the first several weeks and then tapered to avoid rebound anxiety with benzodiazepine withdrawal when antidepressant effects are noted. Patients do not usually require benzodiazepines during maintenance treatment of depression, and every attempt should be made to wean patients off benzodiazepines for long-term maintenance.

Psychotic or **delusional depression** usually requires a combination of antidepressant and antipsychotic medications during the acute and continuation phases, but there are no reported studies on maintenance treatment of psychotically depressed patients. The standard of care is to discontinue the antipsychotic after four to six months and maintain the patient on the antidepressant alone. The antipsychotic should be tapered slowly over at least one month, maybe longer. The patient should be aware that psychotic symptoms may emerge. If any early signs of psychosis are evident, the antipsychotic should be increased slightly and then maintained at the lowest possible dose.

For the acute treatment of psychotic depression, the combination of TCAs and antipsychotics has been best studied in Antipsychotics such as chlorpromazine (Thorazine) should be avoided in combination with the TCAs, because the anticholinergic burden is high with these agents combined and the combination may be associated with cognitive impairment or delirium. The combination of nortriptyline (a secondary TCA) and perphenazine (Trilafon, a midpotency antipsychotic) has been shown to be effective and well tolerated.[105] A meta-analysis demonstrated efficacy of the combination of antidepressants and antipsychotics better than either agent alone and of comparable efficacy to ECT.[106] The more dopaminergic antidepressants (amoxepine, clomipramine) may exacerbate extrapyramidal side effects. Combinations of SSRIs and antipsychotics have also been reported as efficacious.

The treatment of bipolar depression is discussed in Chapter 5.

Post-psychotic depression is a depressive episode that occurs after recovery from a psychotic episode in a primary psychotic disorder such as schizophrenia or schizoaffective disorder. These episodes have been shown to respond well to imipramine, amitriptyline, and trazodone.[107,108,109] Maintenance treatment with antidepressants in psychotic disorders has not been systematically studied.

SAD may respond to any of the antidepressants. However, the treatment of choice for SAD is light therapy (discussed in the acute treatment section). Fluoxetine is also effective in SAD. Because SAD is a cyclic disorder with episodes occurring at approximately the same time every year, recurrences can be predicted and therefore anticipated. Treatment (antidepressants or light) may be initiated at the earliest signs of depression or shortly before the anticipated time of onset and continued until the anticipated time of remission. Treatment during the continuation phase should be at the same dose used to achieve remission. In a sense this is prophylactic treatment, although the treatment does not need to be maintained throughout the year.

Premenstrual dysphoric disorder is also a cyclic exacerbation of depressive and physical symptoms around the later half of the luteal phase of the menstrual cycle. Most studies of premenstrual dysphoric disorder use continuous treatment throughout the month. Medications shown efficacious by placebo-controlled, randomized studies for acute treatment of this condition are fluoxetine, clomipramine, d-fenfluramine, and light.[110,111,112,113,114,115,116,117] While most studies involved continuous treatment, a few have provided treatment beginning on day 14 of the menstrual cycle and proceeding to menses. This strategy, however, is probably not useful with fluoxetine, since the half-life is so long and the medication takes four weeks to reach steady-state. The majority of patients relapse with discontinuation of the medication, and remit again with reinstitution of therapy, so long-term treatment is probably indicated for these patients. Long-term treatment with fluoxetine has demonstrated efficacy at preventing recurrence.[118]

Patients with a **high risk for suicide**—those with active suicidal ideation with or without a plan, history of previous suicide attempt, impulsivity, substance abuse, chronic medical illness, or family history of affective disorder or suicide—should be prescribed a medication that is not lethal in overdose. The safest medications in overdose are SSRIs, bupropion, venlafaxine, and trazodone. TCAs and MAOIs are best avoided in this group.

Dysthymia responds better to the SSRIs and MAOIs than to the TCAs.[119] Because dysthymia is by definition a chronic, unremitting illness, the need for long-term treatment is obvious. If patients develop an MDE on antidepressant therapy, the antidepressant dose may be increased or if already at the maximum (or maximum tolerated) dose, augmented with a second agent. Patients should then be maintained on the regimen on which remission was achieved.

COMORBID PSYCHIATRIC CONDITIONS

Obsessive-compulsive disorder (OCD) and MDD frequently coexist. Fortunately, the treatment for both conditions is similar. The treatment of choice for OCD is a serotonergic agent such as clomipramine or an SSRI, usually at a higher dose than that needed for depression. Depressed patients with comorbid OCD should therefore be treated with higher doses of SSRI or clomipramine than usual for depression.

Generalized anxiety disorder and **panic disorder** may also be comorbid with depression. As for OCD, the treatment is similar for both conditions. For patients with any comorbid anxiety disorder or associated anxiety symptoms, initial starting doses of antidepressants should be less (half) than the typical starting dose.

Substance abuse is frequently comorbid with depression. Dual diagnosis patients are especially difficult to treat since the substance abuse confounds the clinical picture and may also contribute to development and maintenance of depression. Patients with primary MDD may use alcohol or other drugs in attempts to self-medicate.

Eating disorders, anorexia nervosa and bulimia nervosa, are also frequently comorbid with depression. The SSRIs have been shown to be efficacious in eating disorders. Appetite suppression is frequently a side effect of the SSRIs, but this is not usually a problem. Patients are less likely to be compliant with a TCA or MAOI given the side effects of weight gain and edema. Bupropion should not be used in this population due to the increased risk of seizures, which is dependent on body weight.

Personality disorders may complicate the treatment of any disorder. The implications of comorbidity with **personality disorders** is reviewed by Shea et al.[120] The incidence of personality disorders in depressed patients is at least 30–40%. Inpatient samples tend to have higher rates of dramatic (Cluster B) personality disorders, particularly borderline and histrionic, while inpatient populations tend to have more anxious-fearful (Cluster C) personality disorders, such as obsessive-compulsive, avoidant, and dependent. The etiological relationship between personality disorders and depression remains unclear, and it has been speculated that personality disorders predispose to the development of depression; personality pathology represents a subclinical form of depression or other axis I pathology; or comorbidity results from chance or nonetiologic factors. There is agreement that these patients have poorer outcomes with antidepressant medications than nonpersonality disordered patients; they respond slower and have more residual symptoms.

Borderline personality disorder patients are impulsive and have chronic suicidality. One study demonstrated preferential response to the MAOI phenelzine over imipramine and placebo.[121] Other studies have demonstrated that those patients with moderately severe schizotypal symptoms respond to antipsychotics.[122,123,124] There is also evidence demonstrating that impulsive and aggressive behavior in the context of character pathology may respond to fluoxetine, lithium, carbamazepine, or valproate.[125,126,127] For impulsive conditions, only medications that are safe in overdose should be prescribed.

Personality disordered patients frequently have only short-lived responses to medications, and maintenance treatment with the agent that produced remission does not have the same prophylactic effect that it does in other patients.

COMORBID MEDICAL CONDITIONS

Patients with underlying **cardiac disease** should be tried first on an agent with no known cardiac toxicity such as an SSRI, bupropion, or venlafaxine. The TCAs and trazodone should be avoided as first-line agents and should only be used with caution in patients who are intolerant of or nonresponsive to other classes of antidepressants.

Hepatic disease may impair metabolism of drugs metabolized by the cytochrome P450 system. Serum levels of drugs should be monitored when appropriate, and for drugs that do not have standards for efficacy, lower doses may be required.

Renal disease may impair excretion of drug and therefore increase the levels of active drug. Recommendations for hepatic disease apply here as well.

The TCAs, bupropion, and the SSRIs all decrease the seizure threshold to variable degrees and should be used with caution in patients with underlying **seizure disorders**, although they are not contraindicated. Patients should be monitored closely for seizure activity and may require increased anticonvulsant levels. Since many of these agents also alter anticonvulsant levels, anticonvulsant levels must be monitored closely with initiation and titration of the antidepressant. Agents that do not alter the seizure threshold are venlafaxine, trazodone, and nefazodone.

SPECIAL POPULATIONS

PEDIATRICS

There is no good evidence for the efficacy of antidepressants in maintenance treatment in children and adolescents. Rosenberg and associates describe in detail the use of antidepressants in children and adolescents.[128] The special considerations involved in using some of these agents in this population are reviewed briefly here.

TCAs have proven safe for use in children. However, due to reports of sudden death with desipramine and imipramine in children, EKGs should be monitored. Baseline EKG should be obtained before initiating treatment, and a follow-up EKG should be obtained prior to each dose increase. Plasma levels should also be checked when steady-state is achieved at a new dose and every few months thereafter. Cardiac toxicity is dose-related. Rapid dose increases may also precipitate seizures in children. Blood pressure and pulse should be monitored as well. The FDA has established guidelines for the safe use of TCAs in children and adolescents.

SSRIs may be safely used in children. Considerations for adults apply to this population as well. Recent studies suggest that SSRIs produce a therapeutic effect on depression in this population.[129]

MAOIs may be especially useful in the pediatric population because of the predominance of atypical features in children as well as the increased risk for bipolar disorder in patients in whom depression first presents in childhood or adolescence. These agents require dietary restrictions, but it may be difficult for children and adolescents to follow the guidelines.

Trazodone is not recommended for routine use in children and adolescents as there is limited data in this population.

Bupropion is not approved by the FDA for use in patients less than 18 years old. There are no data on its use for depression in children.

PREGNANCY AND LACTATION

There is concern about the teratogenic effects of antidepressants since they cross the placenta and are present in the fetus during development. However, none of the antidepressants has been demonstrated convincingly to have teratogenic effects, although there is some evidence to suggest that these agents are not safe during pregnancy, particularly during organogenesis in the first trimester. The little data in this area have been reviewed extensively.[130,131,132]

There have been no controlled studies of psychotropics in pregnant women and little retrospective uncontrolled data with the newer antidepressants. There is no definitive evidence for teratogenicity with the TCAs, and the secondary TCAs are considered relatively safe in pregnancy. Clomipramine is category C due to fetotoxic effects at supratherapeutic doses in mice.

MAOIs have been shown to be teratogenic in animals although there is no supporting evidence in humans. These medications should be avoided, however, due to the risk of hypertensive crisis that could lead to vascular compromise for both mother and fetus.

The SSRIs, bupropion, and trazodone are classified as category B because there are no controlled studies in pregnant women. The retrospective data do not indicate an unusually high risk with fluoxetine. There are little to no data for sertraline, bupropion, and trazodone.

Symptoms associated with antidepressant use and withdrawal have been noted in neonates of mothers taking antidepressants at the time of parturition and during lactation. TCA use during the third trimester may be associated with neonatal toxicity or withdrawal symptoms including tremor, myoclonus, irritability, seizures, tachycardia, heart failure, respiratory distress, cyanosis, and urinary retention. Goldberg recommended tapering TCAs one month prior to estimated date of confinement to avoid withdrawal in the neonate.[132]

Antidepressants are secreted into breast milk, resulting in detectable levels in nursing infants of lactating mothers who are exposed to these drugs.[133] The drug levels present in the nursing infant are variable, depending on the drug and maternal metabolism. The SSRIs, especially, are secreted at high levels in breast milk. The clinical significance of this exposure is uncertain.

In addition to concern about congenital malformations, there is also concern about behavioral teratogenicity. Psychotropics probably have an effect on neuronal development; the consequences of this on later behavior and psychopathology are unknown.

Physicians should counsel all female patients of reproductive age who are taking antidepressants, especially those in maintenance treatment, about the risks and benefits of continuing their psychotropic medication during pregnancy and should guide the patient in pregnancy planning. Although the use of any antidepressant during pregnancy is not recommended, especially during the first trimester, the risk of maternal depression for the fetus must be weighed against the risk of possible teratogenesis or behavioral teratogenesis. Maternal depression may put the fetus in jeopardy by exposing it to poor nutrition, high-risk behavior, and possible death by suicide. If the patient is at very high risk for recurrence or severe illness, the risk of recurrence may be greater than the possible risk of medication effects to the fetus, so the patient may be better off continuing the medication throughout the pregnancy, or at least restarting it at the beginning of the second trimester.

Psychotropics should be tapered prior to conception if possible, or at least as soon as the patient is aware of the pregnancy, if the decision to stop medication is made. At least, a respite from the medication during the first trimester may be attempted. Adjunctive psychotherapy may be helpful during pregnancy to delay recurrence until medications can be restarted safely. Treatment strategy during pregnancy may not be to achieve or maintain remission but simply to ameliorate the most threatening symptoms.

Of the antidepressants, SSRIs may be the safest class during pregnancy. Therefore, if a patient is to remain on antidepressant therapy during pregnancy, is not already on an SSRI, and has not failed a trial of an SSRI, switching to an SSRI during pregnancy may be warranted.

GERIATRICS

Maintenance treatment of depression in the elderly has not been systematically studied despite the high incidence of depression and suicidality and the increased morbidity and mortality it accounts for in this age group. This topic was recently reviewed by Reynolds and the NIH Consensus Conference.[134,135]

The body of evidence for efficacy and necessity of maintenance treatment in the elderly is less robust than for adults. Georgotas et al. demonstrated the efficacy of the MAOI phenelzine in maintenance treatment of recurrent MDD in elderly patients, but they were unable to show efficacy of nortriptyline in this group.[99] There are limited data from open trials suggesting efficacy of maintenance treatment in late life. Preliminary results from a randomized, double-blind, placebo-controlled study of nortriptyline in a three-year maintenance study show that nortriptyline significantly decreases recurrence.[136] Maintenance studies of SSRIs in the elderly have not yet been reported.

Despite the lack of convincing evidence for the efficacy of maintenance therapy in this population, maintenance treatment is recommended for most elderly patients. Patients with a first episode after age 60 and those with more than three previous episodes should have maintenance treatment. Maintenance dose should be the same as that required to attain acute response.

In the elderly,

☐ Initiate therapy with smaller doses than in adults and increase by smaller increments and at greater intervals. Shorter half-life agents are preferred, because the elderly are more susceptible to adverse effects. Drugs may accumulate due to impaired hepatic and renal function, physical illness, and medications. End organ sensitivity may also be higher.

☐ TCAs may be used safely in this population, although they are generally less well tolerated in the elderly. The secondary TCAs (nortriptyline and desipramine) are recommended in the elderly due to their lesser anticholinergic effects. Because many of the side effects are dose-related or related to the rate of increase, initial doses should be lower (25 mg desipramine or 10 mg nortriptyline) and rate of increase slower with smaller increments (25 mg desipramine or 10 mg nortriptyline every 7–10 days). Since elderly patients still require the same therapeutic levels for efficacy as do younger patients, doses should still be pushed to adequate levels. One mistake commonly made in treating the elderly is to maintain the dose at subtherapeutic blood levels.

☐ Elderly patients must be carefully monitored, given that they are more likely to have comorbid medical problems and be on multiple concomitant medications that may make TCA use more complicated. Patients with cardiac disease may be more vulnerable to the tachycardia or modest decrease in cardiac conduction associated with TCA use, therefore EKGs must be monitored and cardiac status assessed routinely. Orthostatic hypotension may be more serious in this population as it predisposes to falls that may result in hip fractures, which carry a 20% mortality rate and 50% morbidity in the elderly.[137]

☐ Caution must be exercised when treating patients on other anticholinergic medications, since the anticholinergic effects are additive and may precipitate delirium. Medications that are also metabolized by the hepatic microsomal P450 2D6 system may alter the levels of TCAs or may have their levels altered by TCAs, either increasing or decreasing their effect. Medications that are highly protein bound, such as digoxin and warfarin, may be displaced by TCAs, thus effectively increasing their free levels and also the likelihood of digoxin toxicity and elevated prothrombin time.

The SSRIs are generally better tolerated than the TCAs in the elderly. However, there are also concerns with the use of these medications. The elderly may have alterations in the hepatic metabolism of drugs and also decreased renal elimination, both of which may contribute to decreased clearance and increased accumulation of medication.

The MAOIs have not been recommended for use in the elderly. However, newer evidence points to their safety in the elderly with careful monitoring of blood pressure and adherence to diet and medication restrictions.

Bupropion has often been preferred in the elderly due to its lack of cardio-vascular side effects compared with the TCAs. There have been no reported studies of maintenance treatment with bupropion or any of the other newer antidepressants in late life.

SUMMARY

Depression is a lifelong illness for the majority of sufferers and carries a high cost in terms of functional disability and diminished quality of life. Maintenance treatment is indicated for patients with depressive disorders who have had three or more previous depressive episodes or severe episodes that carry a high risk for suicide or drastic life consequences. There are many antidepressants currently available that have proven efficacy in both acute and maintenance treatment of depression. Choice of agent depends on symptom profile, side-effect profile, medical and psychiatric comorbidity, and concomitant medications among other considerations. Guidelines for maintenance treatment should be followed.

REFERENCES

1. Angst, J. (1992). How recurrent and predictable is depressive illness? In Montgomery, S., Rovillan, F. (Eds.), *Long-Term Treatment of Depression* (pp. 1–13). New York: John Wiley & Sons, Ltd.
2. Reiger, D.A., Farmer, M.E., Rae, D.S., et al. (1990). Comorbidity of mental disorders: Alcohol and other drug abuse: Results from the Epidemiologic Catchment Area (ECA) Study. *JAMA*, 264:2511–2518.
3. Kessler, R.C., McGonagle, K.A., Zhao, S., et al. (1994). Lifetime and 12-month prevalence of DSM-III-R psychiatric disorders in the United States: Results from the National Comorbidity Survey. *Arch Gen Psychiatry*, 51:8–19.
4. Greenberg, P.E., Stiglin, L.E., Finkelstein, S.N., et al. (1993). The economic burden of depression. *J Clin Psychiatry*, 54(11):405–428.
5. McCombs, J.S., Nichol, M.B., Stimmel, G.L., et al. (1990). The cost of antidepressant drug therapy failure: A study of antidepressant use patterns in a medicaid population. *J Clin Psychiatry*, 51(Suppl 6):60–69.
6. Zis, A.P., Goodwin, F.K. (1979). Major affective disorder as a recurrent illness: A critical review. *Arch Gen Psychiatry*, 36:835–839.
7. Keller, M.B. (1994). Depression: A long-term illness. *Br J Psychiatry*, 165(Suppl 26):9–15.
8. Keller, M.B., Lavori, P., Mueller, T.I., et al. (1992). Time to recovery, chronicity, and levels of psychopathology in major depression: A five-year prospective follow up of 431 subjects. *Arch Gen Psychiatry*, 49:809–816.
9. Keller, M.B., Klerman, G.L., Lavori, P.W., et al. (1984). Long-term outcome of episodes of major depression: Clinical and public health significance. *JAMA*, 252:788–792.
10. Keller, M.B., Shapiro, R.W., Lavori, W., et al. (1982). Relapse in major depressive disorder: Analysis with life table. *Arch Gen Psychiatry*, 39:911–915.
11. Keller, M.B., Lavori, P.W., Lewis, C.E., et al. (1983). Predictors of relapse in major depressive disorder. *JAMA*, 250:3299–3304.
12. Keller, M.B., Lavori, W., Rice, J., et al. (1986). The persistent risk of chronicity in recurrent episodes of nonbipolar major depressive disorder: A prospective follow-up. *Am J Psychiatry*, 143:24–28.
13. Angst, J. (1988). Clinical course of affective disorders. In Helgson, T., Daly, R.J. (Eds.), *Depressive Illness: Prediction of Course and Outcome* (pp. 1–44). Berlin: Springer.
14. Coryell, W., Endicott, J., Keller, M. (1990). Outcome of patients with chronic affective disorder: A five-year follow-up. *Am J Psychiatry*, 147:1627–1633.
15. Angst, J. (1985). Verlauf und Ausgang affektiver und schizo-affectiver Erkrankungen. 2. Weitbrecht-Symposium, Bonn.
16. Wells, K.B., Stewart, A., Hays, R.D., et al. (1989). The functioning and well-being of depressed patients: Results from the medical outcome study. *JAMA*, 262:914–919.
17. Wells, K.B., Burnam, M.A. (1991). Caring for depression in America: Lessons learned from early findings of the medical outcomes study. *Psychiatric Med*, 9:503–519.
18. Guze, S.B., Robins, E. (1970). Suicide and primary affective disorder. *Br J Psychiatry*, 117:437–438.
19. Black, D.W., Winokur, G., Nasrallah, A. (1987). Suicide in subtypes of major affective disorder: A comparison with general population suicide mortality. *Arch Gen Psychiatry*, 44:878–880.
20. National Center for Health Statistics: Vital Statistics of the United States, 1988, Vol. II, Mortality, Part A. (1991). Washington, DC: U.S. Public Health Service.
21. Parkin, D. Stengel, E. (1965). Incidence of suicidal attempts in an urban community. *Br Med J*, 2:133–138.

22. Miller, N.S., Mahler, J.C., Gold, M.S. (1991). Suicide risk associated with drug and alcohol dependence. *J Addictive Diseases*, 10:49–61.
23. Fawcett, J., Scheffner, W. Clark, D., et al. (1987). Clinical predictors of suicide in patients with major affective disorders: A controlled prospective study. *Am J Psychiatry*, 144:35–40.
24. Beck, A.T., Brown, G., Berchick, R.J., et al. (1990). Relationship between hopelessness and ultimate suicide: A replication with psychiatric outpatients. *Am J Psychiatry*, 147:190–195.
25. Kreitman, N. (1988). Suicide, age, and marital status. *Psychological Med*, 18:121–128.
26. Conwell, Y, Rotenberg, M., Caine, E.D. (1990). Completed suicide at age fifty and over. *J Am Geriatrics Society*, 38:640–644.
27. Conwell, Y. (1995). Suicide among elderly persons. *Psychiatric Services*, 46:563–564.
28. Isometsä, E.T., Heikkinen, M.E., Martunen, M.J., et al. (1995). The last appointment before suicide: Is suicide intent communicated? *Am J Psychiatry*, 152:919–922.
29. Katon, W., Schulberg, H. (1992a). Epidemiology of depression in primary care. *Gen Hosp Psychiatry*, 14:237–247.
30. Nielsen, A.C., III, Williams, T.A. (1980). Depression in ambulatory medical patients. *Arch Gen Psychiatry*, 37:999–1004.
31. Hohman, A.A., et al. (1991). Psychotropic medication prescription in ambulatory care DICP. *Ann Pharmacother*, 25:85–89.
32. Katon, W., et al. (1992b). Adequacy and duration of antidepressant treatment in primary care. *Med Care*, 30:67–76.
33. Spitzer, R.L. (1994). Utility of a new procedure for diagnosing mental disorders in primary care: The PRIME-MD 1000 study. *JAMA*, 272:1749–1756.
34. Beck, A., Ward, C., Mendelson, H., et al. (1961). An inventory for measuring depression. *Arch Gen Psychiatry*, 4:561–571.
35. Zung, W.W.W. (1965). A self-rating depression scale. *Arch Gen Psychiatry*, 12:63.
36. Derogatis, L.R., Lipman, R.S., Rickels, K. (1973). The Hopkins symptom checklist (HSCL): A measure of primary symptom dimensions in psychological measurement. In Pichot, P. (Ed.), *Modern Problems in Pharmacopsychiatry*. Basel: Karger.
37. Rush, A.J., Giles, D.E., Schlesser, M.A., et al. (1985). The inventory for depressive symptomology (IDS): Preliminary findings. *Psychiatry Res*, 18:65–87.
38. Radloff, L.S., (1977). The CES-D scales: A self-report depression scale for research in the general population. *Appl Psychol Meas*, 1:385–401.
39. American Psychiatric Association. (1994). *Diagnostic and Statistical Manual of Mental Disorders* (4th ed.). Washington, DC: American Psychiatric Press.
40. Maier, W., Lichterman, D. (1993). The genetic epidemiology of unipolar depression and panic disorder. *Int Clin Psychopharm*, 8(Suppl 1):27–33.
41. *Practice Guideline for Major Depressive Disorder in Adults*. (1993). Washington, DC: American Psychiatric Press.
42. Janicak, P.G., Davis, J.M., Preskorn, S.H., et al. (1993). *Principles and Practice of Psychopharmacotherapy*. Baltimore: Williams & Wilkins.
43. Montgomery, S.A. (1995). Rapid onset of action of venlafaxine. *Int Clin Psychopharm*, 10(Suppl 2):21–27.
44. Rudolph, R., Entsuah, R., Derivan, A. (1991). Early clinical response in depression to venlafaxine hydrochloride. *Biol Psychiatry*, 29(115):630S.
45. Rickels, D. (1991). Venlafaxine: A new potent antidepressant agent with punative fast onset of action. *Biol Psychiatry*, 1:345–346.
46. Stein, G., Bernadt, M. (1993). Lithium augmentation therapy in tricyclic-resistant depression: A controlled trial using lithium in low and normal doses. *Br J Psychiatry*, 162:634–640.

47. Joffe, R.T., Levitt, A.J., Bagby, R.M., et al. (1993). Predictors of response to lithium and triiodothyronine augmentation of antidepressants in tricyclic non-responders. *Br J Psychiatry*, 163:574–578.
48. Howland, R.H. (1993). Thyroid dysfunction in refractory depression: Implications for pathophysiology and treatment. *J Clin Psychiatry*, 54(2):47–54.
49. Joffe, R.T., Singer, W. (1992). Thyroid hormone use to enhance the effects of drugs. *Clin Neuropharm*, 15(Suppl 1):389A–390A.
50. Nakamura, T., Nomura, J. (1992). Comparison of thyroid function between responders and nonresponders to thyroid hormone supplementation in depression. *Jap J Psychiatry Neurol*, 46:905–909.
51. Wallace, A.E., Kofoed, L.L., West, A.N. (1995). Double-blind, placebo-controlled trial of methylphenidate in older depressed, medically ill patients. *Am J Psychiatry*, 152:929–931.
52. Rosenthal, N.E. (1993). Diagnosis and treatment of seasonal affective disorder. *JAMA*, 270:2717–2720.
53. Thase, M.E. (1990). Relapse and recurrence in unipolar major depression: Short-term and long-term approaches. *J Clin Psychiatry*, 51(Suppl 6):51–57.
54. Solomon, D.A., Bauer, M.S. (1993). Continuation and maintenance pharmacotherapy for unipolar and bipolar mood disorders. *Psych Clin N Amer*, 16:515–540.
55. Kasper, S. (1993). The rationale for long-term antidepressant therapy. Special issue: Affective disorders: Current and future perspectives. *Int Clin Psychopharm*, 8:225–235.
56. Hirschfeld, R.M.A., Schatzberg, A.F. (1994). Long-term management of depression. *Am J Med*, 97(Suppl 6A):33–38.
57. Montgomery, S.A. (1994). Long-term treatment of depression. *Br J Psychiatry*, 164(Suppl 26):31–36.
58. Hirschfeld, R.M.A. (1994). Guidelines for the long-term treatment of depression. *J Clin Psychiatry*, 55(Suppl 12):59–67.
59. Kupfer, D.J. (1991). Long-term treatment of depression. *J Clin Psychiatry*, 52(Suppl 5):28–34.
60. Kupfer, D.J., Frank, E. (1992). The minimal length of treatment for recovery. In Montgomery, S.A., Rovillan, F. (Eds.), *Long-Term Treatment of Depression* (pp. 33–52). Chichester, England: John Wiley & Sons, Ltd.
61. Tollefson, G.D. (1993). Adverse drug reactions/interactions in maintenance therapy. *J Clin Psychiatry*, Suppl 54:48–58.
62. Montgomery, S.A., Montgomery, D.B. (1992). Prophylactic treatment in recurrent unipolar depression. In Montgomery, S.A., Rovillan, F. (Eds.), *Long-Term Treatment of Depression* (pp. 53–79). Chichester, England: John Wiley & Sons. Ltd.
63. Consensus Development Panel (1985). NIMH/NIH Consensus Development Conference Statement: Mood disorders, pharmacologic prevention of recurrences. *Am J Psychiatry*, 142:469–476.
64. Frank, E., Kupfer, D.J., Perel, J.M., et al. (1993). Comparison of full-dose versus half-dose pharmacotherapy in the maintenance treatment of recurrent depression. *J Affective Disorders*, 27:139–145.
65. Robinson, D.S., Lerfald, S.C., Bennett, B., et al. (1991). Continuation and maintenance treatment of major depression with the monoamine oxidase inhibitor phenelzine: A double-blind placebo controlled discontinuation study. *Psychopharmacol Bull*, 27:31–39.
66. Frank, E., Kupfer, D.J., Perel, J.M., et al. (1990). Three-year outcomes for maintenance therapies in recurrent depression. *Arch Gen Psychiatry*, 47:1093–1099.
67. Kupfer, D.J., Frank, E., Perel, J.M., et al. (1992). Five-year outcome for maintenance therapies in recurrent depression. *Arch Gen Psychiatry*, 49:769–773.
68. Perel, J.M. (1988). Compliance during tricyclic antidepressant therapy: Pharmacokinetic and analytical issues. *Clin Chem*, 34:881–887.

69. Frank, E., Perel, J.M., Mallinger, A.G., et al. (1992). Relationship of pharmacologic compliance to long-term prophylaxis in recurrent depression. *Psychopharmacol Bull*, 28:231–235.
70. Frank E., Kupfer, D.J., Siegel, L. R. (1995). Alliance not compliance: A philosophy of outpatient care. *J Clin Psychiatry*, 56(Suppl 1):11–16.
71. Greden, J.F. (1993). Antidepressant maintenance medications: When to discontinue and how to stop. *J Clin Psychiatry*, 54(Suppl 8):39–45.
72. Dilsaver, S.C., Greden, J.F. (1984). Antidepressant withdrawal phenomena. *Biol Psychiatry*, 19:237–256.
73. Dilsaver, S.C. (1988). Monoamine oxidase inhibitor withdrawal phenomena: Symptoms and pathophysiology. *Acta Psychiatr Scand*, 78:1–7.
74. Mallya G., White, K., Gunderson, C. (1993). Is there a serotonergic withdrawal syndrome? *Biol Psychiatry*, 33:851–852.
75. Coppen, A., Ghose, K., Montgomery S., et al. (1978). Continuation therapy with amitriptyline in depression. *Br J Psychiatry*, 133:28–33.
76. Glen, A.I.M., Johnson, A.L., Shepherd, M. (1984). Continuation therapy with lithium and amitriptyline in unipolar depressive illness: A randomized double-blind controlled trial. *Psychol Med*, 14:37–50.
77. Rouillan, F., Serrurier, D., Miller, H.D., et al. (1991). Prophylactic efficacy of maprotiline in unipolar depression relapse. *J Clin Psychiatry*, 52:423–431.
78. Prien, R.F., Klett, C.J., Caffey, E.M. (1973). Lithium carbonate and imipramine in the prevention of affective episodes. *Arch Gen Psychiatry*, 29:420–425.
79. Kane, J.M., Quitkin, F.M., Rifkin, A., et al. (1982). Lithium carbonate and imipramine in the prophylaxis of unipolar and bipolar II illness. *Arch Gen Psychiatry*, 39:1065–1069.
80. Prien, R.F., Kupfer, D.J., Mansky, P.A., et al. (1984). Drug therapy in the prevention of recurrences in unipolar and bipolar affective disorders: Report of the NIMH Collaborative Study group comparing lithium carbonate-imipramine combination. *Arch Gen Psychiatry*, 41:1096–1104.
81. Glassman, A.H., Roose, S.P. (1987). Cardiovascular effects of tricyclic antidepressants. *Psychiatric Ann*, 17:340–347.
82. Boehnert, M.T., Lovejoy, F.H., Jr. (1985). Value of the QRS duration vs. the serum drug level in predicting seizures and ventricular arrhythmias after an acute overdose of tricyclic antidepressants. *N Eng J Med*, 313:474–479.
83. Foulke, G.E., Albertson, T.E. (1987). QRS interval in tricyclic antidepressant overdose: Inaccuracy as a toxicity indicator in emergency setting. *Ann Emerg Med*, 16:160–163.
84. Reynolds, C.F., III, Frank, E., Perel, J.M., et al. (1992). Comorbid pharmacotherapy and psychotherapy in the acute and continuation treatment of elderly patients with recurrent major depression: A preliminary report. *Am J Psychiatry*, 1992:148:1687–1692.
85. Wehr, T.A., Goodwin, F.K. (1987). Can antidepressants cause mania and worsen the course of affective illness? *Am J Psychiatry*, 144:201–204.
86. Altshuler, L.L., Post, R.M., Leverich, G.S., et al. Antidepressant-induced mania and cycle acceleration: A controversy revisited. *Am J Psychiatry*, 152:1130–1138.
87. Montgomery, S.A., Dufour, H., Brian, S., et al. (1988). The prophylactic efficacy of fluoxetine in unipolar depression. *Br J Psychiatry*, 153(Suppl 3):69–76.
88. Doogan, D.P., Caillard, V. (1992). Sertraline in the prevention of depression. *Br J Psychiatry*, 160:217–222.
89. Montgomery, S.A., Dunbar, G. (1993). Paroxetine is better than placebo in relapse prevention and the prophylaxis of recurrent depression. *Int Clin Psychopharm*, 8:189–195.
90. Nemeroff, C.B., DeVane, C.L., Pollock, B.G. (1996). Newer antidepressants and the cytochrome P450 system. *Am J Psychiatry*, 153:311–320.
91. Gitlin, M.J. (1994). Psychotropic medications and their effects on sexual function: Diagnosis, biology, and treatment approaches. *J Clin Psychiatry*, 55:406–413.

92. Rothschild, A.J. (1995). Selective serotonin reuptake inhibitor-induced sexual dysfunction: Efficacy of a drug holiday. *Am J Psychiatry*, 152:1514–1516.
93. Teicher, M., Glod C., Cole, J. (1990). Emergence of intense suicidal preoccupation during fluoxetine treatment. *Am J Psychiatry*, 147:207–210.
94. Wirshing, W., VanPutten, T., Rosenberg, J., et al. (1992). Fluoxetine, akathisia and suicidality: Is there a causal connection? *Arch Gen Psychiatry*, 49:580–581.
95. Beasley, C.M., Dornseif, B.E., Poltz, J.A., et al. (1991). Fluoxetine versus trazodone: Efficacy and activating-sedating effects. *J Clin Psychiatry*, 52:294–299.
96. Mann, J., Kapur, S. (1991). The emergence of suicidal ideation and behavior during antidepressant pharmacotherapy. *Arch Gen Psychiatry*, 48:1027–1033.
97. Fava, M., Rosenbaum, J. (1991). Suicidality and fluoxetine: Is there a relationship? *J Clin Psychiatry*, 52:108–111.
98. Sternbach, H. (1991). The serotonin syndrome. *Am J Psychiatry*, 148(6):705–713.
99. Georgotas, A., McCue, R.E., Coopen, T.B. (1989). A placebo-controlled comparison of nortriptyline and phenelzine in maintenance therapy of elderly depressed patients. *Arch Gen Psychiatry*, 46:783–786.
100. Robinson, D.S., Lerfald, S.C., Bennett, B., et al. (1991). Continuation and maintenance treatment of major depression with the monoamine oxidase inhibitor phenelzine: A double-blind placebo controlled discontinuation study. *Psychopharmacol Bull*, 27:31–39.
101. Linden, C.H., Rumack, B.H., Strehlke, C. (1984). Monoamine oxidase inhibitor overdose. *Ann Emerg Med*, 13:1137–1144.
102. Kaplan, R.F., Feinglass, N.G., Webster, W., et al. (1986). Phenelzine overdose treated with dantrolene sodium. *JAMA*, 255:642–644.
103. Dilsaver, S.C. (1988). Monoamine oxidase inhibitor withdrawal phenonema: Symptoms and pathophysiology. *Acta Psychiatr Scand*, 78:1–7.
104. Bergeron, R., Blier, P. (1994). Cisapride for the treatment of nausea produced by selective serotonin reuptake inhibitors. *Am J Psychiatry*, 151:1084–1086.
105. Spiker, D.G., Weiss, J.C., Dealy, R.S., et al. (1985). The pharmacological treatment of delusional depression. *Am J Psychiatry*, 142:430–436.
106. Wolfersdorf, M., Barg, T., Konig, F., et al. (1995). Paroxetine as antidepressant in combined antidepressant-neuroleptic therapy in delusional depression: Observation of clinical use. *Pharmacopsychiatry*, 28:56–60.
107. Siris, S.G., Morgan, V., Fagerstrom, R., et al. (1987). Adjunctive imipramine in the treatment of postpsychotic depression: A controlled trial. *Arch Gen Psychiatry*, 44:533–539.
108. Prusoff, B.A., Williams, D.H., Weisman, M.M., et al. (1979). Treatment of secondary depression in schizophrenia. *Arch Gen Psychiatry*, 36:569–575.
109. Singh, A.N., Saxena, B., Nelson, H.L. (1978). A controlled clinical study of trazodone in chronic schizophrenic patients with pronounced depressive symptomatology. *Curr Ther Res*, 23:485–501.
110. Stone, A. B., Pearlstein, T. B., Brown, W. A. (1991). Fluoxetine in the treatment of late luteal phase dysphoric disorder. *J Clin Psychiatry*, 52:290–293.
111. Wood, S.H., Mortola, J.F., Chan, Y., et al. (1992). Treatment of premenstrual syndrome with fluoxetine: A double-blind, placebo controlled, crossover study. *Obstet Gynecol*, 80:339–344.
112. Menkes, D.B., Taghavi, F., Mason, P.A., et al. (1992). Fluoxetine treatment of severe premenstrual syndrome. *Br Med J*, 305:346–347.
113. Menkes, D.B., Taghavi, F., Mason, P.A., et al. (1993). Fluoxetine's spectrum of action in premenstrual syndrome. *Int Clin Psychopharm*, 8:95–102.
114. Sundblad, C., Modigh, K., Andersch, B., et al. (1992). Clomipramine effectively reduces premenstrual irritability and dysphoria: A placebo-controlled trial. *Acta Psychiatr Scand*, 85:39–47.
115. Sundblad, C., Hedberg, M.A., Eriksson, E. (1993). Clomipramine administered during the

luteal phase reduces the symptoms of premenstrual syndrome: A placebo-controlled trial. *Neruopsychopharm*, 9:133–145.

116. Brzezinski, A.A., Wurtman, J.J., Wurtman, R.J., et al. (1990). d-Fenfluramine suppresses the increased calorie and carbohydrate intakes and improves the mood of women with premenstrual depression. *Obstet and Gynecol*, 76:296–301.

117. Parry, B.L., Mahan, A.M., Mostofi, N., et al. (1993). Light therapy of late luteal phase dysphoric disorder: An extended study. *Am J Psychiatry*, 150:1417–1419.

118. Pearlstein, T.B., Stone, A.B. (1994). Long-term fluoxetine treatment of late luteal phase dysphoric disorder. *J Clin Psychiatry*, 55:332–335.

119. Howland, R.A. (1991). Pharmacotherapy of dysthymia: A review. *J Clin Psychopharm*, 11:83–92.

120. Shea, M.T., Widiger, T.A., Klein, M.H. (1992). Comorbidity of personality disorders and depression: Implications for treatment. *J Consulting Clin Psychol*, 60:857–868.

121. Parsons, B., Quitkin, F.M., McGrath, P.J., et al. (1989). Phenelzine, imipramine, and placebo in borderline patients meeting criteria for atypical depression. *Psychopharm Bull*, 25:524–534.

122. Soloff, P.H., George, A., Nathan, R.S., et al. (1989). Amitriptyline versus haloperidol in borderlines: Final outcomes and predictors of response. *J Clin Psychopharm*, 9:238–246.

123. Cowdry, R.W., Gardner, D.L. (1988). Pharmacotherapy of borderline personality disorder: Alprazolam, carbamazepine, trifluroperazine and tranylcypromine. *Arch Gen Psychiatry*, 45:802–803.

124. Goldberg, S.C., Schulz, S.C., Schulz, P.M., et al. (1986). Borderline and schizotypical personality disorders treated with low-dose thiothixene versus placebo. *Arch Gen Psychiatry*, 43:680–686.

125. Coccaro, E.F., Astill, J.L., Herbert, J.L., et al. (1990). Fluoxetine treatment of impulsive aggression in DSM-III-R personality disorder patients. *J Clin Psychopharm*, 10:373–375.

126. Cornelius, J.R., Soloff, P.H., Perel, J.M., et al. (1990). Fluoxetine trial in borderline personality disorder. *Psychopharm Bull*, 26:151–154.

127. Norden, M.J. (1989). Fluoxetine in borderline personality disorder. *Prog Neuro-Psychopharm Biol Psychiatry*, 13:885–893.

128. Rosenberg, D., Holttum, J., Gershon, S. (1994). *Textbook of Pharmacotherapy for Child and Adolescent Psychiatric Disorders*. New York: Brunner/Mazel, Inc.

129. Ryan, N.D., Varma, D. (1998). *Biol Psychiatry*, 44:336–340.

130. Cohen, L.S., Heller, V.L., Rosenbaum, J.F. (1989). Treatment guidelines for psychotropic drug use in pregnancy. *Psychosomatics*, 30(1):25–33.

131. Miller, L. (1991). Clinical strategies for the use of psychotropic drugs during pregnancy. *Psychiatric Med*, 9:275–298.

132. Goldberg, H.L., Nissim, R. (1994). Psychotropic drugs in pregnancy and lactation. *Int J Psychiatry in Med*, 24:129–149.

133. Wisner, K.L., Perel, J.M. (1988). Psychopharmacologic agents and electroconvulsive therapy during pregnancy and the puerperium. In Cohen, R.L. (Ed.), *Psychiatric Consultation in Childbirth Settings: Parent- and Child-Oriented Approaches*. New York: Plenum Medical Book Company.

134. Reynolds, C.F. (1994). Treatment of depression in late life. *Am J Med*, 97(Suppl 6A):39–46.

135. NIH Consensus Conference. (1992). Diagnosis and treatment of depression in late life. *JAMA*, 268:1018–1024.

136. Reynolds, C.F., III, Frank, E., Perel, J.M., et al. (1992). Combined pharmacotherapy and psychotherapy in the acute and continuation treatment of elderly patients with recurrent major depression: A preliminary report. *Am J Psychiatry*, 149:1687–1692.

137. Frymoyer, J.W. (1994). *Orthopedic Knowledge Update Psychiatry*. Rosemont, IL: American Academy of Orthopedieons, 527.

BIPOLAR ILLNESS

MANIC-DEPRESSIVE DISORDER

Bipolar illness is an illness characterized by affective instability resulting in periods of major depression or mania. The *Diagnostic and Statistical Manual of Mental Disorders*, fourth edition, (DSM-IV) criteria for major depression, mania, hypomania, and mixed episode are presented in Tables 5–1 through 5–4.

SUBTYPES

The DSM-IV divides bipolar illness into bipolar I, bipolar II, rapid cycling, and mixed episode. To diagnose bipolar I disorder, a patient must have experienced at least one manic episode. The diagnosis of bipolar II disorder requires the presence of a hypomanic episode that is characterized by the same features of a manic episode but of lesser severity. In addition to subsequent manic episodes, a bipolar patient may experience depressive or mixed episodes and possibly interepisode disturbances of mood, including irritability and lability. *Irritability* is defined as being quick to anger; *lability* is defined as rapid fluctuations between mood states (angry, sad, happy, etc.) not due to external stimuli.

145

TABLE 5-1. CRITERIA FOR MAJOR DEPRESSIVE EPISODE

A. Five (or more) of the following symptoms have been present during the same two-week period and represent a change from previous functioning; at least one of the symptoms is either depressed mood or loss of interest or pleasure.

Note: Do not include symptoms that are clearly due to a general medical condition or mood-incongruent delusions or hallucinations.

(1) depressed mood most of the day, nearly every day, as indicated by either subjective report (e.g., feels sad or empty) or observation made by others (e.g., appears tearful). Note: In children and adolescents, can be irritable mood

(2) markedly diminished interest or pleasure in all, or almost all, activities most of the day (as indicated by either subjective account or observation made by others)

(3) significant weight loss when not dieting or weight gain (e.g., a change of more than 5% of body weight in a month) or decrease or increase in appetite nearly every day. Note: In children, consider failure to make expected weight gains.

(4) insomnia or hypersomnia nearly every day

(5) psychomotor agitation or retardation nearly every day (observable by others, not merely subjective feelings of restlessness or being slowed down)

(6) fatigue or loss of energy nearly every day

(7) feelings of worthlessness or excessive or inappropriate guilt (that may be delusional) nearly every day (not merely self-reproach or guilt about being sick)

(8) diminished ability to think or concentrate, or indecisiveness, nearly every day (either by subjective account or as observed by others)

(9) recurrent thoughts of death (not just fear of dying), recurrent suicidal ideation without a specific plan, or a suicide attempt or a specific plan for committing suicide

B. The symptoms do not meet criteria for a mixed episode.

C. The symptoms cause clinically significant distress or impairment in social, occupational, or other important areas of functioning.

D. The symptoms are not due to the direct physiological effects of a substance (e.g., a drug of abuse, a medication) or a general medical condition (e.g., hypothyroidism).

E. The symptoms are not better accounted for by bereavement, i.e., after the loss of a loved one, the symptoms persist for longer than two months or are characterized by marked functional impairment, morbid preoccupation with worthlessness, suicidal ideation, psychotic symptoms, or psychomotor retardation.

Adapted with permission from the *Diagnostic and Statistical Manual of Mental Disorders*, 4th ed. (p. 329). Copyright 1994 by American Psychiatric Association.

In rapid cycling bipolar illness, a patient cycles between periods of depression and mania with three or more such "cycles" per year. These patients may lack the period of interepisode "euthymic" mood that characterizes nonrapid cyclers. As rapid cycling is more common in patients who have suffered with bipolar illness for many years, it may represent a progression of the underlying pathologic process.

TABLE 5–2. CRITERIA FOR MANIC EPISODE

A. A distinct period of abnormally and persistently elevated, expansive, or irritable mood, lasting at least one week (or any duration if hospitalization is necessary).

B. During the period of mood disturbance, three (or more) of the following symptoms have persisted (four if the mood is only irritable) and have been present to a significant degree:

   (1) inflated self-esteem or grandiosity
   (2) decreased need for sleep (e.g., feels rested after only three hours of sleep)
   (3) more talkative than usual or pressure to keep talking
   (4) flight of ideas or subjective experience that thoughts are racing
   (5) distractibility (i.e., attention too easily drawn to unimportant or irrelevant external stimuli)
   (6) increase in goal-directed activity (either socially, at work or school, or sexually) or psychomotor agitation
   (7) excessive involvement in pleasurable activities that have a high potential for painful consequences (e.g., engaging in unrestrained buying sprees, sexual indiscretions, or foolish business investments)

C. The symptoms do not meet criteria for a mixed episode.

D. The mood disturbance is sufficiently severe to cause marked impairment in occupational functioning or in usual social activities or relationships with others, or to necessitate hospitalization to prevent harm to self or others, or there are psychotic features.

E. The symptoms are not due to the direct physiological effects of a substance (e.g., a drug of abuse, a medication, or other treatment) or a general medical condition (e.g., hyperthyroidism).

Note: Maniclike episodes that are clearly caused by somatic antidepressant treatment (e.g., medication, electroconvulsive therapy, light therapy) should not count toward a diagnosis of bipolar I disorder.

Adapted with permission from the *Diagnostic and Statistical Manual of Mental Disorders*, 4th ed. (p. 332). Copyright 1994 by American Psychiatric Association.

The last subtype of bipolar illness is mixed episode in which a patient has a constellation of symptoms that fulfill criteria for both a manic and a depressive episode simultaneously.

Bipolar I illness affects approximately 1% of the population while bipolar II illness affects 0.5% of the population, making these disorders less common than unipolar depression. Rapid cycling patients comprise between 15–20% of all bipolar patients.[1]

The median age of onset of bipolar disorder is between 19 and 21 years.[2,1] While bipolar I illness affects males and females equally, bipolar II illness affects females predominantly. Females are more likely to initially present with a depressive episode, while males are more likely to present with an initial manic episode.

TABLE 5–3. CRITERIA FOR HYPOMANIC EPISODE

A. A distinct period of persistently elevated, expansive, or irritable mood, lasting throughout at least 14 days, that is clearly different from the usual nondepressed mood.

B. During the period of mood disturbance, three (or more) of the following symptoms have persisted (four if the mood is only irritable) and have been present to a significant degree:

   (1) inflated self-esteem or grandiosity
   (2) decreased need for sleep (e.g., feels rested after only three hours of sleep)
   (3) more talkative than usual or pressure to keep talking
   (4) flight of ideas or subjective experience that thoughts are racing
   (5) distractibility (i.e., attention too easily drawn to unimportant or irrelevant external stimuli)
   (6) increase in goal-directed activity (either socially, at work or school, or sexually) or psychomotor agitation
   (7) excessive involvement in pleasurable activities that have a high potential for painful consequences (e.g., engaging in unrestrained buying sprees, sexual indiscretions, or foolish business investments)

C. The episode is associated with an unequivocal change in functioning that is uncharacteristic of the person when not symptomatic.

D. The disturbance in mood and the change in functioning are observable by others.

E. The episode is not severe enough to cause marked impairment in social or occupational functioning or to necessitate hospitalization, and there are no psychotic features.

F. The symptoms are not due to the direct physiological effects of a substance (e.g., a drug of abuse, a medication, or other treatment) or a general medical condition (e.g., hyperthyroidism).

Note: Hypomaniclike episodes that are clearly caused by somatic antidepressant treatment (e.g., medication, electroconvulsive therapy, light therapy) should not count toward a diagnosis of bipolar II disorder.

Adapted with permission from the *Diagnostic and Statistical Manual of Mental Disorders*, 4th ed. (p. 238). Copyright 1994 by American Psychiatric Association.

DIFFERENTIAL DIAGNOSIS

When a patient presents with a first episode of mania, before being given the diagnosis of bipolar disorder, organic etiologies that can present as mania should be ruled out. A list of these is given in Table 5–5.

Organic mania, also known as secondary mania, may occur in patients at any age with no previous history of bipolar or other affective illness. The major etiologies responsible for secondary mania include drug-induced, metabolic, and infectious. Treatment in secondary mania is directed at

TABLE 5–4. CRITERIA FOR MIXED EPISODE

A. The criteria are met both for a manic episode and for a major depressive episode nearly every day during at least a one-week period.

B. The mood disturbance is sufficiently severe to cause marked impairment in occupational functioning or in usual social activities or relationships with others or to necessitate hospitalization to prevent harm to self or others, or there are psychotic features.

C. The symptoms are not due to the direct physiological effects of a substance (e.g., a drug of abuse, a medication, or other treatment) or a general medical condition (e.g., hyperthyroidism).

Note: Mixedlike episodes that are clearly caused by somatic antidepressant treatment (e.g., medication, electroconvulsive therapy, light therapy) should not count toward a diagnosis of bipolar I disorder.

Adapted with permission from the *Diagnostic and Statistical Manual of Mental Disorders*, 4th ed. (p. 335). Copyright 1994 by American Psychiatric Association.

removal of the causative agent or treatment in the underlying abnormality. An organic mania is especially likely in patients who present with a first episode of mania after age 60.

NATURAL COURSE

The natural course of bipolar illness is that of a *lifelong illness with multiple, recurrent episodes of depression and/or mania*. Zis and Goodwin reviewed nine longitudinal studies of affective illness, from Kraepelin in 1921 through Angst and Grof in 1976, to determine the rate of relapse in both unipolar and bipolar affective disorders.[3] Bipolar patients have more than one episode of depression and/or mania and have a larger number of recurrent episodes than their unipolar counterparts. It is interesting to note that between 5 to 10 years frequently elapse between age of first onset of symptoms and age of first treatment, including hospitalization.

Bipolar patients recover to varying degrees from an acute episode as illustrated by Carlson et al., who followed 53 patients with a 14.7-year mean duration of bipolar illness and found that patients had a median of greater than five episodes.[4] Their report is unique in that their center was an initial referral site for patients seeking treatment with lithium and thus may reflect the natural course of the untreated illness. They concluded that the prognosis of bipolar illness varies from acute exacerbations with complete recovery to a slow, insidious course. A "pure" bipolar I patient, by definition, recovers completely from a single episode of illness to a pre-illness level of functioning. Atypical forms also exist in which patients do not recover completely or present with intra- or interepisode symptoms that may be

TABLE 5–5. REPORTED CAUSES OF SECONDARY MANIA

Drugs	Corticosteroids, isoniazid, procarbazine hydrochloride, lysergic acid diethylamide (LSD), sympathomimetics, levodopa, cyproheptadine hydrochloride, thyroxine, l-glutamine, tolmetin, alprazolam, metrizamide, propafenone, captopril, yohimbine, procainamide, alcohol intoxication
Drug withdrawal	Clonidine hydrochloride
Metabolic	Hemodialysis, postoperative state, hyperthyroidism, vitamin B_{12} deficiency, Cushing's syndrome
Infection	Influenza Q fever, post-St. Louis type A encephalitis, cryptococcoses, HIV, neurosyphilis
Neoplasm	Meningiomas, gliomas, thalamic metastases
Epilepsy	Complex partial seizures with right temporal focus
Surgery	Right hemispherectomy
Cerebrovascular accident	Thalamic stroke
Other	Cerebellar atrophy, head trauma, multiple sclerosis, Wilson's disease

From Cassem, N.H. (1991). *Massachusetts General Hospital Handbook of General Hospital Psychiatry*, 3rd ed. St. Louis: Mosby. Reprinted with permission.

labeled as "schizoaffective." For purposes of this discussion, these patients are considered atypical bipolar patients.

Keller et al. followed 173 bipolar patients for five years to determine the predictive value of each patient's index episode (depression, mania, or mixed/cycling).[5] The rate of recovery from the index episode was greatest for the manic patients, intermediate for the depressed patients, and slowest for the mixed/cycling patients (i.e., patients with atypical forms of bipolar illness). Examining the patients five years after the index episode, the authors found that the mixed/cycling patients were the least likely to recover fully from their index episode and had a shorter time to relapse compared with the manic patients. With regard to recurrences of bipolar illness, again the patients with mixed/cycling index episode were the most likely to relapse. In summary, mixed/cycling (i.e., atypical) bipolar patients have the worst course and prognosis overall.

Tohen et al. followed 24 first-episode manic patients in treatment for four years after recovery from their first episode.[6] After six months, 20% of patients suffered a depressive episode. When they included these first-episode patients with a previously studied cohort of 51 multiple-episode patients, they found a relapse rate of 30% at six months.[7]

COST OF BIPOLAR ILLNESS

Bipolar illness extracts a tremendous cost, both monetary and emotional, from patients, their families, and society. Affective disorders overall, including bipolar disorder, cost $20.8 billion in 1985 and $30.4 billion in 1990.[8] With the advent of lithium as a treatment for bipolar disorder, the overall cost of treatment of a bipolar patient has decreased by approximately one-half.[9] Reifman and Wyatt estimated that over 10 years of lithium use has saved approximately $4 billion.[10]

Coryell et al. reported on the psychosocial functioning of patients they had followed with bipolar and unipolar illness for five years.[11] While bipolar patients appeared to have attained a slightly higher level of education than their unipolar counterparts and a slightly higher level of income, income level and percent employment for bipolar patients had dropped at the end of five years, although *not* as much as for unipolar patients. Only one-half of bipolar patients had married at the end of five years, compared with normal control subjects, although those who did marry reported a level of satisfaction similar to that of normals. In other words, one-half of the bipolar patients studied continued to exhibit lower psychosocial functioning five years after their index episode of depression or mania.

Patients with bipolar disorder are at high risk for suicide. In a series of patient cohorts followed for 30 years, 1 in 10 bipolar patients committed suicide[12,13] and one-fourth of patients attempted suicide during the course of their illness.[14] Mueller-Oerlinghausen et al. reviewed the mortality data for over 800 bipolar patients and found that the mortality rate was two to three times that of the general population and the majority of these patients were treated at some point in their illness with lithium.[15] Other authors have reported a suicide rate five times in excess of the general population.[16] In comparison to unipolar disorder, bipolar patients are 7.5 times more likely to commit suicide.[13] Lithium has been shown to decrease the mortality rate of bipolar patients in several reports.[17,18,19] A 1995 NIMH report on bipolar disorder stated that lithium treatment extends the life expectancy of bipolar patients by an average of seven years.

An additional cost to society is that of a decreased level of psychosocial functioning in bipolar patients, both intra- and interepisode. Harrow et al. in a naturalistic follow-up study concluded that bipolar patients have a greater degree of impairment than unipolar patients.[20] In their study, 40% of bipolar patients had chronic impairments in work and social functioning. In contrast, 60% of the unipolar patients had only minimal psychosocial impairments. A review of the data from those patients with poor psychosocial outcomes revealed a high incidence of persisting psychotic or affective symptomatology. Again, most of these patients appeared to suffer from atypical forms (i.e., mixed/cycling) of bipolar illness that may have directly contributed to their poorer psychosocial outcome. Coryell et al. noted that at the end of a five-year follow-up period, bipolar patients had diminished levels of income and significant deficits in all areas of psychosocial function, even those patients who had been in remission for the previous two of the five years.[11]

ACUTE AND CONTINUATION PHARMACOLOGICAL TREATMENT OF MANIA

Before proceeding to our discussion of the maintenance pharmacotherapies for bipolar disorder, it is helpful to consider briefly the pharmacological management of acute mania. Side effects of the various agents, dosages used, the role of monitoring, clinically relevant drug-drug interactions, and methods of drug discontinuation are discussed in the section on maintenance pharmacotherapies. Chemical structures, chemical names, and cost of the preparations are given in the sections concerning maintenance therapy.

LITHIUM

Lithium monotherapy is an effective treatment for acute manic symptoms in approximately 60–80% of cases. The major drawback of lithium monotherapy for an acute manic episode is the 9- to 14-day delay of onset of action before major symptom response. The serum level of lithium necessary for antimanic response is 0.8–1.2 mEq/L.

ANTIPSYCHOTICS

Antipsychotics are effective agents in the treatment of acute mania and their use predates that of lithium. The advantage of antipsychotics is their apparent more rapid onset of action compared with lithium. Prien et al. compared lithium alone with chlorpromazine alone for the treatment of acute mania and found that chlorpromazine was superior in treating the highly active or psychotic patient, but that both drugs were equally effective in treating mildly active patients.[21] The authors also reported that the patients who received antipsychotics reported feeling more sluggish and fatigued than those who received lithium. Shopsin et al. compared lithium with chlorpromazine in the treatment of acute schizophrenic patients and found that chlorpromazine was clearly more effective in treating both thought disorder symptoms and aberrant behaviors.[22] They also reported that lithium treatment may worsen psychotic symptoms (compared with chlorpromazine). A major disadvantage to antipsychotic use is the increased risk of extrapyramidal side effects, including tardive dyskinesia.

Clozapine may be an alternative for treatment-resistant mania in both typical and atypical bipolar illness. Calabrese et al. reported "marked improvement" over 13 weeks in 18 of 25 acutely manic patients (72%) who had previously failed or could not tolerate lithium, anticonvulsants, or neuroleptics. Clozapine therapy, however, should only be instituted by a psychiatrist familiar with its use.[23]

ANTIPSYCHOTICS AND LITHIUM

Given the more rapid onset of antimanic action of antipsychotics, their greater efficacy in calming the acutely agitated manic patient, and their availability in intramuscular preparations, they are usually the agent of first choice in treating an acute mania with associated behavioral disturbance. Lithium should be added to the treatment regimen as early as possible in the acute treatment phase with the intent of tapering the antipsychotic, because of the increased prevalence and persistence of tardive dyskinesia in bipolar patients.[24,25]

CARBAMAZEPINE

Carbamazepine is generally as effective in the treatment of acute mania as lithium, although superiority to lithium has not been demonstrated. Lerer et al. assigned 29 bipolar-manic patients to acute treatment with either lithium or carbamazepine for four weeks.[26] Lithium levels were maintained close to 1.0 mEq/L; carbamazepine levels were maintained in the range of 8–12 μg/ml. While both groups demonstrated improvement in manic symptoms, lithium treatment appeared to be superior but did not reach statistical significance. In patients who have failed acute lithium treatment, one may consider acute treatment with carbamazepine. As with lithium, carbamazepine is available only in an oral preparation.

VALPROATE

Two studies (Pope et al., 1990; Bowden et al., 1994) have demonstrated an efficacy of valproate equivalent to that of lithium in the treatment of acute mania.[27,28] Pope et al. administered valproate or placebo to 36 acutely manic patients who had failed a lithium trial or were unable to tolerate lithium side effects.[27] The valproate group noted "substantial antimanic effects" one to four days after beginning the trial. It was also noted that the valproate patients required less lorazepam than the placebo group for agitation. Bowden et al. reported similar results in their placebo-controlled study of valproate versus lithium.[28] In a later study Bowden et al. noted a favorable treatment response of valproate serum levels between 45 to 100–125 mg/ml in acutely manic patients.[29]

While there is no evidence currently that valproate is superior to lithium overall in treatment of bipolar disorder, a history of head injury and/or abnormal electroencephalogram (EEG) may predict a favorable response to valproate.[30]

In addition to valproate's more rapid onset of antimanic activity with standard dosing, an alternative "loading dose" strategy may promote even more rapid antimanic effects. Keck et al., noting that antimanic activity occurred within several days of reaching a serum concentration at or above 50 mg/L, devised a "loading strategy" to achieve therapeutic serum concentrations within 24 hours of the first valproate dose.[31] Patients were given divalproex sodium 20 mg/kg/day in divided doses for five days. In the Keck study of 19 patients, the loading strategy was well tolerated by the 15 of 19 patients who completed the study, and significant antimanic effects were noted after three days.

An intravenous preparation of valproate is available and may offer an alternative for the acute treatment of mania in hospital settings.

BENZODIAZEPINES

Limited data exist on the use of benzodiazepines, particularly clonazepam and lorazepam, in the treatment of acute mania. Chouinard et al. compared clonazepam with lithium in 11 patients in a double-blind, crossover study design of 10-day duration and reported that clonazepam at a mean dose of 10.4 mg/day was superior to lithium in treating motor overactivity and logorrhea.[32] Bradwejn et al. compared clonazepam with lorazepam in a two-week, double-blind study in 24 patients with acute mania and found lorazepam to be superior, producing a marked improvement in symptomatology.[33] Sixty-one percent of patients in the lorazepam group responded, compared with 18.3% in the clonazepam group. An additional advantage of lorazepam is the availability of an intramuscular preparation. The results of these two studies aside, clinical experience is lacking with regard to benzodiazepine treatment of acute mania. Rather, these agents appear to function as agents of chemical restraint. Currently in the treatment of acute mania, benzodiazepines are generally reserved for use as an adjunctive treatment for behavioral disturbance in the highly agitated manic patient. In this role, they may be a safer option than antipsychotics, yet equally effective.[34]

CALCIUM-CHANNEL BLOCKERS

The results of several studies suggest that calcium-channel blockers (i.e., diltiazem, isradipine, nicardipine, nifedipine, verapamil) may be effective as mood-stabilizers in the treatment of acute mania. Verapamil 160 mg/day has been shown to be superior to placebo in the treatment of acute mania in several double-blind, crossover studies and to have similar efficacy to lithium in doses of 320 mg/day.[35,36,37]

OTHER COMBINATION STRATEGIES

In patients who cannot tolerate or have failed lithium treatment in the past, either an anticonvulsant (carbamazepine or valproate) or a calcium-channel blocker may be used in conjunction with an antipsychotic in the treatment of an agitated, acutely manic patient. As with lithium, the agitated, acutely manic patient may be started on neuroleptic treatment and then have an anticonvulsant added to the regimen within several days.

ROLE OF ECT

Electroconvulsive therapy (ECT) has been clearly shown to be efficacious in the treatment of acute mania. Mukherjee et al. reviewed 50 years of data concerning the use of ECT in acute mania.[38] They found an overall response rate of 80%. The treatments themselves are considered to be as safe as lithium treatment, have an equal or greater degree of efficacy, and an equivalent time to antimanic response (i.e., two weeks). Electroconvulsive treatments for mania are administered three times per week for a maximum of 10 to 15 treatments and are, at least initially, given as bilateral treatments. ECT is generally reserved for patients who have failed pharmacological treatments and is therefore viewed as a second- or third-line therapy. A study of ECT in a group of 24 treatment-refractory patients demonstrated a 54% response rate.[39]

The predictors of response to acute treatment are similar to those for maintenance pharmacological treatment and are discussed in that section.

ACUTE AND CONTINUATION PHARMACOLOGICAL MANAGEMENT OF DEPRESSION

The overwhelming majority of the data available for acute treatment of depression concerns unipolar depression. For a review of this material, see Chapter 4 on the acute and continuation pharmacotherapy of major depression. The use of antidepressants for maintenance pharmacotherapy of bipolar disorder is reviewed later in this chapter.

MAINTENANCE PHARMACOLOGICAL TREATMENT IN BIPOLAR DISORDER

The goals of maintenance pharmacotherapy of bipolar disorder are to prevent recurrence, decrease mortality and morbidity, and slow progression of the disorder. The ongoing use of a mood-stabilizing agent in the maintenance treatment of bipolar disorder to prevent recurrence is commonly accepted. Lithium is the agent of first choice and the sole drug most commonly used for this purpose. Patients who fail lithium therapy or who cannot tolerate its side-effect profile, should next be given a trial of one of the anticonvulsants, carbamazepine or valproate. Failure of these three agents, alone and in two-drug combinations, may necessitate a trial of a less-studied therapy such as a calcium-channel blocker or clozapine.

The choice of a maintenance regimen may be predicated by the index episode (i.e., whether the initial episode was either a mania or a major depression). Shapiro et al. found an association between the index episode and responsiveness to choice of maintenance regimen. Patients who presented with a depressive episode were more successfully treated with a combination of lithium and imipramine than with either agent alone. Patients who presented with a manic episode responded equally well to lithium monotherapy or the lithium/imipramine combination therapy.[40]

DURATION OF TREATMENT

The necessary duration of maintenance pharmacotherapy for bipolar illness is currently believed to be lifelong. Discontinuation of maintenance lithium therapy carries with it a significant risk of relapse, but the degree of risk may be modified by gradual discontinuation versus sudden discontinuation. Faedda et al. followed 64 clinically stable bipolar patients who were having their lithium discontinued on clinical grounds.[41] The patients were tapered off lithium either rapidly (less than two weeks) or gradually (over two to four weeks) and the cohort was followed prospectively for five years. Seventy-five percent of all the patients suffered a recurrence within the five-year period, and bipolar I patients were 1.5 times more likely to suffer a recurrence than bipolar II patients. With regard to speed of lithium taper, rapidly tapered patients predominantly suffered their recurrences of depression or mania earlier than the gradually tapered patients. The authors noted in their discussion that 66% of the patients were having their lithium tapered because they had experienced "prolonged well-being," yet 75% of them went on to recurrence within five years. This strongly supports the necessity of lifelong maintenance treatment with lithium.

A related issue in maintenance lithium treatment is the phenomenon of "lithium-discontinuation-induced refractoriness" that has been seen clinically and has been reported by Post et al. in 1992 and Post in 1993.[42,43] The scenario: A bipolar patient who has been stable on lithium therapy for a period of years has the medication discontinued for clinical reasons. The patient then proceeds to relapse and when lithium therapy is re-instituted, it is ineffective in treating the patient's symptoms. While the reports of this phenomenon are anecdotal and nothing can yet be said regarding its incidence, we have seen evidence of this phenomenon in several bipolar patients at our center.

While the majority of data regarding duration of treatment is derived from studies of lithium therapy, the results are also believed to apply to such other mood-stabilizing agents as carbamazepine and valproate.

FAILURE RATE OF MOOD-STABILIZERS

The natural course of bipolar illness as described includes recurrence of some degree of affective symptoms even in the presence of a mood stabilizer. This phenomenon has been studied, and while most of the data apply directly to failure of lithium, they are believed to apply to other mood-stabilizing agents as well.

The failure of lithium as a *panacea* in the maintenance treatment of bipolar disorder is well established. Prien et al. followed 117 bipolar patients in a double-blind fashion for two years and reported a 55% failure rate for lithium monotherapy.[44] Harrow et al. followed a group of bipolar patients who had presented to their center with acute mania for longer than one-and-a-half years.[20] They noted that while on lithium monotherapy, 42% of the patients had a relapse or recurrence of mania within the follow-up period, and 30% of the patients experienced a major depression during the follow-up year. Peselow et al. reviewed the data on 1,200 patients followed for five years with bipolar illness at their center and concluded that lithium therapy alone prevented relapse in 83% of patients at one year, 52% at two years, and 37.5% at five years.[45] In other words, *17% of patients at one year, 48% of patients at two years, and 62.5% of patients at five years will suffer a recurrence of bipolar illness on lithium therapy alone.* Of those patients who had failed lithium monotherapy and were subsequently treated with combination therapy, their relapse rate was less than that for lithium alone.

FACTORS AFFECTING COMPLIANCE

Factors affecting patient compliance with maintenance lithium pharmacotherapy include the patients' tolerance of side effects and their awareness of the recurrent nature of their illness. The role of their physicians is to maintain the drug at an effective serum concentration while continuing to educate the patient regarding the necessity of continued lithium therapy, and when possible, to treat side effects either by adjunctive medications like propranolol or inositol or through carefully monitored dose reduction. Similar principles apply to maintenance therapy with anticonvulsants. A recent study followed 140 bipolar patients prospectively for one year after either a manic or mixed episode and found that 51% (71) were noncompliant with their medications during that period. The most common reason given by the patients for their noncompliance was "denial of need." Comorbid substance abuse was another factor associated with medication noncompliance. This underscores the need for ongoing psychoeducation with the bipolar patient regarding the need for ongoing compliance with medication.[46]

LITHIUM

Lithium is the first-choice agent for acute treatment of bipolar disorder and the agent most studied for maintenance therapy. Lithium is available in an oral preparation as either a liquid (lithium citrate) or a tablet (lithium carbonate). The pharmacokinetic properties of lithium are reviewed in Table 5–6; available preparations of lithium, including a slow-release form, are given in Table 5–7, and costs of the various lithium preparations in Table 5–8. There have been more than 10 double-blind, placebo-controlled studies that have demonstrated the efficacy of lithium treatment for bipolar illness. These are summarized in Table 5–9.

PREDICTORS OF RESPONSE

Grof et al. outlined the predictors of response to lithium therapy.[47,48]

Most important, the patient must carry a diagnosis of a primary affective disorder with an episodic course. They noted that the observations of an increasing failure rate of lithium therapy may in fact be due not to the drug itself, but rather to the use of lithium for conditions other than bipolar illness, such as aggressivity, schizoaffective illness, and character disorders. They also note that a family history of bipolar illness and an "optimal" score on personality testing are predictive of a good response to lithium treatment. The authors also provide an additional listing of variables that appear to

text continues on page 160

TABLE 5–6. PHARMACOKINETIC PROPERTIES OF LITHIUM

Absorption	Peak Serum Levels	Serum Half-Life	Principle Route of Excretion
Gastrointestinal	2–4 hours	20–24 hours	Renal

From Rosenberg, D.R., Holttum, J., Gershon, S. (1994). *Textbook of Pharmacotherapy for Child and Adolescent Psychiatric Disorders* (p. 240). Philadelphia: Brunner/Mazel. Reprinted with permission.

TABLE 5–7. AVAILABLE PREPARATIONS OF LITHIUM

Generic	Trade Name	Strength
Lithium carbonate	Eskalith	300 mg
Lithium carbonate	Lithium carbonate	300 mg
Lithium carbonate	Lithonate	300 mg
Lithium carbonate	Lithotabs	300 mg
Lithium carbonate, slow release	Eskalith CR	450 mg
Lithium carbonate, slow release	Lithobid	300 mg
Lithium citrate syrup	Cibalith	8mEq/5 ml (equal to one 300 mg tablet)

From Rosenberg, D.R., Holttum, J., Gershon, S. (1994). *Textbook of Pharmacotherapy for Child and Adolescent Psychiatric Disorders* (p. 258). Philadelphia: Brunner/Mazel. Reprinted with permission.

TABLE 5–8. AVAILABLE PREPARATIONS AND COSTS FOR LITHIUM

Compound	Trade Name	Nonparenteral Preparations	Average Dose/Day	Average Cost/Day
Lithium carbonate	Eskalith	Tablets: 300 mg	1800 mg	$1.08
Lithium carbonate	Lithium carbonate	Tablets: 300 mg	1800 mg	$0.54
Lithium carbonate	Lithonate	Tablets: 300 mg	1800 mg	$0.48
Lithium carbonate	Lithotabs	Tablets: 300 mg	1800 mg	$0.60
Lithium carbonate, slow release	Eskalith CR	Tablets: 450 mg	1350 mg	$1.17
Lithium carbonate, slow release	Lithobid	Tablets: 300 mg	1800 mg	$1.56
Lithium citrate syrup	Cibalith	8 mEQ/5ml (equal to one 300 mg tablet)	1800 mg	$0.17

From *Red Book Annual Pharmacist Reference, 1996.* Copyright 1996 by Medical Economics, Montvale, NJ. Reprinted with permission.

TABLE 5-9. MAINTENANCE TREATMENT FOR BIPOLAR DISORDER WITH LITHIUM

Study	Symptom-free intervals[1]	Length of study (months)	Total number of patients	Outcome
Baastrup et al. (1970)	Undefined	5	50	Li > Plc
Mekia (1970)	Undefined	24	19	Li > Plc
Coppen et al. (1971)	Undefined	4–28	39	Li > Plc
Hullin et al. (1972)	Undefined	6	36	Li > Plc
Cundall et al. (1972)	Undefined	12	16	Li > Plc
Persson (1972)	6 months	24	24	Li > Plc
Stallone et al. (1973)	Undefined	24–28	52	Li > Plc
Prien et al. (1973a)[2]	Undefined	24	205	Li > Plc
Prien et al. (1973b)	Undefined	24	44	Li > IMI = Plc
Fieve et al. (1976)	Undefined	15–17	53	Li > Plc
Quitkin et al. (1981)	6 weeks	30	75	Li = Li + IMI
Kane et al. (1982)	6 months	11	22	Li > IMI = Plc
Prien et al. (1984)	2 months	24	117	Li = Li + IMI > IMI

IMI = imipramine, Li = lithium, Plc = placebo, CBZ = carbamazepine.
[1] Mostly patients from lithium clinics who were euthymic and then randomized to the treatment conditions.
[2] Patients were manic during their index episode.
From Kasper, S. (1993). The rational for long-term antidepressant therapy. *Int Clin Psychopharmoco*, 8:225–235. Copyright 1993 by Rapid Science Publishers. Reprinted with permission.

have no correlation with lithium responsiveness: sex, age at onset, age at onset of treatment, number of previous episodes, plasma and platelet MAO concentrations and measurements of red blood cell lithium concentration. The more atypical clinical features that are present decrease the patient's responsiveness to lithium. In other words, *"the most typical" bipolar patient is the most responsive to lithium treatment.*

LITHIUM DOSING

What is the effective serum level of lithium necessary for successful maintenance therapy while minimizing the incidence of adverse reactions to the drug? While laboratories commonly report a normal serum range for lithium of 0.6 to 1.2 mEq/L, and the commonly accepted serum level necessary for treatment of acute mania is between 0.8 and 1.2 mEq/L, the necessary level for maintenance therapy is less well established. Several studies have attempted to address this question and we review them below.

Gelenberg et al. studied 94 bipolar patients in a double-blind fashion, assigning them to receive either standard dose therapy (with a serum lithium concentration of 0.8 to 1.0 mEq/L) or low dose therapy (with resulting serum lithium concentrations of 0.4 to 0.6 mEq/L.[49] Fifty-three percent of the low dose group experienced a recurrence of their illness compared with 32% of the standard dose group, a risk of recurrence 2.6 times greater in the lower serum concentration group than in the standard group. The median time to recurrence was 24 weeks for the low dose group and 29 weeks for the standard dose group. The reports of side effects, not surprisingly, were higher in the standard serum concentration group and included polyuria, tremor, weight gain, diarrhea, and metallic taste in the mouth. The authors of the study concluded that while the lower serum level of lithium is better tolerated, the standard level of 0.8 to 1.0 mEq/L, with its associated side effects, should be the goal for maintenance therapy and that patient education is necessary to increase patient compliance with the standard dose regimen.

Keller et al. re-examined the question of standard versus low dose lithium regimens for maintenance therapy, and in particular, their relationship with subsyndromal (i.e., subclinical or subtle) symptoms of mania or depression.[50] Ninety-four patients with bipolar disorder were assigned to either low dose or standard dose lithium therapy (as described above) in a double-blind manner. Fifty-three percent of the low dose patients suffered a recurrence of bipolar illness compared with 32% of the standard dose group, yielding a risk of recurrence 2.6 times greater in the low dose group. These results confirmed those of Gelenberg et al.[49] With regard to the predictive value of subsyndromal or subtle symptoms of bipolar illness, of the patients in the low dose group who experienced hypomanic symptoms, 67% proceeded to suffer a recurrence of mania. Of the patients in the low dose group who reported subclinical depressive symptoms, 37% went on to suffer a major depressive episode. Overall, 76% of patients who developed subsyndromal hypomanic symptoms and 39% who developed subsyndromal depressive symptoms proceeded to suffer a recurrence. Patients in both low and standard dose groups were twice as likely to develop subsyndromal depressive than hypomanic symptoms, but patients with subsyndromal hypomanic symptoms were two times as likely to suffer a relapse compared with those patients with subsyndromal depressive symptoms.

These studies reveal that standard (0.8 to 1.0 mEq/L) level lithium therapy is more than twice as effective in preventing recurrence of bipolar illness, although a significant proportion of these patients' illness will recur, and in one-third to three-quarters of patients, the development of subsyndromal symptoms of hypomania or depression herald the development of a full major depressive or manic episode. Patients need to be educated with regard to recognizing subsyndromal symptoms so that they may be treated early before a full-blown recurrence of bipolar illness develops. A so-called hypomanic or depressive "alert" should be aggressively managed by first obtaining a serum lithium level to verify that the drug concentration is in the therapeutic range, and second by increasing the daily dosage of lithium while continuing to monitor the serum concentration. If a rapid response to a hypomanic alert is accompanied by an increase in lithium dosage, many of these recurrences can be averted.

MONITORING LITHIUM THERAPY

Before lithium therapy is initiated, especially long-term therapy, the accepted work-up includes serum blood urea nitrogen (BUN) and creatinine, nematology profile, thyroid panel, pregnancy test, and electrocardiogram, as well as a complete medical history and physical examination.

Serum lithium levels should be obtained five to seven days after a dose increase. The level most commonly obtained is the serum trough that is drawn 12 hours after a dose. Typically, the level is drawn in the morning after the patient has taken the evening dose and prior to taking the morning dose. Slow-release lithium preparations produce serum levels approximately 30% greater than an equivalent dosage of the standard lithium preparation. During initiation of lithium therapy or during dosage adjustments, lithium levels should be obtained weekly. Once a patient has reached a stable serum lithium concentration, his or her level should be checked every month for three months, then every two months for the next six months, and then once every six months thereafter. Clinical evidence of the new onset of side effects or the question of lithium toxicity should prompt obtaining a serum lithium level sooner.

During the first six months of lithium therapy, serum BUN and creatinine should be followed every two to three months as measures of renal function. In patients on maintenance lithium therapy, renal function should be checked every six months. In our center, we obtain 24-hour urine creatinine clearances every six months on our lithium-treated patients. While this test is slightly more inconvenient for the patient compared with a serum BUN/Cr, it is more sensitive in revealing small declines in renal function. Overall, our patients have been compliant with this test. A final note: Different laboratories have different standards and procedures for testing creatinine clearance, so one should be aware of his or her laboratory's method and should attempt to use the same laboratory each time, if possible, to avoid confusion in interpreting results.

Thyroid function should be followed every three months for the first six months of lithium treatment. After an initial thyroid panel, one need only follow the serum TSH level. During maintenance therapy, the TSH should be obtained every six months.

In patients in whom serum lithium levels do not appear to correlate with the clinical presentation, an intraerythrocyte level of lithium may be obtained. This assay of the *intracellular* concentration of lithium, as opposed to the serum concentration, may be used to measure compliance with lithium treatment over the previous three weeks in much the same way as hemoglobin A-1C measures glucose control in a diabetic on insulin therapy.[51] In the future, nuclear magnetic resonance (N.M.R.) spectroscopy may provide an alternative mechanism for measuring lithium's activity in the brain as recently evidenced in a report using such scanning to measure brain lithium concentrations in patients with bipolar disorder.[52] This technique is currently limited by a lack of information on the therapeutic range of brain lithium concentrations and by the lack of N.M.R. for lithium in most centers.

In summary, monitoring serum lithium concentrations provides the clinician with a method of both increasing the effectiveness of lithium treatment and minimizing the occurrence of lithium intoxication/toxicity. Serum monitoring does not, however, replace clinical monitoring of a patient's degree of affective symptomatology and side effects.

Lithium has a low therapeutic index (i.e., the difference between the therapeutic and toxic serum concentrations is small) and lithium toxicity can present with myriad possible symptoms. A comprehensive listing is given in Table 5–10.

PREDICTORS OF RELAPSE/RECURRENCE ON LITHIUM

A greater number of previous bipolar episodes, the presence of rapid cycling or a mixed presentation, and comorbidity with either a personality disorder (DSM-IV Axis II) or personality traits are predictive of failure of maintenance lithium therapy. While the number of prior episodes of depression or mania is not a predictor of future episodes, it does appear clinically to be predictive of diminished responsiveness to lithium. Bipolar variants, rapid cycling, and mixed presentation, as discussed, have a diminished responsiveness to lithium monotherapy and usually require adjunctive mood-stabilizing agents. Patients with comorbid personality disorders or traits who fail lithium monotherapy and proceed to other agents may not have truly "failed" the lithium trial; rather, their baseline level of characterological symptomatology may be misperceived as residual or recurrent symptoms of bipolar disturbance, and the patients are labeled as lithium failures.

MANAGEMENT OF ADVERSE DRUG REACTIONS ON LITHIUM

Side effects may occur in two-thirds of patients on lithium and may vary in degree of clinical relevance. They are listed in Table 5–11. As discussed, they represent the major reason for noncompliance with lithium. Effective management of side effects, therefore, aids in preventing recurrence

TABLE 5–10. SYMPTOMS AND SIGNS OF LITHIUM TOXICITY

Gastrointestinal symptoms Anorexia Nausea Vomiting Diarrhea Constipation Dryness of the mouth Metallic taste	**Mental symptoms** Difficulty swallowing Slowing of thought Confusion Somnolence Restlessness–disturbed behavior Stupor Coma

Neuromuscular symptoms and signs
General muscle weakness
Ataxia
Tremor
Muscle hyperirritability
   Fasciculation (increased by tapping muscle)
   Twitching (especially of facial muscles)
   Clonic movements of whole limbs
   Choreoathetotic movements
   Hyperactive deep tendon reflexes
	Cardiovascular system
	Pulse irregularities
	Fall in blood pressure
	Electrocardiographic changes
	Peripheral circulatory failure
	Circulatory collapse
	
	Miscellaneous
	Polyuria
	Polydypsia
	Glycosuria

Central nervous system Anesthesia of skin Incontinence of urine and feces Slurred speech Blurring of vision Dizziness Vertigo Epileptiform seizures Electroencephalographic changes	General fatigue Lethargy and a tendency to sleep (drowsiness) Dehydration Skin rash–dermatitic lesions Weight loss Weight gain Alopecia Quincke's edema

of bipolar illness. Some of the more common side effects of lithium are discussed below.

The **tremor** caused by lithium is a postural tremor with a frequency of 8 to 10 Hz. It affects the hands predominantly and is usually symmetric. Patients usually complain of the tremor when it interferes with activities requiring fine motor movements of the hands (writing, crocheting, etc.). Beta-blockers such as propranolol and atenolol are the treatments of choice for those patients in whom the tremor interferes with function. Propranolol is usually given in starting doses of 10–20 mg two to three times per day and increased to a maximum dose of 120 mg/day; atenolol is given usually at 50 mg once per day and increased to a maximum dose of 50–100 mg once or twice per day. When using these agents as antihypertensives, concomitant asthma or diabetes is a relative contraindication, and the clinician must carefully monitor the patient for hypotension when titrating the drug to a therapeutic dose.

Weight gain is seen in some patients with lithium treatment. Patients may report gains of 5 to 15 kg over a few months to several years. While part of

TABLE 5-11. SIDE EFFECTS OF LITHIUM AND THEIR MANAGEMENT

Side Effect	Management
Gastrointestinal	Give lithium after meals, give smaller doses more often, try slow-release preparation, lower the dosage
Tremor	Lower the dosage, give propranolol (40–100 mg/day), consider adding a benzodiazepine
Polyuria-diabetes insipidus	Try slow-release preparation, lower the dosage, add amiloride (5–10 mg/day), careful monitoring of lithium levels
Acne	Benzoyl peroxide (5–10%) topical solution, erythromycin (1.5–2%) topical solution
Muscular weakness, fasciculations, headaches	Usually resolve with first few weeks of treatment
Hypothyroidism	Levothyroxine (0.05 mg qd), follow TSH level and increase to 0.2 mg qd as needed
T wave inversion	Benign, no treatment needed
Cardiac dysrhythmias	Usually must discontinue lithium
Psoriasis, alopecia areata	Dermatology consult, reversible if lithium stopped
Weight gain	Difficult to treat, diet; may be partially reversible if lithium stopped
Edema	Consider spironolactone (50 mg po qd); if severe, monitor lithium levels; resolves when lithium stopped
Leukocytosis	Benign, no treatment needed

Adapted from Kaplan, H. Sadock (1995). *Comprehensive Textbook of Psychiatry*, 6th ed. Copyright 1995 by Williams & Wilkins, Baltimore. Reprinted with permission.

this weight gain is secondary to "water weight" (edema) and, in severe cases, may respond to judicious use of diuretics (see below), the remainder appears to be due to a poorly understood effect of lithium on carbohydrate metabolism and glucose tolerance.

Polyuria is the most common side effect of lithium therapy and is found in 20 to 25% of patients. Lithium may produce polyuria by inducing a nephrogenic diabetes insipidus-like syndrome causing patients to produce large volumes of dilute urine. The method of treatment has three steps: hold lithium doses for three to four days; begin a low dose of a thiazide or potassium-sparing diuretic (i.e., hydrochlorothiazide 25–50 mg/day); then re-start lithium at a lower dose and titrate to within therapeutic serum concentrations. An alternative treatment regimen may involve adding inositol, a metabolite whose intracellular levels in the brain and other tissues are reduced as a direct consequence of lithium treatment.[53,54] Bersudsky et al. reported that inositol treatment (1 g three times per day) resolved polyuria/polydipsia in 9 of 14 patients on lithium therapy; 5 reported dramatic resolution of polyuria while 4 reported a mild-to-moderate improvement.[55] The efficacy of inositol treatment has been confirmed in several other studies.[56,57] These reports suggest that inositol may be useful at a dose of 1 to 3 g three times per day for the treatment of lithium-induced polyuria.

Gastrointestinal disturbances, usually diarrhea or nausea, are common with lithium therapy. They usually resolve by administering lithium after mealtimes or by switching preparations (e.g., lithium carbonate to lithium citrate or long-acting preparation). Of course, other causes of diarrhea should be ruled out, such as infection. A patient on stable maintenance lithium therapy who presents with diarrhea, with or without accompanying fever and other manifestations of an infection, must have his or her lithium serum concentration followed closely as these processes may perturb drug homeostasis, causing either too high or too low a serum lithium concentration.

Acne and **other dermatological conditions** have been associated with lithium therapy, usually in a dose-dependent fashion. Management includes the standard dermatologic preparations (i.e., topical antibiotics or topical steroids) or switching to an alternative lithium preparation (switching citrate form for carbonate form or vice versa). Inositol, at a dose of 1 to 2 g tid, may have a role in the treatment of lithium-induced psoriasis.

MANAGEMENT OF DRUG-DRUG INTERACTIONS INVOLVING LITHIUM

Lithium may potentially interact with many commonly prescribed medications. A list of these agents and their interactions with lithium is given in Table 5–12. Some of the more common interactions are discussed in the following text.

Coadministration of diuretics with lithium may either increase or decrease the serum lithium concentration depending on the class of diuretic used. Loop diuretics (furosemide), thiazide diuretics, and potassium-sparing diuretics (triamterene) may increase the serum lithium level. Osmotic diuretics (mannitol and urea) will decrease serum lithium levels by increasing renal excretion of the drug.

The use of nonsteroidal anti-inflammatory agents (NSAIDs, ibuprofen, etc.) in a patient on lithium may cause the serum lithium level to increase, possibly to toxic levels. As these agents are becoming increasingly available in over-the-counter preparations, the physician must caution the patient carefully regarding their use. In some cases, where a nonsteroidal agent is indicated in a fixed dosage, the serum lithium level may be monitored closely and adjusted accordingly. Sulindac is the only NSAID that does not significantly increase serum lithium levels when coadministered with lithium.

TABLE 5–12. LITHIUM DRUG INTERACTIONS

Increase serum lithium levels
Antibiotics
Carbamazepine
Diuretics
Nonsteroidal anti-inflammatory agents

Decrease serum lithium levels
Acetazolamide
Caffeine
Osmotic diuretics
Theophylline

Interact with lithium to produce sedation and/or confusional states
Alcohol
Antihypertensives
Antipsychotics (especially haloperidol)

ANTIPSYCHOTICS

While research data support the use of antipsychotics in the treatment of acute mania, the question of maintenance antipsychotic use has not been rigorously studied. Clinical experience, however, has demonstrated the value of maintenance antipsychotics in some patients refractory to other agents, in severely agitated or persistently psychotic patients with an euthymic or stable mood, or in patients who are noncompliant with oral therapy and require a depot medication. The literature also notes this use.[58] One study that addressed this issue found that 52 of 77 patients (68%) hospitalized for bipolar manic or bipolar mixed episodes were still receiving antipsychotic medication six months after discharge. Risk factors for ongoing antipsychotic use in this study included male sex, history of medication noncompliance in the month preceding hospitalization, and increased severity of manic symptoms.[59] Important considerations in the use of antipsychotics for maintenance therapy are discussed in Chapter 6 on schizophrenia. Of particular concern in bipolar patients on chronic antipsychotic therapy is the increased risk of tardive dyskinesia. Therefore, the risks of less effective treatment of symptoms must be weighed against the risk of the movement disorder.

A clozapine trial may be indicated in mixed bipolar patterns (i.e., dysphoric mania) with psychosis who have failed lithium, anticonvulsant, and traditional neuroleptic therapy. Suppes et al. followed seven such patients openly for three to five years on clozapine. While marked functional and symptomatic improvement was noted in all, six of the seven who remained on clozapine required no further hospitalizations. Another follow-up study reported similar results.[60,61]

Another role for antipsychotics in maintenance treatment is in the rapid treatment after onset of subsyndromal symptoms of mania. Clinically, we have used a low dose of a medium-potency antipsychotic (thioridazine 50 mg/day) for several days at hour of sleep when bipolar patients have reported the onset of hypomanic symptoms (decreased need for sleep, increased irritability, increased energy) together with an increase in their daily lithium dose. A benzodiazepine may also be used for this purpose, as discussed below.

CARBAMAZEPINE

Carbamazepine (Figure 5–1) is an anticonvulsant used in the treatment of trigeminal neuralgia and epilepsy and was initially noted in these patients to ameliorate comorbid psychiatric symptoms. It is also useful as a mood stabilizing agent in bipolar disorder. While the available data are favorable and support its use as a second-line agent for patients who have failed lithium, it is limited to smaller and less-definitive trials than those concerning the use of lithium.

There have been 16 open studies and four double-blind studies of carbamazepine in bipolar disorder.[62] Additionally, five studies examined carbamazepine prophylaxis versus lithium[63,64,65] or placebo.[66] They are listed in Table 5–13.

No significant differences were found between carbamazepine and lithium although the side-effect profile of carbamazepine was more easily tolerated. Watkins et al., however, noted a decreased period of remission in carba-

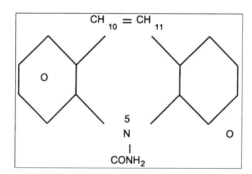

FIG. 5–1. Carbamazepine.

TABLE 5–13. CONTROLLED TRIALS OF LONG-TERM TREATMENT OF
UNIPOLAR DEPRESSION AND BIPOLAR DISORDER WITH CARBAMAZEPINE

Study	Medication	Total Number of Patients	Outcome
Ballenger and Post (1978)	CBZ, Plc	10	CBZ: 70% improved
Okuma et al. (1981)	CBZ, Plc	22	CBZ: 60% improved
Placidi et al. (1986)[1]	CBZ, Li	56	CBZ or Li: 66% improved
Watkins et al. (1987)	CBZ, Li	37, unipolar, bipolar	CBZ: 84% improved, Li: 84% improved
Lusznat et al. (1988)	CBZ, Li	40, mania or hypomania	CBZ: 45% improved, Li: 25% improved

CBZ = carbamazepine, Li = lithium, Plc = placebo, UP = unipolar, BP = bipolar.
[1] About half the patients were diagnosed as affective disorder with schizophrenic features.
From Kasper, S. (1993). The rationale for long-term antidepressant therapy. *Int Clin Psychopharmacol*, 8:225–235. Copyright 1993 by Rapid Science Publishers. Reprinted with permission.

mazepine patients compared with lithium (3.3 versus 9.3 months).[67] A single study compared carbamazepine with placebo and found it to be superior in maintenance treatment.[66] Taken together, these studies suggest that carbamazepine may be of benefit in the maintenance treatment of bipolar disorder, although the superiority of its use as monotherapy versus as an adjunct to lithium cannot be determined currently from the data. We would consider a trial of carbamazepine in a bipolar patient who has failed lithium treatment or as an adjunct to lithium in a patient with breakthrough symptoms on a therapeutic dose.

Like lithium, carbamazepine is available only as an oral preparation as shown in Table 5–14. Peak serum concentrations occur four to eight hours after a dose. The half-life of the drug varies with duration of treatment. Initially, the half-life is between 18 to 55 hours but decreases to 5–26 hours after several weeks of use due to induction of hepatic metabolism. Dosages in bipolar disorder range between 200–1,600 mg/day. To initiate therapy in an outpatient, 200 mg–300 mg/day in divided doses is given initially and then increased by 200 mg every three to four days. We tend to keep patients at low doses of carbamazepine for the first one to two weeks, if clinically feasible, as this lessens the initial side effects of fatigue and gastrointestinal distress until hepatic enzyme induction occurs. Doses can be increased more rapidly on an inpatient unit. Although formal studies of therapeutic serum concentration do not exist for carbamazepine in bipolar disorder, we strive for a serum blood level at the midrange or slightly above the therapeutic

TABLE 5–14. AVAILABLE PREPARATIONS AND COSTS OF ANTICONVULSANTS

Drug	Available Preparations	Average Cost/Day
Carbamazepine	**Generic** 200 mg scored tablets 100 mg scored tablets, chewable	$0.90
	Tegretol 200 mg scored tablets 100 mg scored tablets, chewable 100 mg/5 ml oral suspensions	$1.51
Valproic Acid	**Generic** 250 mg capsules 250 mg/5 ml oral syrup	$0.84
	Depakene 250 mg capsules 250 mg/5 ml oral syrup	$4.91
Divalproex (enteric coated)	**Generic** 125, 250, 500 mg unscored tablets	$1.14
	Depakote 125, 250, 500 mg unscored tablets "Sprinkles," can be put directly on food	$2.68

range for seizure disorder, a point at which a balance between therapeutic effect and side effects occurs. In patients who have had acute symptoms stabilized on carbamazepine, maintenance treatment should maintain the serum level that was effective during the acute treatment period.

Reports in the literature indicate that carbamazepine may become less effective over time.[68,42] The mechanism for this has yet to be established and its true prevalence is not yet known. Therefore, the clinician treating a bipolar patient with carbamazepine must monitor closely not only the serum concentration, but also the clinical picture as well and educate the patient on self-monitoring for the advent of subsyndromal symptoms of depression or mania.

MONITORING OF CARBAMAZEPINE THERAPY

As with lithium treatment, a precarbamazepine workup should include a thorough history and physical examination, an electrocardiogram, pregnancy test, serum chemistries, baseline hematologic parameters, and thyroid studies. In addition, liver function tests should be obtained.

Monitoring serum concentration is the sole available method of drug monitoring. Therapeutic levels for the treatment of bipolar illness have not been worked out as they have for seizure disorders. Serum levels are generally kept between 4 to 12 μg/ml in bipolar patients as this is the accepted range for seizure patients. A level is generally drawn as a morning trough, approximately 12 hours after the evening dose and before the morning dose. Following a change in dosage, a serum level should be checked in five days. Because of its high level of binding to serum proteins, a routine serum level may be inaccurate in conditions in which the patient's serum protein concentrations are abnormally increased or decreased. In these patients, a free serum carbamazepine level provides a more accurate measurement of active drug concentration.

In patients beginning a course of maintenance carbamazepine therapy, the serum concentration, as well as a complete blood count, platelet count, and differential, should be checked every two weeks for the first two months of treatment. After two months, all should be checked no less than every three months.

PREDICTORS OF RELAPSE

No formal studies exist regarding prediction of relapse on carbamazepine as they do with lithium. Based on clinical experience, however, the predictors described for lithium apply to carbamazepine.

MANAGEMENT OF ADVERSE DRUG REACTIONS

Adverse drug reactions with carbamazepine are divided into idiosyncratic and dose-related. They are listed in Table 5–15. Idiosyncratic drug reactions are rare, potentially life-threatening, and may occur at any point in treatment, although they most commonly occur within the first three to six months. They include agranulocytosis, hepatic failure, Stevens-Johnson

TABLE 5–15. SIDE EFFECTS OF CARBAMAZEPINE

Common	Uncommon
Diplopia	Agranulocytosis and aplastic anemia
Drowsiness	Hyponatremia and water intoxications
Incoordination	Liver toxicity
Nystagmus	Neurotoxicity
Nausea	Mania
Leukopenia	Exacerbation/precipitation of behavior problems
Skin rashes	Hypocalcemia
	Stevens-Johnson Syndrome
	Pancreatitis

syndrome, and pancreatitis. The physician should educate the patient to monitor for the development of new physical symptoms and report them to the physician.

Dose-related side effects are common and include fatigue, nausea, blurred vision, and ataxia. These symptoms may appear transiently at initiation of carbamazepine treatment or with dosage increase and usually respond to a decrease in dosage. They may be more severe in adolescents and the elderly. Less commonly, one may see skin rashes, hyponatremia, mild elevations of liver function tests, and slight leukopenia or thrombocytopenia. Obtaining baseline laboratory studies at the beginning of treatment allows the physician to monitor any new laboratory abnormalities closely and, as many are benign, they do not necessarily indicate the need for discontinuation of carbamazepine therapy.

Carbamazepine may be fatal in overdose, especially in dosages exceeding 6 gm. Symptoms of overdose include impaired consciousness, seizures, ophthalmoplegia, nystagmus, and respiratory failure. Agranulocytosis is a rare but potentially fatal side effect of carbamazepine therapy. Any patient presenting with unexplained fever and symptoms of an infectious process should have a white blood cell count obtained immediately.

MANAGEMENT OF DRUG-DRUG INTERACTIONS

Like valproate, carbamazepine is highly protein bound in the blood and is metabolized by the liver. Concomitant use of carbamazepine with other highly protein bound drugs may either increase the serum concentration of carbamazepine or the other drugs. The most common of these interactions are given in Tables 5–16 and 5–17. Concomitant use of carbamazepine and these agents requires close monitoring of carbamazepine serum concentrations and surveillance for signs of drug toxicity.

VALPROIC ACID

Valproate is also an anticonvulsant used in the treatment of bipolar disorder (Figure 5–2). It is available in two forms: valproic acid and sodium valproate. Within three to eight hours of ingestion, peak serum concentrations are attained (regardless of the preparation) and the half-life of the medication in the serum is 6 to 16 hours. Valproate is available in oral preparations either in capsules or a sprinkle preparation. Costs of the various oral preparations are given in Table 5–14. An intravenous preparation is also available.

Like carbamazepine, an appropriate serum concentration for bipolar patients has not been determined, and like carbamazepine, the therapeutic

TABLE 5–16. ANTICONVULSANT DRUG INTERACTIONS

Effects Increased by	Effects Decreased by Anticonvulsants
Cimetidine	Birth control pills
Chloramphenicol	Cortisol
Chlorpheniramine	Coumarin
Disulfiram	Dexamethasone
Erythromycin	Diazepam
Isoniazid	Digoxin
Methylphenidate	Neuroleptics
Phenothiazine	Phenylbutazone
Propoxyphene	Prednisolone
Sulthiame	Tricyclic antidepressants
Tricyclic antidepressants	Warfarin

TABLE 5–17. CARBAMAZEPINE DRUG
INTERACTIONS

Decreases Serum Half Life
Haloperidol
Phenytoin
Theophylline

Increases Serum Concentrations
Lithium

Decreases Serum Levels by Simultaneous Administration
Phenobarbital
Phenytoin
Primidone

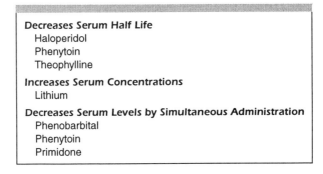

FIG. 5–2. Valproic acid.

range for treatment of epilepsy, 50 μg/ml–100μg/ml, is used. Valproate treatment is initiated in divided doses (250 mg bid or tid) and the dosage is increased by 250 mg every few days as tolerated while closely following serum concentrations. One generally should check a serum level after five days on either 500 mg or 750 mg/d to establish a baseline and then increase as tolerated. The therapeutic range is a serum concentration of 50 to 100 μg/ml with a target level between 80 μg/ml and 95 μg/ml in otherwise healthy adult patients.

Valproic acid appears to have superior efficacy to lithium in both the acute and maintenance treatment of the rapid cycling variant of bipolar disorder.[69,70] Puzynski and Klosiewicz followed a small group of bipolar patients for two to three years and found that valproate monotherapy reduced the number, severity, and duration of depressive and manic episodes.[71] A general rule in the treatment of patients with rapid cycling bipolar disorder is to achieve mood-stabilizer monotherapy with one of the anticonvulsants initially by pushing the serum concentration as high as tolerated before adding a second (or third) mood stabilizer. The unfavorable alternative is to proceed immediately to combination therapy before completing an adequate trial of monotherapy.

MONITORING VALPROATE THERAPY

As with the other mood-stabilizers, valproate therapy requires monitoring of the serum concentration of the drug, as well as monitoring of hematologic and hepatic parameters. Serum concentrations should be checked five days after a dosage adjustment as a trough, 12 hours after the evening dose and before the morning dose. Once a stable concentration has been achieved, levels should be checked, and the patient evaluated clinically, at a minimum of every six months. Measurements of free serum valproate are also available for more accurate determination of drug concentration in medically complex patients. Hematological and hepatic measurements should be obtained at baseline prior to implementation of valproate treatment and should be followed at a minimum of every six months or sooner if clinical symptoms indicate.

PREDICTORS OF RELAPSE

Again, no controlled studies have been carried out to determine predictors of relapse/recurrence of bipolar illness with valproate treatment. It is generally believed, as with carbamazepine, that the predictors of relapse discussed for lithium hold for valproate.

MANAGEMENT OF ADVERSE DRUG REACTIONS

As with carbamazepine, side effects of valproate can be divided into idiosyncratic and dose-related. They are listed in Table 5–18. Also as

TABLE 5–18. VALPROIC ACID SIDE EFFECTS AND INTERACTIONS

Side Effects		Interactions	
Common	**Uncommon**	**Decreases Effect of**	**Increases Effects of**
GI upset	Liver toxicity	Hepatically	Carbamazepine
Increased	Hyperammonemia	metabolized	Phenytoin
appetite/	Blood dyscrasias	drugs	
weight gain	Alopecia		
Sedation	Decreased serum		
Tremor	carnitine		
	Neural tube defects		
	Pancreatitis		
	Hyperglycinemia		
	Menstrual irregularity		

with carbamazepine, **idiosyncratic side effects** of valproate are rare but potentially fatal and include agranulocytosis, hepatic failure, and pancreatitis. Therefore, any new physical symptoms should be sought and worked up as necessary. Also, the patient should be educated to monitor for any new physical symptoms.

Dose-related side effects are common and include **anorexia, nausea, vomiting, diarrhea, tremor,** and **sedation**. These are usually present transiently at the beginning of treatment and often resolve without intervention. Patients may also complain of **weight gain** and **transient hair loss**. Tremor or gastrointestinal symptoms that fail to resolve may be treated with a beta-blocker (propranolol or atenolol in doses given above in lithium section) or an H_2-blocker (i.e., ranitidine 150 mg once or twice per day). **Leukopenia** or **thrombocytopenia** may also occur in mild forms on valproate therapy but are generally reversible upon dosage decrease or drug discontinuation. These hematological abnormalities may occur at any point in the course of therapy.

MANAGEMENT OF DRUG-DRUG INTERACTIONS

Like carbamazepine, valproate is highly protein bound and is largely metabolized by hepatic enzymes. Medications that may affect or be affected by valproate are also given in Table 5–18. Two important interactions with valproate include fluoxetine that causes an increase in valproate concentration through inhibition of its metabolism and aspirin that increases the free, active concentration of valproate by displacing it from its serum protein binding.

COMBINATION THERAPIES

What of the patient who fails monotherapy with one or more of the mood-stabilizers? Initial failure of lithium treatment would prompt treatment with one of the anticonvulsants either alone or in combination with lithium. If the patient were then stabilized and maintained successfully for a period of six months, one could attempt to taper the lithium.

There are limited data available on combination therapies. However, Ketter et al. reported a single case of a rapid-cycling bipolar patient who was maintained successfully on both carbamazepine and valproate after he had failed trials of each agent alone.[72] The authors argue that the success of combination therapy in this particular case is due to the synergistic effect of the two agents. Whether this finding can be generalized to other patients is not known, but it may be attempted in the difficult-to-treat patient.

CALCIUM-CHANNEL BLOCKERS

Abnormalities in intracellular calcium metabolism have been discovered in bipolar patients and a therapeutic role for the calcium-channel blockers (i.e., antagonists) has been hypothesized in bipolar illness. The chemical structures of these agents are given in Figure 5–3. Only limited data exist on the value of these agents and what are available focuses on one agent in particular, verapamil. Giannini et al. performed a year-long, double-blind study comparing verapamil and lithium in a crossover fashion.[73] They found that bipolar patients achieved mood stabilization more quickly on verapamil than on lithium and that after crossover, the initial lithium treatment group evidenced further improvement on verapamil whereas the initial verapamil group had no additional benefit from lithium. While this study is small (20 patients) and its results have not been confirmed in other studies, it presents verapamil as a promising agent in bipolar patients who failed with the other mood stabilizers. Given the lack of widespread use of this drug as a mood stabilizer, we recommend consultation with a psychiatrist experienced in its use.

BENZODIAZEPINES

As previously discussed, there is a use for the benzodiazepines, particularly lorazepam and clonazepam, in the symptomatic treatment of acute mania. Their role in maintenance treatment is less well defined and has been looked at in two studies with conflicting results. Aronson et al. treated five bipolar patients who had been refractory to lithium treatment

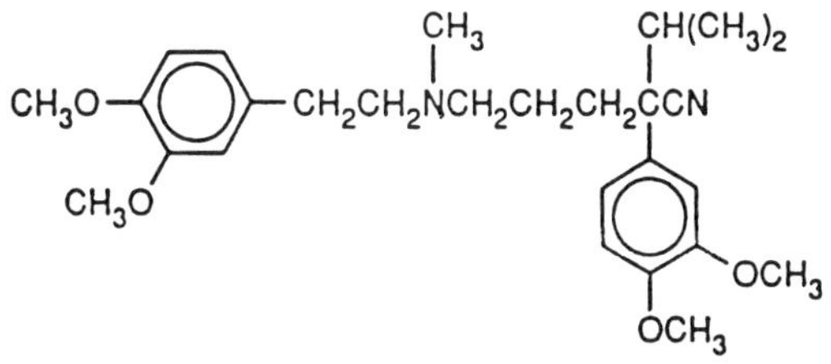

verapamil

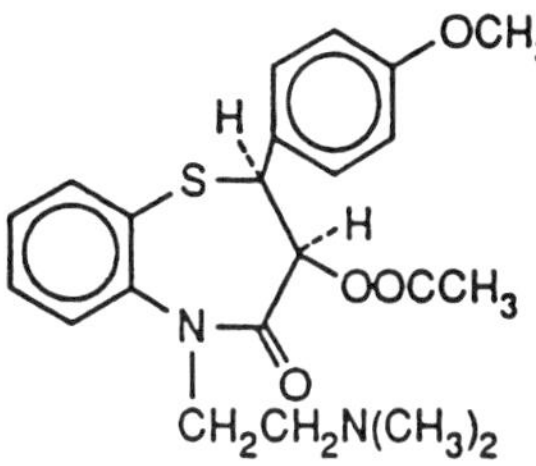

diltiazem

FIG. 5–3. Chemical structures of calcium-channel blockers.

with clonazepam monotherapy.[74] All the patients relapsed quickly (2 to 15 weeks), and the study was terminated. Sachs et al. reported success with modifying the treatment regimen of bipolar patients on maintenance lithium plus haloperidol to lithium plus clonazepam.[75]

In our clinical experience, clonazepam as an adjunct to a mood stabilizer may be helpful in those bipolar patients with comorbid anxiety symptoms or baseline mild-to-moderate agitation. A several day course of clonazepam at hour of sleep (0.5 to 1.0 mg) may also be helpful in maintenance therapy of patients who report subsyndromal symptoms of mania.

Treatment of bipolar patients with benzodiazepines requires knowledge of their associated risks: dependency and drug-induced agitation/dysphoria. Patients who have been treated with benzodiazepines at doses of 2 to 4 mg or greater of clonazepam or lorazepam must have the drug tapered to avoid risk of withdrawal, if discontinuation is clinically indicated. This risk is greatest with alprazolam, a benzodiazepine with a half-life of only 12 hours.

ANTIDEPRESSANTS

Psychiatry appears to have a continually expanding armamentarium of antidepressant drugs. Most studies of these drugs have been in the treatment of unipolar depression, and it is in no way clear that we may extrapolate those results to the treatment of bipolar depression. The unipolar depression studies are discussed in Chapter 4. An additional risk of antidepressant treatment in bipolar depression is the risk of inducing mania. Currently no class of antidepressant has been shown to be free of this risk. We therefore recommend that concomitant use of a mood stabilizer be considered in bipolar depressed patients. Next, we review the current state of knowledge regarding antidepressant use in bipolar disorder.

SELECTIVE SEROTONIN REUPTAKE INHIBITORS

While these agents have become the first-line therapy for depressive symptoms in outpatient unipolar depression given their favorable side-effect profile and low risk of toxicity, there are no controlled studies to date on their use as maintenance agents in bipolar depression. It has been our clinical experience that these agents offer no advantage over more traditional antidepressant agents in treating major depressive episodes. They may have use, however, in the treatment of subsyndromal depressive symptoms.

TRICYCLIC ANTIDEPRESSANTS

The tricyclic antidepressants have been found to be superior to placebo for the treatment of bipolar depression in seven controlled studies reviewed by Zornberg and Pope.[76] As discussed, these agents are commonly administered with a mood stabilizer, usually lithium.

MONOAMINE OXIDASE INHIBITORS

Himmelhoch et al. reported that the monoamine oxidase inhibitor tranylcypromine was superior in efficacy to imipramine in the treatment of bipolar depressed patients who exhibited symptoms of anergia, motor retardation, hyperphagia, and hypersomnia.[77] They employed a double-blind design in the study of 56 depressed patients with either bipolar illness type I or II and found tranylcypromine superior to imipramine with greater improvement in symptomatology, higher global response, and a lower attrition rate. The authors went on to report a crossover study of the same patients who either failed to respond or could not tolerate the medication. These results were published by Thase et al. and demonstrated that while 9 of the 12 patients who crossed over from imipramine to tranylcypromine showed a positive treatment response, only one of four of the patients crossed over from tranylcypromine to imipramine showed a positive treatment response.[78] They again concluded that the monoamine oxidase inhibitors appeared to be efficacious in the treatment of anergic bipolar depression and appeared to have superior efficacy to tricyclic antidepressants.

BUPROPION

Sachs et al. performed a double-blind prospective study of bupropion versus desipramine in 15 bipolar depressed patients for both acute treatment (eight weeks) and maintenance treatment (one year).[79] The authors found no difference in efficacy between the two drugs for acute treatment. However, during the maintenance phase, there was an increased incidence of mania/hypomania in the desipramine group compared with the bupropion group (50 vs. 11%). They concluded that bupropion was an equally effective agent in depression compared with tricyclics and appeared less likely to induce a hypomanic or manic episode.

OTHER ANTIDEPRESSANTS

Recent arrivals to the antidepressant market include venlafaxine, nefazodone, and mirtzapine. These agents have differing modes of action than the agents discussed previously. There are currently no data available from clinical trials on the use of these agents in either the acute or maintenance treatment of bipolar depression.

MANAGEMENT OF DRUG-MEDICAL ILLNESS INTERACTIONS

THYROID DISEASE AND LITHIUM

Thyroid disease, usually hypothyroidism, occurs in 5 to 35% of patients on maintenance lithium therapy and thyroid function usually returns to normal when lithium is discontinued. Hypothyroidism develops more commonly in women after one-half to one-and-a-half years of lithium therapy and may contribute to the development of rapid cycling.[80] Lithium treatment may be continued in these patients if clinically indicated by initiating thyroid hormone supplementation in the form of levothyroxine (T_4). The development of hypothyroidism in a bipolar patient may be heralded not only by the classic signs and symptoms (fatigue, cold intolerance, constipation, weight gain, thin hair, doughy skin, bradycardia, etc.), but also by the onset of depressive symptoms or rapid cycling.

RENAL DISEASE AND LITHIUM

Historically, a concern of long-term lithium maintenance therapy has been the possibility of adverse effects on renal function. Indeed, several case reports have been published reporting the onset of end-stage renal disease in patients taking lithium. Recent investigations have shown the long-term effects of lithium on renal function to be minimal. Hetmar et al. reported that patient age, preexisting renal disease, and number of episodes of lithium intoxication were predictors of decline in renal function in lithium-treated patients, while the duration of the treatment was not predictive.[81] They also noted an increased association between twice-a-day dosing and renal complications (compared with once-a-day dosing). Walker, in a comprehensive review of the literature, reported that lithium caused a progressive impairment in urinary concentrating ability, especially in those with a history of episodes of acute lithium intoxication or concurrent neuroleptic use.[82] He noted that avoidance of lithium toxicity was the most important factor in the long-term preservation of renal function and that stable maintenance therapy with lithium had little effect on glomerular filtration rate. Patients with impaired urinary concentrating ability and concurrent polyuria should be followed more closely as they are at increased risk for episodes of lithium intoxication due to the possibility of increased renal loss of fluids.[82]

SPECIAL POPULATIONS

RAPID CYCLING BIPOLAR DISORDER

The rapid cycling variant of bipolar disorder occurs in 15 to 20% of bipolar patients at some point in their illness.[83,70] Its association with hypothyroidism and female predominance has been described above.[84] Rapid cycling does not appear to be genetically mediated and may represent a transient phase of bipolar illness.[85] Antidepressant monotherapy is associated with the onset of rapid cycling and is a factor in its continuation.[86]

Rapid cycling may represent a more treatment refractory form of bipolar illness. Wehr et al. reported that 63% of 51 "treatment refractory" rapid cycling patients referred to their cluster were truly treatment refractory.[86] The remaining 37% achieved symptom remission with combination treatment with both an antidepressant and a mood stabilizer. Clinically, this population may require more than one mood stabilizing agent. Alternative strategies for refractory patients may include high dose levothyroxine[80] or clozapine.[87,88,89]

PREGNANCY/LACTATION

Relapse of bipolar illness is common in pregnancy and the postpartum period, with an incidence of 60%. However, exposure of the fetus to the three main mood stabilizing agents (lithium, carbamazepine, and valproate) during the first trimester may result in birth defects.[90] Lithium exposure carries with it a 4 to 12% risk of major congenital abnormalities, the classic one being Ebstein's anomaly. Carbamazepine exposure is associated with developmental delay, craniofacial defects, and neural tube defects, while valproate is associated with a 1 to 2% incidence of neural tube defects. Management of the pregnant bipolar patient involves a careful risk-versus-benefit analysis of risks of treatment to fetus versus risks of nontreatment to mother and fetus. Ideally, one would discontinue mood stabilizers the entire first trimester. However, this may not always be possible. In that event, the pregnant patient (and family) should receive extensive counseling regarding the risks of treatment to the fetus, and the patient should undergo extensive fetal monitoring throughout the course of the pregnancy including measurement of serum alpha-fetoprotein. Frequent measurements of serum drug concentrations are also required through the course of pregnancy given its effects on hepatic and renal metabolism, resulting in either increased or decreased drug concentrations in the serum. Verapamil may be an alternative to the above agents given its better safety profile in pregnancy.

TREATMENT OF THE ELDERLY

Treatment of the elderly bipolar patient follows similar guidelines to those of the adult bipolar with several caveats. First, lithium levels above 0.7 mEq/L are poorly tolerated. Elderly patients should be maintained on lower serum concentrations of lithium, which fortunately produce equivalent mood stabilizing effects. Second, lithium-induced side effects, particularly diarrhea and tremor, are more common in the elderly population. Finally, an elderly patient being started or maintained on lithium requires a periodic thorough medical history and physical examination, including electrocardiogram and laboratory studies.

While studies are lacking regarding the use of carbamazepine and valproate in the elderly bipolar patient, clinical experience tells us to follow similar guidelines to those with lithium as outlined previously for treatment of the elderly bipolar patient.

TREATMENT OF ADOLESCENTS

Lithium is the agent of first choice in adolescents with bipolar disorder as it is in adults. But it appears to be less effective in this population due to the tendency of adolescent bipolar illness to present as mixed mania or as mania with severe psychotic symptoms.

Strober et al. looked at responses to lithium maintenance therapy in adolescents and found that 62.5% of adolescents with bipolar illness completed one-and-a-half years of lithium therapy without relapse compared with 92.3% patients in the nonlithium group who relapsed within the same time period.[91]

Therapeutic serum concentrations of lithium and the rules of monitoring are the same for adolescents as they are for adults. Side effects in adolescents are similar to those of adults and are managed in a similar fashion.

Evidence on the use of other agents is largely anecdotal, and such treatment should be carried out by a psychiatrist with experience in treating adolescents with bipolar illness.

REFERENCES

1. Weissman, M.M., Leaf, P.J., Tishler, G.L., et al. (1988). Affective disorders in five United States communities. *Psychological Medicine*, 18:141–153.
2. Burke, K.C., Burke, J.D., Regier, D.A., et al. (1990). Age at onset of selected mental disorders in five community populations. *Arch Gen Psychiatry*, 47:511–518.
3. Zis, A.P., Goodwin, F.K. (1979). Major affective disorder as a recurrent illness: A critical review. *Arch Gen Psychiatry*, 36:835–839.
4. Carlson, G.A., Katin, J., Davenport, Y.B., et al. (1974). Follow-up of 53 bipolar manic-depressive patients. *Br J Psychiatry*, 124:134–139.
5. Keller, M.B., Lavoci, P.W., Coryell, W., et al. (1993). Bipolar I: A five-year prospective follow-up. *J Nerv Mental Dis*, 181(4):238–245.
6. Tohen, M., Waternaux, C.M., Tsuang, M.T., et al. (1990a). Four-year follow-up of twenty-four first episode manic patients. *J Affec Disorders*, 19(2):79–86.
7. Tohen, M., Waternaux, C.M., Tsuang, M.T. (1990b). Outcome in mania. A 4-year prospective follow-up of 75 patients utilizing survival analysis. *Arch Gen Psychiatry*, 47(12):1106–1111.
8. Rice, D.P., Miller, L.S. (1995). The economic burden of affective disorders. *Br J Psychiatry*, (Suppl)27:34–42.
9. Cusano, P.P., Mayo, J., O'Connell, R.A. (1977). The medical economics of lithium treatment for manic-depressives. *Hosp Comm Psychiatry*, 28(3):169–173.
10. Reifman, A., Wyatt, R.J. (1980). Lithium: A brake in the rising cost of mental illness. *Arch Gen Psychiatry*, 37(4):385–388.
11. Coryell, W., Scheftner, W., Keller, M., et al. (1993). The enduring psychosocial consequences of mania and depression. *Am J Psychiatry*, 150(5):720–727.
12. Winokur, G., Tsuang, M. (1975). The Iowa 500: Suicide in mania, depression, and schizophrenia. *Am J Psychiatry*, 132:650–651.
13. Morrison, J.R. (1982). Suicide in or psychiatric practice population. *J Clin Psychiatry*, 43:348–352.

14. Regier, D.A., Hirschfeld, R.M.A., Goodwin, F.K., et al. (1988). The NIMH depression awareness, recognition and treatment program. *Am J Psychiatry*, 145:1351–1357.
15. Muller-Oerlinghausen, B., Ahrens, B., Grof, E., et al. (1992). The effect of long-term lithium treatment on the mortality of patients with manic-depressive and schizoaffective illness. *Acta Psychiatr Scand*, 86:218–222.
16. Vestergaard, P., Aagaard, J. (1991). Five-year mortality in lithium-treated manic-depressive patients. *J Affec Disorders*, 21(1):33–38.
17. Coppen, A., Standish-Barry, H., Bailey, J., et al. (1990). Long-term lithium and mortality. *Lancet*, 335:1347.
18. Coppen, A., Standish-Barry, H., Bailey, J., et al. (1991). Does lithium reduce the mortality of recurrent mood disorders? *J Affec Disorders*, 23:1–7.
19. Mueller-Oerlinghausen, B., Ahrens, B., Volk, J., et al. (1991). Reduced mortality of manic-depressive patients in long-term lithium treatment: An international collaborative study by IGSLI. *Psychiatry Res*, 36:329–331.
20. Harrow, M., Goldberg, J.F., Grossman, L.S., et al. (1990). Outcome in manic disorders: A naturalistic follow-up study. *Arch Gen Psychiatry*, 47:665–671.
21. Prien, R.F., Caffey, E.M., Klett, C.J. (1971). A comparison of lithium carbonate and chlorpromazine in the treatment of acute mania. *Arch Gen Psychiatry*, 26:146–153.
22. Shopsin, B., Kim, S.S., Gershon, S. (1971). A controlled study of lithium vs. chlorpromazine in acute schizophrenics. *Br J Psychiatry*, 119:435–440.
23. Calabrese, J.R., Kimmel, S.E., Woyshville, M.J. (1996). Clozapine for treatment-refractory mania. *Am J Psychiatry*, 153:759–764.
24. Yassa, R., Nair, V., Schwartz, G. (1984). Tardive dyskinesia and the primary psychiatric diagnosis. *Psychosomatics*, 25(2):135–138.
25. Mukherjee, S., Rosen, A.M., Caracci, G., et al. (1986). Persistent tardive dyskinesia in bipolar patients. *Arch Gen Psychiatry*, 43:342–346.
26. Lerer, B., Moore, N., Meyendorff E., et al. (1987). Carbamazepine versus lithium in mania: A double-blind study. *J Clin Psychiatry*, 48:89–93.
27. Pope, H.G., Jr., McElroy, S.L., Keck, P.E., Jr., et al. (1990). Valproate in the treatment of acute mania: A placebo controlled study. *Arch Gen Psychiatry*, 48(1):62–68.
28. Bowden, C.L., Brugger, A.M., Swann, A.C., et al. (1994). Efficacy of dinolproex vs. lithium and placebo in the treatment of mania. The Depokate Mania Study Group. *JAMA*, 271:918–924.
29. Bowden, C.L., Janicak, P.G., Orsulak, P. (1996). Relation of serum valproate concentration to response in mania. *Am J Psychiatry*, 153:765–770.
30. Stoll, A.L., Banov, M., Kolbrener, M., et al. (1994). Neurologic factors predict a favorable valproate response in bipolar and schizoaffective disorders. *J Clin Psychopharmacol*, 14(5):311–313.
31. Keck, P.E., Jr., McElroy, S.L., Tugrul, K.C., et al. (1993). Valproate oral loading in the treatment of acute mania. *J Clin Psychiatry*, 54(8):305–308.
32. Chouinard, G., Young, S.N., Annable, L. (1983). Antimanic effect of clonazepam. *Biol Psychiatry*, 18:451–466.
33. Bradwejn J., Shriqui C., Koszycki. D., et al. (1990). Double-blind comparison of the effects of clonazepam and lorazepam in acute mania. *J Clin Psychopharmacol*, 10(6):403–408.
34. Lenox, R.H., Newhouse, P.A., Creelman, W.L., et al. (1992). Adjuncture treatment of manic agitation with lorazepam versus haloperidol: A double-blind study. *J Clin Psychiatry*, 53(2):47–52.
35. Dubovsky, S.L., Franks, R.D., Lifschitz, M., et al. (1982). Effectiveness of verapamil in the treatment of a manic patient. *Am J Psychiatry*, 139:502–504.
36. Dubovsky, S.L., Franks, R.D. (1983). Intracellular calcium ions in affective disorders: A review and an hypothesis. *Biol Psychiatry*, 18:781–797.

37. Giannini, A.J., Houser, W.L., Jr., Loiselle, R.H., et al. (1984). Antimanic effects of verapamil. *Am J Psychiatry*, 141:1602–1603.
38. Mukherjee, S., Sackeim, H.A., Schnur, D.B. (1994). Electroconvulsive therapy of acute manic episodes: A review of 50 years' experience. *Am J Psychiatry*, 151:169–176.
39. Mukherjee, S., Sackeim, H.A., Lee, C. (1988). Unilateral ECT in the treatment of manic episodes. *Convulsive Therapy*, 4:74–80 [B].
40. Shapiro, D.R., Quitkin, F.M., Fleiss, J.L. (1989). Response to maintenance therapy in bipolar illness: Effect of index episode. *Arch Gen Psychiatry*, 46:401–405.
41. Faedda, G.L., Tondo, L., Baldessarini, R.J., et al. (1993). Outcome after rapid vs. gradual discontinuation of lithium treatment in bipolar disorders. *Arch Gen Psychiatry*, 50:448–455.
42. Post, R.M., Leverich, G.S., Altschuler, L., et al. (1992). Lithium-discontinuation-induced refractoriness: Preliminary observations. *Am J Psychiatry*, 149:1727–1729.
43. Post, R.M. (1993). Issues in the long-term management of bipolar affective illness. *Psychiatry Ann*, 23:86–93.
44. Prien, R.F., Kupfer, D.J., Mansky, P.A., et al. (1984). Drug therapy in the prevention of recurrences in unipolar and bipolar affective disorders: Report of the NIMH Collaborative Study Group comparing lithium carbonate, imipramine, and a lithium carbonate-imipramine combination. *Arch Gen Psychiatry*, 41:1096–1104.
45. Peselow, E.D., Fieve, R.R., Difiglia, C., et al. (1994). Lithium prophylaxis of bipolar illness: The value of combination treatment. *Br J Psychiatry*, 164:208–214.
46. Keck, P.E., McElroy, S.L., Strakowski, S.M. (1997) Compliance with maintenance treatment in bipolar disorder. *Psychopharmacol Bull*, 33(1):87–91.
47. Grof, P., Hux, M., Grof, E., et al. (1983). Prediction of response to stabilizing lithium treatment. *Pharmacopsychiatry*, 16:195–200.
48. Grof, P., Alda, M., Grof, E., et al. (1993). The challenge of predicting response to stabilizing lithium treatment: The importance of patient selection. *Br J Psychiatry*, 163(Suppl 21):16–19.
49. Gelenberg, A.J., Kane, J.M., Keller, M.B., et al. (1989). Comparison of standard and low serum levels of lithium for maintenance treatment of bipolar disorder. *N Engl J Med*, 321:1489–1493.
50. Keller, M.D., Lavori, P.W., Kane, J.M., et al. (1992). Subsyndromal symptoms in bipolar disorder: A comparison of standard and low serum levels of lithium. *Arch Gen Psychiatry*, 49(5):371–376.
51. Harvey, N.S., Kay, R. (1991). Compliance during lithium treatment, intra-erythrocyte lithium variability and relapse. *J Clin Psychopharmacol*, 11:362–367.
52. Gyulai, L., Wicklund, S.W., Greenstein, R., et al. (1991). Measurement of tissue lithium concentration by lithium magnetic resonance spectroscopy in patients with bipolar disorder. *Biol Psychiatry*, 29:1161–1170.
53. Hallcher, L.M., Sherman, W.R. (1980). The effect of lithium ion and other agents on the activity of myo-inositol-1-phosphatase from bovine brain. *J Biol Chemistry*, 255:10896–10901.
54. Allison, J.H., Stewart, M.A. (1971). Reduced brain inositol in lithium-treated rats. *Nature New Biology*, 233:267–268.
55. Bersudsky, Y., Vinnitsky, I., Grisaru, N., et al. (1992). The effects of inositol on lithium-induced polyuria-polydypsia in rats and humans. *Human Psychopharmacol*, 7:403.
56. Kofman, O., Sherman, W.R., Kady, V., et al. (1992). Restorations of brain myo-inositol levels in rats increases latency to lithium-pilocurpine seizures. *Psychopharmacology*, 110(1–2):229–234.
57. Grisaru, N., Belmaker, R.H. (1994). Letter, *Br J Psychiatry*, 164:133.
58. Sernyak, M.J., Woods, S.W. (1993). Chronic neuroleptic use in manic-depressive illness. *Psychopharmacol Bull*, 29:375–381.
59. Keck, P.E., McElroy, S.L., Strakowski, S.M., et al. (1996). Factors associated with maintenance antipsychotic treatment of patients with bipolar disorder. *J Clin Psychiatry*, 57(4):147–151.

60. Suppes, T., McElroy, S.L., Gilbert, J. (1992). Clozapine in the treatment of dysphoric mania. *Biol Psychiatry*, 32:270–280.
61. Zarate, C.A. Tohen, M., Banov, M.D., et al. (1995). Is clozapine a mood stabilizer? *J Clin Psychiatry*, 56(3):108–112.
62. Prien, R.F., Gelenberg, A.J. (1989). Alternatives to lithium for preventive treatment of bipolar disorder. *Am J Psychiatry*, 146:840–848.
63. Coxhead, N., Silverstone, T., Cookson, J. (1992). Carbamazepine versus lithium in the prophylaxis of bipolar affective disorder. *Acta Psychiatr Scand*, 85:114–118.
64. Lusznat, R.M., Murphy, D.P., Nunn, C.M. (1988). Carbamazepine vs. lithium in the treatment and prophylaxis of mania. *Br J Psychiatry*, 153:198–204.
65. Small, J.G., Klapper, M.H., Milstein, V., et al. (1991). Carbamazepine compared with lithium in the treatment of mania. *Arch Gen Psychiatry*, 48(10):915–921.
66. Okuma, T., Inanaga, K., Otsuki, S., et al. (1981). A preliminary double-blind study of the efficacy of carbamazepine in prophylaxis of manic-depressive illness. *Psychopharmacologia* (Berlin), 73:95–96.
67. Watkins, S.E., Callender, K., Thomas, D.R., et al. (1987). The effect of carbamazepine and lithium on remission from affective illness. *Br J Psychiatry*, 150:180–182.
68. Frankenburg, F.R., Tohen, M., Cohen, B.M., et al. (1988). Long-term response to carbamazepine: A retrospective study. *J Clin Psychopharmacol*, 8(2):130–132.
69. Calabrese, J.R., Delucchi, G.A. (1990). Spectrum of efficacy of valproate in 55 patients with rapid-cycling bipolar disorder. *Am J Psychiatry*, 147(4):431–434.
70. Calabrese, J.R., Markovitz, P.J., Kimmel, S.E., et al. (1992). Spectrum of efficacy of valproate in 78 rapid-cycling bipolar patients. *J Clin Psychopharmacol*, 12(Suppl 1):535–565.
71. Puzynski, S., Kosiewkz, L. (1984). Valproic acid amide as a prophylactic agent in affective and schizoaffective disorders. *Psychopharmacol Bull*, 20:151–159.
72. Ketter, T.A., Pazzaglia, P.J., Post, R.M. (1992). Synergy of carbamazepine and valproic acid in affective illness: Case report and review of the literature. *J Clin Psychopharmacol*, 12(4):276–281.
73. Giannini, A.J., Tarasjewski, R., Loiselle, R.H. (1987). Verapamil and lithium in maintenance therapy of manic patients. *J Clin Psychopharmacol*, 27:980–982.
74. Aronson, T.A., Shukla, S., Hirschowitz, J. (1989). Clonazepam treatment of five lithium-refractory patients with bipolar disorder. *Am J Psychiatry*, 146:77–80.
75. Sachs, G.S., Weilburg, J.B., Rosenbaum, J.F. (1990). Clonazepam vs. neuroleptics as adjuncts to lithium maintenance. *Psychopharmacol Bull*, 26:137–143.
76. Zornberg, G.L., Pope, H.G., Jr. (1993). Treatment of depression: Bipolar disorder: New directions for research. *J Clin Psychopharmacol*, 13:397–408.
77. Himmelhoch, J.M., Thase, M.E., Mallinger, A.G., et al. (1991). Tranylcypromine versus imipramine in anergic bipolar depression. *Am J Psychiatry*, 148(7):910–916.
78. Thase, M.E., Mallinger, A.G., McKnight, D., et al. (1992). Treatment of imipramine-resistant recurrent depression, IV: A double-blind crossover study of tranylcypromine for anergic bipolar depression. *Am J Psychiatry*, 149(2):195–198.
79. Sachs, G.S., Lafer, B., Stoll, A.L., et al. (1994). A double-blind trial of bupropion versus desipramine for bipolar depression. *J Clin Psychiatry*, 55(9):391–393.
80. Bauer, M.S., Whybrow, P.C., Winokur, A. (1990a). Rapid cycling bipolar affective disorder: I. Association with grade I hypothyroidism. *Arch Gen Psychiatry*, 47:427–432.
81. Hetmar, O., Poulsen, U.J., Ladefoged, J., et al. (1991). Lithium: Long-term effects on the kidney: A prospective follow-up study ten years after kidney biopsy. *Br J Psychiatry*, 158:53–58.
82. Walker, R.G. (1993). Lithium nephrotoxicity. *Kidney Int*, 44(Suppl.42):593–598.
83. McElroy, S.L., Keck, P.E., Pope, H.G., et al. (1988). Valproate in the treatment of MPID-cycling bipolar disorder. *J Clin Psychopharmacol*, 8:275–279.

84. Bauer, M.S., Whybrow, P.C. (1990b). Rapid cycling bipolar affective disorder: II. Treatment of refractory rapid cycling with high-dose levothyroxine: A preliminary study. *Arch Gen Psychiatry*, 47:435–440.

85. Coryell, W., Endicott, J., Keller, M. (1992). Rapidly cycling affective disorder: Demographics, diagnosis, family history and course. *Arch Gen Psychiatry*, 49:126–131.

86. Wehr, T.A., Sack, D.A., Rosenthal, N.E., et al. (1988). Rapid cycling affective disorder: Contributing factors and treatment response in 51 patients. *Am J Psychiatry*, 145:179–184.

87. Suppes, T., Phillips, K.A., Judd, C.R. (1994). Clozapine treatment of nonpsychotic rapid cycling bipolar disorder: A report of three cases. *Biol Psychiatry*, 36:338–340.

88. Calabrese, J.R., Meltzer, H.Y., Markovitz, P.J. (1991). Clozapine prophylaxis in rapid cycling bipolar disorder. Letter, *J Clin Psychopharmacol*, 11(6):396–397.

89. Frye, M.A., Altshuler, L.L., Bhran, J.A. (1996). Clozapine in rapid cycling bipolar disorder. Letter, *J Clin Psychopharmacol*, 16(1):87–90.

90. vanGent, E.M., Verhoeven, W.M.A. (1992). Bipolar illness, lithium prophylaxis, and pregnancy. *Pharmacopsychiatry*, 25:187–191.

91. Strober, M., Morrell, W., Lampert C., et al. (1990). Relapse following discontinuation of lithium maintenance therapy in adolescents with bipolar I illness: A naturalistic study. *Am J Psychiatry*, 147(4):457–461.

6

SCHIZOPHRENIA

INTRODUCTION

Schizophrenia is the most severe psychiatric disorder, and a large pro-portion of the chronically and persistently mentally ill suffer from chronic schizophrenia. Patients with schizophrenia fill the state mental hos-pitals, community mental health centers, structured community residences, and the streets. Schizophrenia is a chronic, lifelong debilitating dis-order.

EPIDEMIOLOGY

PREVALENCE

The lifetime prevalence of schizophrenia is approximately 1–2%. A review of 21 studies over 50 years found a lifetime prevalence of 0.9–11.0/1000 general population.[1] The most recent and probably best estimate of the prevalence of schizophrenia in the United States is from the Epidemi-ologic Catchment Area (ECA) study that found a lifetime prevalence of 1.5%.[2]

187

GENDER AND AGE

The prevalence of schizophrenia is approximately equal in males and females. However, there is a gender difference in age of onset of illness. The peak age of onset for males is 18–24, while for women it is age 25–34 with a mean age of onset five years later in women than in men. There is a bimodal distribution for age of onset in women with a second smaller peak after menopause (age 40–45) accounting for 10% of the women.[3] There are several factors that may contribute to this gender difference including the putative protective effect of estrogen that has anti-dopaminergic properties.[4,5] Psychotic symptoms frequently worsen during the premenstrual, post-partum, and post-menopausal periods, coinciding with rapidly falling levels of estrogen. Conversely, symptoms may improve during pregnancy, a high estrogen state. Differing social roles and societal expectations may also contribute to gender differences in age of onset and clinical features.[4,5]

There are also gender differences in clinical features.[6,7,8] Premorbid adjustment is different: Males tend to be more schizoid and aggressive, while females are more shy, less aggressive, and have better social relationships. Males are more likely to have had perinatal complications. The clinical symptom profile is different: Men tend to have more negative symptoms, aggressivity, antisocial behavior, and substance abuse; women tend to have more Schneiderian first-rank symptoms (thought broadcasting, thought insertion, thought withdrawal, and multiple voices commenting on their behavior) and affective and paranoid symptoms with interpersonal conflict and self-destructive behavior. Men use distraction as a primary coping strategy while women use techniques reflecting more adaptive learning and better social skills. Young women generally require lower antipsychotic doses and levels than men, but they may require higher doses postmenopausally. In general, females may demonstrate better social adjustment (more likely to be married, living with families, and employed with higher income), spend less time in hospital, and have less severe psychopathology.

COMORBIDITY WITH SUBSTANCE ABUSE

There is significant comorbidity between schizophrenia and substance abuse. In the ECA study, 47% of patients with schizophrenia or schizoaffective disorder suffer from comorbid substance abuse or dependence; 34% have comorbid alcohol dependency; and 28% suffer from other drug dependency.[2] Patients with schizophrenia are almost five times more likely to suffer from substance abuse or dependence than the general population. Those with current substance abuse are higher users of inpatient psychiatric, jail, and emergency services and incur higher costs.[9] The significance for treatment of substance abuse in schizophrenia is addressed later.

COST

Schizophrenia places a large economic burden not only on the patient, the patient's family, and on society. The economic cost of schizophrenia is comprised of direct and indirect costs. The direct costs of psychiatric treatment include hospitalization, medications, outpatient visits, institutionalization, criminal justice system involvement, and rehabilitation. The indirect costs include lost productivity of patients and their families and wages lost because of suicide. In 1991, the estimated direct cost of schizophrenia was $19 billion and the indirect cost was $46 billion for a total cost of $65 billion.[10] Other analyses have concluded that schizophrenia costs account for 2.5% of the total health care costs.[11]

An estimated 10% of disability recipients suffer from schizophrenia. Many of these patients also receive public assistance in the form of housing, food stamps, and other social welfare services. The estimated cost of public expenditure for schizophrenia in the late 1980s was $15–20 billion annually.[11]

The economic cost to families is also great. Franks (1987) estimated the average cost to an individual family with a schizophrenic child to be over $11,000 per year.[12] The cost of suffering to patients and their families is immeasurable.

NATURAL HISTORY

Schizophrenia is a chronic, lifelong illness in the majority of cases. The course of the illness is marked by intermittent exacerbations of psychosis with a progressive functional decline. Most longitudinal studies indicate that the extent of decline is usually evident within the first 10 years of the illness.[13] Data from the era before effective treatments were available suggest that some patients have spontaneous and complete remission. Kraepelin estimated that 13% of his patients recovered completely and for prolonged periods of time, while Bleuler asserted that 25% recover entirely and persistently.[14] However, the definition of remission and also the validity of the diagnosis is in question; some of these patients may have had bipolar illness, which is more likely to remit.

Early intervention with antipsychotic treatment in first-break schizophrenia improves the long-term course.[13] Shortening the period of acute psychosis by administering medications or electroconvulsive therapy (ECT) improves the long-term prognosis, and patients not treated with medications or ECT on their first hospitalization had a greater number of hospital days during a four- to five-year follow up period.[15] Each subsequent episode may become more difficult to treat, taking longer to respond to medications and requiring higher doses. Also, episode frequency may increase over the course of the illness.

Maintenance antipsychotic treatment has been clearly shown to markedly decrease the rate of relapse compared with placebo, although maintenance treatment does not entirely prevent relapse. In his summary of relapse rates from over 20 years of international studies, Hogarty found that 70% of patients who are not maintained on medications relapse within one year after discharge from hospital.[16] The relapse rate is 10% per month and is reduced 2.5- to 10-fold in patients on antipsychotic medication.[17] This relapse rate is the same for oral and depot antipsychotic administration. There is evidence that the risk of relapse decreases over time from the last episode. However, relapse rates on maintenance antipsychotic medication continue to be less than on placebo even three years after the most recent episode, indicating that long-term maintenance treatment is efficacious.[18]

Even with the best maintenance treatment currently available, patients continue to have a 15% chance of recurrence of a psychotic episode. In addition, most patients suffer chronic social and functional impairment. The addition of psychosocial treatment to a maintenance antipsychotic regimen can decrease the relapse rate over time and improve functioning and quality of life.[19]

MORBIDITY

The course of schizophrenia is marked by a functional decline. Even when patients are not in the midst of a psychotic episode and their symptoms are well controlled, they do not return to their premorbid level of functioning. They tend to experience a downward drift in socioeconomic status, rarely meeting their pre-illness potential. The majority of patients, especially men, are unable to develop and maintain intimate relationships. Many individuals with schizophrenia live in inadequate housing or are homeless. An estimated 14–40% of the homeless in the United States suffer from schizophrenia.[20,21]

MORTALITY

Schizophrenia carries a mortality rate three times higher than the general population; this increased mortality is primarily attributable to unnatural causes of death, particularly suicide, in patients younger than 40 years.[22] Suicide is the leading cause of death in schizophrenia. Studies have reported attempted suicide rates of 18–55% with approximately 10% of patients with schizophrenia completing suicide.[23] Suicidality is more closely linked with depressive symptomatology and major depressive episodes than with psychosis. In fact, several studies have demonstrated that command auditory hallucinations are an infrequent cause of suicide in a schizophrenic population. Patients with schizophrenia who commit suicide have a higher incidence of depressive symptomatology, hopelessness, previous major depressive episodes, previous treatment with antidepressants, and prior suicide attempts.[23] Depressive symptomatology frequently emerges in the post-psychotic period or between episodes, as patients gain understanding about their illness and have insight into the devastating consequences of their chronic relapsing psychotic disorder.

Several reviews of the risk factors for suicide in schizophrenia indicate that while schizophrenia shares some risk factors with affective disorders, there are some risk factors that are unique to schizophrenia.[23,24,25,26] Young males, particularly those with higher premorbid functioning and higher IQ who are early in the course of their illness but who have experienced several psychotic relapses and established a chronic course, seem to be at especially high risk. Those with a history of depressive episodes, treatment for depression, and suicide attempts are at higher risk for suicide. Depressed mood, hopelessness, suicidal ideation, feelings of inadequacy, and fear of continued decline are all associated with suicide in schizophrenia. Lack of social supports including being unmarried, living alone, and being unemployed are also risk factors. There is some debate over whether higher antipsychotic doses may be a risk factor by contributing to depressive symptomatology or akathisia. The high mortality rate may also be accounted for by a higher incidence of many medical conditions, particularly diabetes and autoimmune diseases.

PATHOPHYSIOLOGY

Schizophrenia is a heterogeneous group of central nervous system disorders. Research into the pathophysiology and pathogenesis of schizophrenia has been inconsistent with diverse findings; no single abnormality has been found in the majority of cases. Many studies suggest abnormalities in brain structural and functional anatomy, as well as in neurotransmitter, endocrine, and autoimmune systems.[27]

STRUCTURAL AND FUNCTIONAL BRAIN ABNORMALITIES

Specific volumetric abnormalities have been detected by both postmortem neuropathological examination and MRI studies.[28,29] These include decreased volume of mesial temporal lobe structures such as hippocampus, amygdala, parahippocampal gyrus, entorhinal cortex, decreased volume of temporal lobe, particularly gray matter, decreased volume of superior temporal gyrus, planum temporale, and thalamus.

Newer techniques like positron emission tomography, single proton emission computed tomography, and functional nuclear magnetic resonance imaging demonstrate diminished blood flow in the dorsolateral prefrontal cortex, lack of activation of cerebral blood flow to frontal lobes during frontal lobe cognitive tasks, and relative hypermetabolism in the basal ganglia.[29,30] A few studies have demonstrated abnormal connectivity between hemispheres and between cortical and subcortical regions.

CYTOARCHITECTURE

Histopathological studies suggest a disruption in the neurodevelopmental processes of neuronal migration and pyramidal cell death. Neuronal disarray is evident in the hippocampus, parahippocampal cortex, prefrontal cortex, cingulate gyrus, motor cortex, mediodorsal thalamic nucleus, and nucleus accumbens.[27] The absence of gliosis supports a neurodevelopmental process and argues against a neurodegenerative process.[28]

BIOCHEMICAL ABNORMALITIES

While a functional excess of dopamine was thought to be the primary biochemical abnormality in schizophrenia, research has not consistently supported this hypothesis. A more recent hypothesis proposed that schizophrenia is characterized by low dopamine activity in prefrontal cortex (causing negative symptoms) and excessive dopamine activity in mesolimbic dopaminergic systems (causing positive symptoms).[31]

Other neurotransmitters including serotonin, norepinephrine, acetylcholine, gamma-aminobutyric acid (GABA), glutamate, opiate peptides, cholecystokinin, vasoactive intestinal polypeptide, somatostatin, neurotensin, and other substances, such as prostaglandins and phospholipids, have also been implicated in the pathogenesis of schizophrenia.

ETIOLOGY

Given the range of pathology seen in schizophrenia, it is perhaps no surprise that there are many hypotheses regarding the pathogenesis of schizophrenia.[27]

GENETIC

There is considerable evidence for a genetic influence in schizophrenia. There is a higher concordance rate for schizophrenia between monozygotic (50%) than dizygotic (20%) twins. First degree relatives of schizophrenics have a 5–10 fold greater chance of developing schizophrenia than the general population, and children of two schizophrenic parents have a 35–45-fold greater chance of having schizophrenia, even when adopted into nonschizophrenic families. A high discordance among monozygotic twins indicates that there is also a strong environmental component.

PERINATAL COMPLICATIONS

Obstetrical complications may be a result of abnormal fetal development and may cause hypoxic damage to vital subcortical and limbic regions, thereby increasing vulnerability to the expression of schizophrenia. Transient perinatal hypoxia seems to be a crucial factor and can damage periventricular structures such as amygdala, hippocampus, and basal ganglia.

VIRAL HYPOTHESIS

Viral infections have been associated with schizophrenia. Viral encephalitides may present with psychoses that resemble schizophrenia. Exposure to viral infection during the second trimester of pregnancy is associated with an increased incidence of schizophrenia compared with exposure during the first or third trimester.[32]

DIAGNOSIS

The diagnosis of schizophrenia is a purely clinical one, based upon the history and exam. There are no diagnostic laboratory or radiographic tests.

PREMORBID SYMPTOMS

The majority of patients with schizophrenia have no premorbid behavioral or personality abnormalities, but 25–50% were described as withdrawn, introverted, suspicious, eccentric, or impulsive as children and demonstrated signs of developmental delay.

POSITIVE SYMPTOMS

The positive or productive symptoms of schizophrenia reflect an excess or distortion of normal functions and may be associated with hyper-dopaminergic activity in the mesolimbic system. These include hallucinations, delusions, thought disorder, and bizarre or agitated behavior. These symptoms are associated with acute onset, history of exacerbations and remissions, normal premorbid functioning, relatively normal social functioning during remissions, normal neuropsychological testing, and lack of structural brain abnormalities. These symptoms respond best to dopamine-blocking antipsychotic medications.

NEGATIVE SYMPTOMS

The negative or deficit symptoms of schizophrenia may reflect diminution or absence of normal functions and may be associated with diminished dopaminergic and serotonergic activity in the dorsolateral prefrontal cortex and with hypofrontality. These symptoms include blunted affect, amotivation, avolition, anhedonia, apathy, and alogia (poverty of speech and thought content). These symptoms are associated with insidious onset, premorbid symptoms, chronic deterioration, structural brain abnormalities, and cognitive deficits on neuropsychological testing. These symptoms are less responsive to pharmacotherapy.

DSM-IV DIAGNOSTIC CRITERIA

Table 6–1 lists the DSM-IV criteria for a diagnosis of schizophrenia.

DIFFERENTIAL DIAGNOSIS

Before the diagnosis of schizophrenia can be made, an organic etiology must be ruled out. The diagnosis *psychotic disorder due to a general medical condition* is made if there is a medical condition etiologically related to the psychotic symptoms. Medical conditions that may present with psychotic symptoms and be mistaken for schizophrenia are listed in Table 6–2.

A *substance-induced psychotic disorder* may also be mistaken for schizophrenia. Substances like alcohol, amphetamines, cannabis, cocaine, hallucinogens, inhalants, opioids, phencyclidine, and sedative-hypnotics may cause psychosis during intoxication or withdrawal. Characteristics of substance-induced psychosis are onset of symptoms near the time of intoxication or withdrawal, absence of symptoms before substance use, resolution of

text continues on page 196

TABLE 6-1. CRITERIA FOR SCHIZOPHRENIA

A. *Characteristic symptoms*: Two (or more) of the following, each present for a significant portion of time during a one-month period (or less if successfully treated):

(1) delusions
(2) hallucinations
(3) disorganized speech (e.g., frequent derailment or incoherence)
(4) grossly disorganized or catatonic behavior
(5) negative symptoms, i.e., affective flattening, alogia, or avolition

Note: Only one Criterion A symptom is required if delusions are bizarre or hallucinations consist of a voice keeping up a running commentary on the person's behavior or thoughts, or two or more voices conversing with each other.

B. *Social/occupational dysfunction*: For a significant portion of the time since the onset of the disturbance, one or more major areas of functioning such as work, interpersonal relations, or self-care are markedly below the level achieved prior to the onset (or when the onset is in childhood or adolescence, failure to achieve expected level of interpersonal, academic, or occupational achievement).

C. *Duration*: Continuous signs of the disturbance persist for at least six months. This six-month period must include at least one month of symptoms (or less if successfully treated) that meet Criterion A (i.e., active-phase symptoms) and may include periods of prodromal or residual symptoms. During these prodromal or residual periods, the signs of the disturbance may be manifested by only negative symptoms or two or more symptoms listed in Criterion A present in an attenuated form (e.g., odd beliefs, unusual perceptual experiences).

D. *Schizoaffective and mood disorder exclusion*: Schizoaffective disorder and mood disorder with psychotic features have been ruled out because either (1) no major depressive, manic, or mixed episodes have occurred concurrently with the active-phase symptoms; or (2) if mood episodes have occurred during active-phase symptoms, their total duration has been brief relative to the duration of the active and residual periods.

E. *Substance/general medical condition exclusion*: The disturbance is not due to the direct physiological effects of a substance (e.g., a drug of abuse, a medication) or a general medical condition.

F. *Relationship to a pervasive developmental disorder*: If there is a history of autistic disorder or another pervasive developmental disorder, the additional diagnosis of schizophrenia is made only if prominent delusions or hallucinations are also present for at least a month (or less if successfully treated).

Classification of longitudinal course (can be applied only after at least one year has elapsed since the initial onset of active-phase symptoms):
Episodic with Interepisode Residual Symptoms (episodes are defined by the reemergence of prominent psychotic symptoms); *also specify if*:
with Prominent Negative Symptoms
Episodic with No Interepisode Residual Symptoms
Continuous (prominent psychotic symptoms are present throughout the period of observation); *also specify if*: **with Prominent Negative Symptoms**
Single Episode in Full Remission
Other or Unspecified Pattern

Adapted with permission from the *Diagnostic and Statistical Manual of Mental Disorders*, 4th ed. (pp. 285–286). Copyright 1994 by American Psychiatric Association.

195

TABLE 6–2. DIFFERENTIAL DIAGNOSIS OF SCHIZOPHRENIA

Neurologic Disease or Injury
Extrapyramidal syndromes
  Parkinson's disease
  Huntington's disease
  Fahr's disease
  Wilson's disease
  Post-encephalitic Parkinson's
    disease
Demyelinating diseases
  Multiple sclerosis
  Metachromatic leukodystrophy
CNS infections
  Post-encephalitis
  AIDS
  HSV encephalopathy
  Jakob-Creutzfeld disease
  Tertiary syphilis
Cerebrovascular disorders
  Multi-infarct dementia
  Arteriovenous malformations
  Subdural hematoma
Degenerative disorders
  Alzheimer's disease
  Friedreich's ataxia
  Olivopontocerebellaratrophy
  Pick's disease
Temporal lobe epilepsy
Anatomical
  Posterior fossa cysts
  Hydrocephalus with aqueductal
    stenosis

Trauma
  Particularly temporal lobe
  Collagen vascular diseases
  Systemic lupus erythematosus
Neoplasms

Metabolic or Systemic Disorders
  Vitamin B_{12} deficiency
  Pellagra
  Hypoglycemia
  Hepatic encephalopathy
  Hyperthyroidism
  Lead poisoning
  Uremia
  Cushing's disease

Genetic or Chromosomal Disorders
  XXY karyotype (Klinefelter's
    syndrome)
  XO karyotype (Turner's or Noonan's
    syndrome)
  18q-deletion
  5,q11-q13 triplication
  Acute intermittent porphyria
  Familial basal ganglia calcification
  Holocystinuria
  Phenylketonuria
  Albinism
  Congenital adrenal hyperplasia
  Glucose-6-phosphate dehydro-
    genase deficiency (favism)
  Kartagener's syndrome

Collagen Vascular Diseases
  Systemic lupus erythematosus

symptoms within one month of use, and symptoms characteristic of the type and amount of substance used.

A diagnosis of *schizophreniform disorder* is made when all the criteria for schizophrenia are met except the duration and social/occupational dysfunction criteria. *Schizoaffective disorder* is characterized by the presence of a major affective episode during a substantial portion of the duration of symptoms of schizophrenia but absent for at least two weeks of the illness duration.

Delusional disorder is characterized by nonbizarre delusions in the absence of auditory or visual hallucinations or other hallmark symptoms of schizophrenia in the absence of a major affective disorder and without functional impairment. Delusions may be of the erotomanic, grandiose, jealous, persecutory, somatic, or mixed type.

A *brief psychotic disorder* is marked by delusions, hallucinations, disorganized speech, or grossly disorganized or catatonic behavior lasting between one day and one month in the absence of a major affective disorder and with eventual full return to premorbid level of functioning.

A *manic episode* may be confused with a schizophrenic psychotic episode in the acute presentation but can be differentiated on the basis of illness course and presence of affective symptoms in the absence of psychotic symptoms. A *major depressive episode with psychotic features* may also be confused with a schizophrenic episode.

ACUTE PHARMACOLOGICAL TREATMENT

The acute treatment of psychotic episodes in schizophrenia has been well studied. We refer readers to a comprehensive book by Janicak et al. for a review of these studies and treatment recommendations.[33]

GENERAL PRINCIPLES OF ACUTE TREATMENT

While antipsychotic medications are the mainstay of acute treatment, they are only a part of a comprehensive treatment plan. To be successful, pharmacotherapy must be combined with psychotherapy that includes psychoeducation about the illness and the role of medications. Other psychosocial treatments including social skills training, cognitive rehabilitation, and group therapy are more useful in the maintenance phase of treatment and are discussed further in a later section of this chapter.

Establishing a therapeutic alliance with patients and their families is the key to successful treatment. However, this can often be a difficult task, especially while the patient is acutely psychotic and may be paranoid, incorporates the treatment team into a delusional system, or is too disorganized to understand the treatment. Facilitating a therapeutic relationship requires honesty, empathy, straightforward communication, and patience.

INITIATING TREATMENT

Once the diagnosis of schizophrenia or a schizophreniform disorder is made, treatment with an antipsychotic medication should be initiated. A complete history and physical exam should be performed to assess general health and rule out an organic etiology. The neurological exam should pay particular attention to the motor system and assess for any abnormal movements before starting antipsychotics. Baseline complete blood count with differential and liver function tests should be obtained. A baseline electrocardiogram should be obtained if using a low potency agent or phenothiazine.

ANTIPSYCHOTIC MEDICATIONS

Antipsychotic medications alleviate psychotic symptoms such as hallucinations, delusions, thought disorder, and disorganized, excited, aggressive behavior in any psychotic disorder, not just schizophrenia. There are several classes of antipsychotic agents: phenothiazines, thioxanthenes, butyrophenones, dibenzoxazepines, dibenzodiazepines, dihydroindolones, and diphenylbutyrylpiperidines. They have different chemical structures but share similar pharmacokinetic, pharmacological, and clinical profiles.

MECHANISM OF ACTION

The mechanism of action of antipsychotic agents is primarily blockade of dopamine (DA) receptors. Acute administration of antipsychotic drugs results in post-synaptic DA-receptor blockade and decreased presynaptic dopamine synthesis and release. Chronic administration may lead to tolerance and supersensitivity states in some dopaminergic systems through a process of DA-receptor up-regulation.

There are several dopaminergic pathways in the brain, each with different functions, anatomical connections, and DA-receptor subtypes. The nigrostriatal system includes the substantia nigra, caudate nucleus, and putamen and is primarily involved in movement. This is the tract involved in antipsychotic-induced movement disorders including parkinsonism and tardive dyskinesia. The mesolimbic and mesocortical systems are the ones primarily thought to be involved in psychotic symptomatology. Dopaminergic projections also run from midbrain to frontal and temporal cortical areas comprising the mesocortical system.

While dopamine D2 receptor antagonism was considered the primary goal of antipsychotic therapy, other DA-receptors, particularly D3 and D4, as well as serotonin (5-HT) receptors are now targets for antipsychotic action. Studies suggest that dopamine D3 and D4 receptor blockade is more specific for the mesolimbic and mesocortical systems than D2 receptor blockade. Serotonin 5-HT2 receptors are involved in the regulation of dopamine synthesis and release and 5-HT2 blockade increases dopamine release. Many of the newer atypical agents have both serotonin and dopamine blocking properties, and these agents are more effective for treatment refractory patients, may improve negative symptoms, and carry a lower risk of extrapyramidal side effects (EPS).

Dopamine autoreceptors on the presynaptic cell provide a negative feedback role and may be responsible for the development of tolerance to clinical effects. There are differences in dopamine autoreceptor subtype and distribution in the dopaminergic systems. Blockade of postsynaptic DA-receptors may increase synaptic dopamine, stimulating presynaptic DA-autoreceptors that may lead to a negative feedback loop with decreased dopamine synthesis and firing rate.

Antipsychotics also affect other central neurotransmitter systems accounting for the nonmotor side effects. They block alpha-noradrenergic, muscarinic cholinergic, histamine, and serotonin receptors. They also block reuptake of norepinephrine.

EFFICACY

All the antipsychotics, with the exception of promazine and mepazine, have been clearly shown to be superior to placebo in controlling psychotic symptoms and to have comparable efficacy. These medications are effective in controlling the positive psychotic symptoms in about 75% of patients with schizophrenia. Clozapine, an atypical antipsychotic with D4 and serotonin antagonism, is efficacious in about 30% of treatment refractory patients. Several studies have shown clozapine to be superior to the standard antipsychotics haloperidol and chlorpromazine.[34]

POTENCY

The major difference between the antipsychotics is relative potency at the dopamine D2 receptor as well as affinity for muscarinic, acetylcholine, histamine, and alpha-adrenergic receptors. These differences account for the variability in side-effect profiles (Table 6–3).

The agents with highest affinity for the D2 receptor are termed high potency agents. These agents are more likely to affect the motor system and cause extrapyramidal side effects. The low potency agents have relatively higher affinity for the muscarinic, histaminic, and adrenergic receptors and are more likely to cause sedation and orthostatic hypotension. The midpotency agents may be better tolerated by some patients.

CHOICE OF ANTIPSYCHOTIC

Given the similar efficacy of all the antipsychotics, past history and side-effect profile are the two most reliable guides to choosing an agent.

TABLE 6–3. RELATIVE POTENCIES OF NEUROLEPTICS IN CLINICAL USE AND AT DOPAMINERGIC AND MUSCARINIC CHOLINERGIC NEURORECEPTORS

Compound	Compound	Comparable Dose [mg]*	D_2 Affinity**	mACh Affinity[†]	Elimination Half-Life (hours)	Dose Range (mg/day)	Therapeutic Plasma Levels
Phenothiazines							
Chlorpromazine	Thorazine	100	1	330	16–30	40–1000	90–300 nmol/L
Thioridazine	Mellaril	100	0.72	1300	16	200–800	
Mesoridazine	Serentil	75	1	330	16–27	100–400	1–6.8 nmol/L
Trifluoperazine	Stelazine	5	7.2	35	13	15–40	0.6–6 nmol/L
Fluphenazine	Prolixin	2	24	13	13–58	2.5–10	2.4–8 nmol/L
Perphenazine	Trilafon	10	13	16	9–21	16–64	
Thioxanthenes							
Chlorprothixene	Taractan	100	2.5	–	8–12	100–600	
Thiothixene	Navane	3	42	8.1	34	20–60	
Butyrophenones							
Haloperidol	Haldol	2	4.7	1	12–36	1–15	5–24 ng/ml
Droperidola (parenteral only)	Inapsine	1.1	≈6.2		–	≈8	
Diphenylbutylpiperidine							
Pimozide	Orap	2	≈5.3	–	29–55[‡]	1–10	
Dibenzoxapine							
Loxapine	Loxitane	15	0.26	52	8–30	60–250	
Dibenzodiazepine							
Clozapine	Clozaril	50	0.11	2000	5–16	300–900	>350 ng/ml
Dihydroindolone							
Molindone	Moban	15	0.16	0.062	6.5	50–225	
Benzisoxazole							
Risperidone	Risperdal	2	–	–	20–24	2–10	

*Based on D^2 affinity, pharmacokinetics, and clinical considerations

**Expressed as ratios to chlorpromazine

[†] Expressed as ratios to haloperidol

[‡] Half-life longer (mean 66–111 h) in Tourette's syndrome

Adapted from Bezchlibnyk-Butler, K.Z., Jeffreis, J.J., Martin, B.A. (1998). *Clinical Handbook of Phychotropic Drugs*, 8th rev ed. Copyright 1998 by Hogrefe & Huber Publishers, Seattle, Toronto, Bern, Göttingen. Reprinted with permission. Also adapted from Rosenberg, D.R., Holttum, J., Gershon, S. (1994). *Textbook of Pharmacotherapy for Child and Adolescent Psychiatric Disorders*. Philadelphia: Brunner/Mazel. Reprinted with permission.

Prior treatment history should be considered when choosing an antipsychotic agent. A prior treatment response to a particular agent may predict a good response again. If a patient has not been on an antipsychotic before, the response of a family member might guide treatment. If a patient has previously been maintained on a particular agent and has an increase in symptoms, simply increasing the dose of the same medication may be effective. However, if the patient did not respond to a particular medication or had intolerable side effects, a different agent should be tried.

Severe adverse reactions to a particular agent should preclude the use of this and similar agents in the future. For example, if a patient is prone to developing dystonias with haloperidol and fluphenazine (high potency agents), a lower potency antipsychotic is recommended. If the patient has a history of noncompliance with medications and a depot form of treatment is considered for maintenance, acute treatment with the same agent in an oral form is suggested. There is no evidence from controlled clinical trials that symptom profile or schizophrenia subtype predicts response to a particular type of medication.

DOSING

The primary goal of antipsychotic therapy is to provide optimal symptom reduction with the least possible morbidity with the lowest effective dose. McEvoy et al. describes titrating antipsychotic dose rapidly to the neuroleptic threshold, the point at which mild-to-moderate hypokinesia-rigidity first appears on clinical exam.[35,36,37] They suggest starting with haloperidol 2 mg/day and increasing the dose by 2 mg every two days based on daily examinations for hypokinesia-rigidity until the neuroleptic threshold is reached. The median dose at which neuroleptic threshold is crossed is approximately 4 mg/day of haloperidol, which corresponds with haloperidol levels around 5 ng/ml, the lower boundary of the therapeutically effective range. Higher doses do not lead to greater improvement in psychosis.

Patients usually respond to antipsychotic drugs within one to two weeks. Improvement may be seen for up to six to eight weeks after optimal dose is achieved, so an adequate therapeutic trial must be at least this long. Several reports indicate continued improvement up to 12 to 24 weeks after achieving a steady dose, especially with clozapine, and a 6-month trial is recommended with clozapine before declaring nonresponse.[38]

Antipsychotics are lipophilic drugs and demonstrate a wide variability in absorption and metabolism. Therefore, effective dose may be quite variable between patients and the effective dose range is wide. Dose-to-blood-level ratio may vary by 100-fold between individuals.[39]

There is no convincing evidence that rapid loading with very high doses of neuroleptic (i.e., haloperidol 60 mg/day) also known as "rapid neuroleptization," produces a more rapid response than the neuroleptic threshold dosing strategy. But there is considerable evidence that it is associated with an increased risk of side effects, especially dystonias and EPS.

Antipsychotics are best administered in split daily doses initially to minimize the side effects, some of which are most pronounced at peak serum drug levels. However, with prolonged administration, doses may be administered once daily because of the long half-lives of these agents. Bedtime dosing is preferred because of the tendency to produce sedation.

The dose equivalency of different antipsychotic agents is based on potency at D2 receptors. Equivalent doses of antipsychotics are given in Table 6–3.

ROUTE OF ADMINISTRATION

Generally, oral antipsychotic administration is preferred. However, in some situations, parenteral administration of antipsychotics is indicated (i.e., an agitated or aggressive patient). Onset of action is quicker with intramuscular administration (30 minutes versus 90 minutes for oral). Many antipsychotics are also available for intravenous administration but are rarely used for acute treatment. Once the patient is calmed, the antipsychotic should be switched to oral administration for the remainder of acute treatment.

Parenteral administration of depot forms of antipsychotics is not indicated in the acute treatment of psychosis due to the very long half-life and inflexibility of day-to-day dosing. However, these forms are very important in maintenance treatment.

THERAPEUTIC DRUG MONITORING

There is no clear role for therapeutic drug monitoring in routine antipsychotic treatment. Some antipsychotics appear to demonstrate a linear relationship between level and clinical response, but studies are inconsistent and contradictory, and no clear guidelines have been established. Haloperidol demonstrates a curvilinear relationship between serum level and clinical response. The therapeutic window for haloperidol serum level is 5–15 or 24 ng/ml. Serum levels >30 ng/ml are associated with toxic side effects.[40] Many antipsychotics have active metabolites that have not been well characterized, thus complicating the effort to correlate levels with clinical response.

Clozapine levels may be useful in guiding treatment if a subtherapeutic response is obtained on a standard dose or in the event of severe adverse effects. Greater therapeutic response is associated with clozapine plasma levels greater than 350 ng/ml.

Therapeutic drug monitoring may be clinically useful for monitoring antipsychotic therapy in limited situations. Darby et al. advocate the use of serial haloperidol levels in selected cases, including nonresponsive patients, to monitor for toxicity, determine patient compliance, and maximize clinical response by dose adjustment.[40] Monitoring levels may also be useful in cases where potential drug interactions or coexisting medical conditions might alter blood levels and in ethnic and geriatric populations in which drug metabolism is less predictable. Therapeutic serum levels have only been clearly defined for haloperidol and clozapine.

ANTIPSYCHOTICS

Classes of antipsychotics, pharmacodynamics, and guidelines for use are discussed in the maintenance treatment section.

ADJUNCTIVE AGENTS

Monotherapy with antipsychotics alone is not always sufficient to achieve symptom control. Other classes of medications are frequently used in conjunction with antipsychotics to target specific symptoms.[41]

Benzodiazepines have no antipsychotic effect in conventional doses but do exhibit an antipsychotic effect, especially in schizophrenia with paranoia and hallucinations, at high doses.[42] When used in combination with antipsychotics at standard doses, they potentiate the antipsychotic effect in nonresponsive patients. They are also effective with antipsychotics for acute control of agitation and aggression in psychotic patients. The addition of a benzodiazepine may also decrease the incidence of dystonias and akathisia with an antipsychotic and may help alleviate negative symptoms. Benzodiazepines are first-line agents in the acute treatment of catatonia and may even be necessary in maintenance treatment. Lorazepam is preferred because its pharmacokinetic profile allows for rapid absorption, and it may be administered in either an oral or intramuscular form. Clonazepam may also be useful and has the advantage of a longer half-life and need for less frequent dosing. Possible adverse effects include sedation, ataxia, and cognitive impairment as well as paradoxical behavioral disinhibition. There are no studies of benzodiazepines in maintenance treatment.

Lithium, as an adjunct to antipsychotics, has demonstrated efficacy in treatment refractory schizophrenia in three studies with lithium levels maintained in the standard range 0.5–1.3 mEq/L.[43,44,45] Predictors of response to lithium augmentation include presence of affective symptoms, family history of affective disorder, episodic course, increased symptom severity, and psychotic excitement. While there is some risk of toxicity when lithium is coadministered with antipsychotics (phenothiazines increase intracellular lithium concentrations), there does not appear to be an appreciable increase in clinically apparent lithium toxicity when combined with antipsychotics in patients with schizophrenia.[41] No long-term studies of lithium augmentation of antipsychotics have been carried out.

Carbamazepine augmentation of antipsychotics has demonstrated efficacy in schizophrenia with excitement, psychomotor overactivity, aggression, and behavioral dyscontrol and in patients with subclinical temporal lobe electroencephalogram abnormalities.[46] There is no additive toxic effect with antipsychotics. Carbamazepine can lower plasma antipsychotic levels, so it may be valuable to monitor antipsychotic and carbamazepine levels. The traditional therapeutic range of 8–12 mEq/ml should be employed.

Beta-blockers, specifically propranolol, have been used to treat akathisia. There is some controversy over whether they may also be a useful adjunct to antipsychotics in treating psychotic symptoms.[41] Propranolol should be started at 10–20 mg two or three times a day and increased by no more than 40 mg/day in divided doses to a maximum of 120 mg/day. Maintenance treatment has not been studied.

Antidepressants may be useful in treating depressive episodes and depressive symptoms that occur in at least one-quarter of schizophrenics. Tricyclic antidepressants and monoamine oxidase inhibitors have been most frequently studied and are effective in treating depressive symptoms. Care must be taken to rule out antipsychotic-induced akinesia as this does not respond to antidepressants. Negative symptoms may respond when there is some overlap with depression. A full-dose and full-duration antidepressant trial seems to be required for the treatment of primary depression. Adding a TCA or SSRI causes an increase in antipsychotic plasma levels.

NONPHARMACOLOGICAL SOMATIC TREATMENTS

Treatment refractory or life-threatening psychosis may be treated acutely with electroconvulsive therapy, and it is the treatment of choice for catatonia.

MAINTENANCE PHARMACOLOGICAL TREATMENT

The need for maintenance treatment in schizophrenia has long been recognized; many of the early studies in this area were conducted

30 years ago. However, despite a clear understanding of maintenance therapy and widespread use of maintenance treatment in schizophrenia, many patients continue to have multiple recurrences and a downward course of illness.

INDICATIONS FOR MAINTENANCE THERAPY

The majority of patients with schizophrenia have a chronic course marked by cognitive impairment and functional decline punctuated by recurrent acute psychotic episodes. The goal of maintenance treatment is twofold: to prevent or delay the recurrence of active psychotic symptoms and to minimize interepisode dysfunction and distress.

At what point during the course of illness should maintenance therapy be considered? First-break psychotic episodes may resolve completely without any further recurrences or they may herald a recurrent chronic course. Because some first psychotic episodes remain single episodes without recurrences, it is prudent to treat the initial episode for 6 to 12 months to ensure a complete recovery and then attempt an antipsychotic taper to avoid committing a patient to long-term antipsychotic treatment unnecessarily. If psychotic symptoms recur after the antipsychotic is discontinued, then indefinite maintenance antipsychotic treatment is warranted.

Predictors of recurrence and a chronic course include poor premorbid functioning, structural brain abnormalities, insidious onset, residual symptoms after resolution of positive symptoms, longer duration of illness prior to hospitalization, and history of birth complications. When a first-break episode occurs in combination with any of these predictors, maintenance therapy should be considered even after only the first psychotic episode.

DURATION OF MAINTENANCE TREATMENT

The rate of relapse off antipsychotics is about 10% per month, even if the patient is maintained symptom-free on antipsychotics for two to three years.[18] If followed long enough, almost all patients withdrawn from medication relapse at some point. Even patients whose illness seems to have "burned out" relapse an average of five months after discontinuing antipsychotic medication.[47] Therefore, maintenance therapy should be lifelong.

EFFICACY OF MAINTENANCE ANTIPSYCHOTICS

There is considerable evidence supporting the efficacy of antipsychotics in maintenance treatment of schizophrenia. At least 35 randomized, double-blind, placebo-controlled studies have demonstrated significant superiority of antipsychotics over placebo in preventing recurrences.[48]

Effective maintenance treatment may actually improve the natural course of schizophrenia. There is convincing evidence that treatment with antipsychotics or electroconvulsive therapy improves the long-term course of the illness and that lack of definitive therapy early in a psychotic episode is harmful both in the short and long term.[15,49]

PREDICTORS OF RESPONSE

Maintenance antipsychotic treatment is of variable efficacy in different patient subgroups. Patients with good interepisode recovery benefit most from maintenance medication. Those who do least well in acute treatment tend to benefit the least from maintenance treatment. Patients who require lower doses of antipsychotic medications have fewer relapses than those who require higher doses.[50]

CONTINUOUS MAINTENANCE TREATMENT

Continuous maintenance therapy is the standard form of maintenance treatment and involves continuous administration of the same dose of antipsychotic medications as required for acute treatment without drug holidays. This strategy is designed to prevent recurrences of psychotic episodes by maintaining a constant therapeutic level of antipsychotics in the system. There is some morbidity and risk with continuous medication therapy including continuous side effects and increased risk of tardive dyskinesia (TD).

INTERMITTENT OR TARGETED THERAPY

Because of the morbidity and risk of long-term antipsychotic exposure, an intermittent dosing strategy with targeted treatment or early intervention has been studied. With this approach, the antipsychotic medication is withdrawn after a psychotic episode has resolved and the patient is in a stable phase. The patient is then monitored closely for emergence of prodromal symptoms of another episode, and antipsychotic treatment is initiated again at the first sign of relapse. Patients are thus able to remain medication-free for periods of time, thereby decreasing the cumulative antipsychotic exposure and potentially decreasing the risk of developing TD.

Several studies comparing this intermittent or targeted treatment strategy with standard continuous therapy indicate that it is not as successful as the continuous medication strategy; patients in the intermittent dosing groups suffered more recurrences and required more hospitalizations than patients in the continuous treatment groups.[51,52,53,54,55] Therefore, intermittent or targeted treatment is not recommended.

CONTINUOUS LOW DOSE MAINTENANCE THERAPY

Another strategy to decrease the long-term antipsychotic exposure is low dose continuous treatment. The advantage of the low dose maintenance treatment is that there is a lower incidence of adverse effects, including TD, as well as an improved subjective sense of well-being.[56] When this strategy is used, antipsychotic dose should be increased at the earliest sign of symptom exacerbation to try to prevent a full-blown episode and avoid hospitalization. The low dose strategy should not be considered if a minor relapse would be disruptive to the patient's life, when a severe relapse would be likely, or when there is a high likelihood of suicide during a relapse.[33]

Most studies examining the efficacy of this approach found that the relapse rate was higher in the low dose maintenance group than the high dose group, although one study found no significant difference between the low and standard dose groups.[33,57,58,59]

ORAL VERSUS DEPOT MEDICATIONS

Depot antipsychotics are long-acting forms that are administered intramuscularly and provide a constant therapeutic level for several weeks after a single dose. There are two depot preparations available in the United States: haloperidol decanoate and fluphenazine decanoate. These preparations consist of an antipsychotic esterified to the fatty acid decanoate producing a lipophilic compound delivered in an oil via intramuscular injection. The nonactive esterified antipsychotic is then hydrolyzed, slowly releasing the active compound.

Depot antipsychotics are valuable in treating noncompliant patients, because the drug is administered intramuscularly once every two to four weeks. Depot antipsychotics are also valuable for patients who rapidly metabolize oral antipsychotics or who are unable to achieve therapeutic serum levels of drug with usual doses. Metabolism of the decanoate form is independent of the first-pass effect in the liver. Other advantages of depot antipsychotics are less individual variability in bioavailability, better dose-concentration relationship, and more stable plasma concentrations over time.[60]

In some studies, although not all, the relapse rate on depot antipsychotics is less than on comparable doses of the oral agent, suggesting an important role for depot forms in maintenance treatment.[33]

Fluphenazine decanoate and haloperidol decanoate have equal efficacy in preventing relapse. A major difference is half-life; fluphenazine decanoate has a half-life of 14 days requiring dosing every two to three weeks while haloperidol decanoate has a half-life of 21 days requiring dosing only once every three to four weeks. Haloperidol decanoate may cause fewer and less severe adverse effects, including EPS, than fluphenazine decanoate.[61,62,63]

The standard dose of depot antipsychotics is fluphenazine decanoate 25 mg every two weeks and haloperidol decanoate 200 mg every four weeks. Low dose depot maintenance strategies may be associated with an increased relapse rate but have the advantage of lower subjective psychological distress, reduced risk of TD, and slight improvement in social and occupational functioning.[64]

Dosing of decanoate forms is based on the oral dose required for symptom control. The oral form of fluphenazine or haloperidol should be used to treat the acute episode. Once a steady dose of oral medication is achieved, one that is sufficient to adequately control symptoms and is tolerated by the patient, the comparable dose of decanoate can be calculated. The conversion factors for fluphenazine and haloperidol are listed in Table 6–4 and Figure 6–1.[65,66] Because of their long half-lives, it takes months to achieve steady-state of depot preparations, so the oral form must be continued during the crossover and then gradually tapered. A cross-tapering schedule is presented in Table 6–4 and Figure 6–1.

If symptoms emerge during the crossover or at any time during depot therapy, additional oral medication may be added to acutely treat psychotic symptoms. The additional oral dose can then be converted to the decanoate form for maintenance treatment if needed. Because changes in decanoate medications do not have an immediate effect, the oral form can be used to titrate the dose on a daily basis.

The conventional ideal candidate for depot therapy is the patient who responds well acutely to haloperidol or fluphenazine but has repeated psychotic episodes clearly precipitated by noncompliance with medications. Some authors believe that this approach excludes patients who may benefit from long-acting injectables and propose that first-break episodes and patients in the early stages of their illness might also benefit from depot therapy. By offering these patients depot medications early in their illness, repeated episodes may be avoided, which may be protective in the long term and improve the natural course of the illness and overall outcome.

COMPLIANCE

Compliance with medications is a crucial issue, particularly in the treatment of schizophrenia. Because patients with chronic schizophrenia are

text continues on page 211

TABLE 6–4. YADALAM AND SIMPSON CONVERSION SCHEDULE FOR ORAL TO DECANOATE FLUPHENAZINE

Baseline Oral Dose (mg/day)	Week 0		Week 2		Week 4		Week 6		Week 8		Week 10	
	Oral	Decanoate	Oral	Decanoate	Oral	Decanoate	Oral	Decanoate	Oral	Decanoate	Oral	Decanoate
								Dosages (mg)[a]				
5	4.0	6.25	2.5	6.25	1.0	6.25		6.25				
10	7.5	6.25	5.0	6.25	2.5	12.5		12.5				
20	15.0	6.25	10.0	6.25	7.5	12.5	5.0	12.5	2.5	12.5		12.5
30	25.0	6.25	20.0	12.5	15.0	25.0	10.0	25.0	5.0	25.0		25.0
40	30.0	6.25	25.0	12.5	20.0	25.0	15.0	25.0	10.0	25.0		25.0

[a]Oral dosages administered daily; decanoate dosages administered every two weeks.

From Yadalam, K.G., Simpson, G.M. (1998). Changing from oral to depot fluphenazine. *J Clin Psychiatry*, 49(9):347. Copyright 1988 by Physicians Postgraduate Press. Reprinted with permission.

HALDOL Decanoate Conversion Guidelines — HALDOL Decanoate Dose

Current Oral HALDOL Dose	Conversion Factor	Initial Monthly HALDOL Decanoate Dose*	Month 2 Dosing†	Month 3 Dosing†	Maintenance
Up to 5 mg/day†	10-15x daily oral dose	50-75 mg/month	Same once a month. Titrate based on clinical response.	Same once a month. Titrate based on clinical response.	Same once a month. Titrate based on clinical response.
Up to 10 mg/day†	10-15x daily oral dose	100-150 mg/month	Same once a month. Titrate based on clinical response.	Same once a month. Titrate based on clinical response.	Same once a month. Titrate based on clinical response.
15 mg/day‡	20x daily oral dose	300 mg/month	Reduce dose by 25% to 15x the former daily dose to 225 mg. Titrate based on clinical response.	Reduce original dose by 25% to 10x the former daily dose to 150 mg	Same once a month. Titrate based on clinical response.
20 mg/day‡	20x daily oral dose	400 mg/month	Reduce dose by 25% to 15x the former daily dose to 300 mg. Titrate based on clinical response.	Reduce original dose by 25% to 10x the former daily dose to 200 mg	Same once a month. Titrate based on clinical response.

* Initial dose should not exceed 100 mg. Remainder of dose can be administered within 3-7 days.
† Patients who are stabilized on oral doses ≤10 mg/day who are elderly, or who are debilitated, or who are at risk for relapse. See full Prescribing Information attached.
‡ Patients who are maintained on oral doses >10 mg/day who are tolerant of oral medication, or who are at risk for relapse.
Supplementation with oral haloperidol can be used during periods of dose adjustments.
Please see full Prescribing Information attached.

HALDOL® Decanoate 100
(HALOPERIDOL) INJECTION
Extending Protection From Relapse

¹After month 3 based on conversion strategy on reverse side.

Comparison of Monthly Haloperidol Dosage Totals: Oral vs Depot Dosing

Daily Oral HALDOL® (haloperidol) Dose	Monthly Total (30 days)	vs	Approximate Maintenance HALDOL® Decanoate Depot Dose* Monthly Total (30 days)
up to 5 mg/day	up to 150 mg/month	vs	50-75 mg/month
up to 10 mg/day	up to 300 mg/month	vs	100-150 mg/month
15 mg/day	450 mg/month	vs	150 mg/month
20 mg/day	600 mg/month	vs	200 mg/month

Guidelines for Low-, Standard-, and High-Dose Maintenance HALDOL Decanoate Therapy³

Low Dose	Standard Dose	High Dose
50-100 mg/month	200 mg/month	>200 mg/month

FIG. 6–1. Dosing timeline for HALDOL Decanoate, McNEILAB, Inc. Reprinted with permission from Ortho-McNeil Pharmaceutical, Raritan, NJ.

almost assured of relapsing within a few years of discontinuing medications, the importance of continuing maintenance medications is obvious. However, there are many factors that contribute to the high rate of medication noncompliance in this population. Lack of insight into the illness and the need for treatment is a *symptom* of the illness and frequently interferes with efforts to provide treatment. In addition, the antipsychotic medications have many intolerable side effects including sedation, muscle stiffness, tremors, abnormal involuntary movements, and akathisia.

Several studies have attempted to elucidate factors that predict treatment compliance in an effort to enhance compliance. The following factors were identified as predictors of medication compliance after discharge from hospital: belief that the medication helped, stated willingness to take medication after discharge, optimism, absence of akinesia, history of medication compliance, and voluntary admission.[67]

Strategies to improve treatment compliance target knowledge and understanding of the illness and medications. Psychoeducation about schizophrenia for patients and their families is the first step in promoting understanding of symptoms, their etiology, and their treatment. Explaining the potential benefit of the medications in helping with those symptoms that are most distressing is beneficial. When patients are aware of potential side effects, they are more likely to be tolerant of them. Informing patients about the most common side effects of antipsychotics and offering antidotes if needed helps build a trusting relationship with the patient. Establishing a therapeutic alliance is a key ingredient in building patient cooperation with the treatment plan.

DISCONTINUATION OF ANTIPSYCHOTIC MEDICATION

Several studies examining relapse rates after antipsychotic medication discontinuation demonstrate a clear increase in relapse rates of patients off medication. A review of the relevant literature by Davis (1986)[48] and updated by Janicak et al. (1993)[33] convincingly reveals a highly significant difference ($p < 10^{-107}$) between relapse rates off antipsychotics (55%) and on antipsychotics (21%). The duration of remission does not affect relapse rate. The relapse rates are similar whether antipsychotics are discontinued after two months or after two to three years of treatment (Hogarty and Ulrich, 1977)[18]. Therefore, patients should not have their antipsychotics discontinued even after years without acute exacerbation.

ROLE OF PSYCHOSOCIAL TREATMENT

The addition of psychosocial interventions to maintenance antipsychotics not only further decreases the relapse rate over medication alone, but also increases the length of time until relapse and helps improve adjustment and functioning.[19,68,69] Social skills training focuses on helping the patient cope with challenges and problems in daily life and enabling the patient to function with the least possible support from the therapist. Cognitive rehabilitation attempts to improve cognitive function in areas of the brain that are affected by the illness. Family therapy helps maintain a connection between patients and their families by providing families new coping strategies, problem-solving skills, and education about the illness. Group therapy not only helps patients improve social skills, but also provides camaraderie and helps reduce the isolation often caused by the illness.

MANAGEMENT OF ACUTE EXACERBATIONS

PSYCHOSIS

Psychotic symptoms may emerge or worsen during the course of maintenance antipsychotic therapy. While symptom exacerbations do not necessarily lead to relapse, they should nevertheless be treated aggressively. The antipsychotic dose should be increased until the patient returns to baseline. If the patient is on depot medications, an oral dose of the same medication can be added acutely. Additional antiparkinsonian agents may be necessary with the increased antipsychotic dose. If an increase in antipsychotic dose is not sufficient to quell an exacerbation, an adjunctive agent such as lithium, carbamazepine, valproate, or a benzodiazepine might be added.

DEPRESSION

Post-psychotic depression occurs in 25–80% of schizophrenia patients.[70] Depressive symptoms frequently emerge after psychotic symptoms are adequately treated. Syndromal depression may be difficult to differentiate from the negative symptom syndrome or antipsychotic-induced akinesia or EPS. Patients on antipsychotics are significantly more likely to suffer from depression than those not on antipsychotics, and antipsychotic use correlates significantly with anhedonia, guilt, and suicidal tendencies but not with other depressive symptoms.[71] Post-psychotic depression responds to tricyclic antidepressants in the same way that a primary major depressive episode does. However, tricyclic antidepressants are not effective for negative symptoms or anergia.[72] SSRIs, MAOIs, bupropion, and other newer antidepressants have not been well studied.[73]

Maintenance treatment with antidepressants after resolution of depressive symptoms has been reported in one study.[74] The authors conclude that patients who have an initial response to antidepressants should continue treatment indefinitely.[73]

MANIA

Manic episodes can occur in the context of a schizoaffective disorder. Mood stabilizers that are used in primary bipolar disorder are also effective in treating schizophrenia with manic symptomatology. Lithium, carbamazepine, and valproate all have demonstrated efficacy for manic symptoms in schizophrenia.[73] Clozapine, olanzapine, and risperidone may also be efficacious in treating mood-related symptoms in schizophrenia.

ANTIPSYCHOTIC MEDICATIONS AND ANTIPARKINSONIAN AGENTS

Classes of Antipsychotics

Antipsychotics belong to several different classes with different chemical structures. The *phenothiazines* are tricyclic compounds. Different side chains off the nitrogen atom determine the phenothiazine subtype: aliphatic (i.e., chlorpromazine), piperidine (i.e., thioridazine, mesoridazine), or piperazine (i.e., trifluoperazine, fluphenazine, perphenazine). *Thioxanthenes* are very similar to the phenothiazines with the substitution of carbon for nitrogen in the middle of the three rings. Subtypes are aliphatic (i.e., chlorprothixene) or piperazine (i.e., thiothixene). *Butyrophenones* are structurally quite different from the phenothiazines but are pharmacologically similar to the piperazines. Haloperidol is the only example of an antipsychotic in this class, but droperidol, an anesthetic, also has some antipsychotic properties. The *diphenylbutylpiperidines* are similar to the butyrophenones. Pimozide is the only available representative of this class in the United States. *Dibenzoxazepines* are also tricyclic compounds and are represented by loxapine. The atypical *dibenzodiazepine* clozapine is structurally similar. The *dihydroindolones*, represented by molindone, are structurally quite different from the others (Figure 6–2). Newer atypicals include Risperidone, Olanzapine, and Quetiapine. Available preparations and costs are given in Table 6–5.

PHARMACOKINETICS/PHARMACODYNAMICS

Despite the structural differences, there are several pharmacokinetic factors that the antipsychotics share, although there is some variability between agents. They are well absorbed from the gastrointestinal tract with peak plasma levels achieved 0.5–6 hours after oral administration. Many are also available in injectable forms. Parenteral administration results in

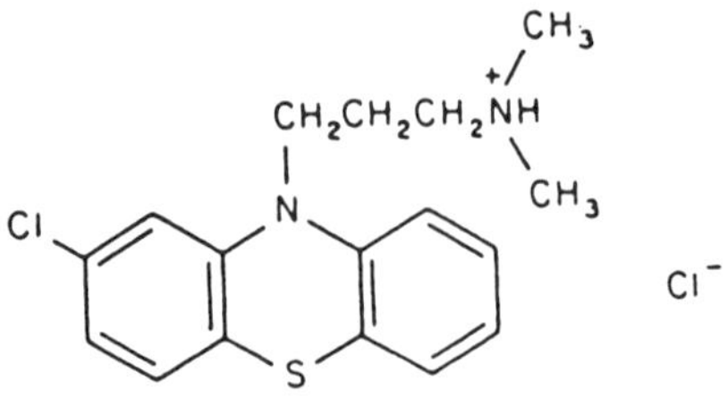

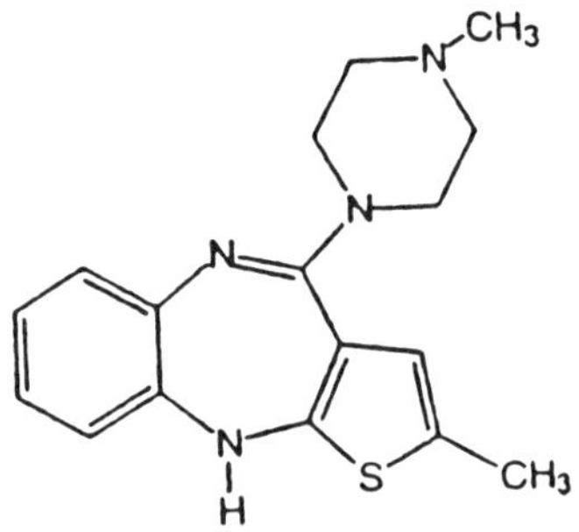

chlorpromazine

olanzapine

FIG. 6–2. *Sample of chemical structures from major neuroleptic classes.*

more reliable, quick, and efficient absorption. Blood levels achieved after a single dose (oral or parenteral) can be quite variable between individuals. These agents are highly lipophilic (except thioridazine and its metabolite mesoridazine) and cross the blood-brain barrier as well as the placental membrane and are also secreted into breast milk. With the exception of mesoridazine, antipsychotics are highly protein bound.

Half-lives of most antipsychotics are in the 10–20 hour range with a few exceptions: molindone has a half-life of 1.5 hours, loxapine has a half-life of 3.4 hours but active metabolites with 9-hour and 30-hour half-lives, and risperidone has a half-life of 3 hours in rapid metabolizers. Many antipsychotics have active metabolites, although for most agents these have not been well characterized. Nevertheless, the onset of action outlasts the half-life of the parent compound, so single daily dosing is usually sufficient. With chronic use, biological and clinical effects can last for months.

Antipsychotics are metabolized in the liver by the microsomal P450 system. Different agents are metabolized by different subtypes of the microsomal enzymes and some inhibit these enzyme systems. This is discussed in more detail in the section on drug-drug interactions. Antipsychotic metabolites are finally excreted in the urine.

TABLE 6–5. AVERAGE COST AND AVAILABLE PREPARATIONS OF ANTIPSYCHOTIC DRUGS

Drug	Trade Name	Enteral Preparations	Injectable	Generic	Average Dose/Day	Average Cost/Day
Chlorpromazine	Thorazine	Tablet: 10, 25, 50, 100, 200 mg; Concentrate: 30, 100 mg/ml	Yes	Yes	400 mg	($0.36)*
Chlorprothixene	Taractan	Tablet: 10, 25, 50, 100 mg	Yes	No	100 mg	$—
Clozapine	Clozaril	Tablet: 25, 100 mg	No	No	300 mg	$12.12
Droperidol**	Inapsine	Injectable: 2.5 mg/ml	No	No	2.5 mg	N/A
Fluphenazine	Prolixin	Tablet: 1, 2.5, 5, 10 mg; Concentrate: 5 mg/ml	No	Yes	5 mg	($0.70)
Haloperidol	Haldol	Tablet: 0.5, 1, 2, 5, 10, 20 mg; Concentrate: 2 mg/ml	Yes	Yes	6 mg	$3.02 ($0.08)
Loxapine	Loxitane	Capsules: 5, 10, 25, 50 mg	Yes	Yes	100 mg	($2.42)
Mesoridazine	Serentil	Tablet: 10, 25, 50, 100 mg; Concentrate: 25 mg/ml	Yes	No	100 mg	$1.10
Molindone	Moban	Tablet: 5, 10, 25, 50, 100 mg; Concentrate: 20 mg/ml	No	No	100 mg	$2.55
Olanzapine	Zyprexa	Tablet: 5, 7.5, 10 mg	No	No	10 mg	$8.19
Perphenazine	Trilafon	Tablet: 2, 4, 8, 16 mg	Yes	Yes	16 mg	($1.01)
Pimozide***	Orap	Tablet: 2 mg	No	No	2 mg	$0.17
Risperidone	Risperdal	Tablet: 1, 2, 3, 4 mg	No	No	6 mg	$7.90
Thioridazine	Mellaril	Tablet: 10, 15, 25, 50, 100, 150, 200 mg; Concentrate: 30, 100 mg/ml	No	Yes	200 mg	$1.20 ($0.16)
Thiothixene	Navane	Capsules: 1, 2, 5, 10, 20 mg; Concentrate: 5 mg/ml	Yes	Yes	20 mg	($0.54)
Trifluoperazine	Stelazine	Tablet: 1, 2, 5, 10 mg; Concentrate: 10 mg/ml	Yes	No	20 mg	$3.58 ($1.14)

For comparison, all average doses are the lowest effective *adult* maintenance dose reported by the manufacturer for hospitalized psychotic patients. Cost is based on bid dosing (unless otherwise indicated) at the average wholesale price and availability reported by Medi-Span for April 1996.

*Cost of generics.

**For sedation—not approved for psychiatric indications.

***For Tourette's disorder—-not approved for psychosis.

Adapted from Bezchlibnyk-Butler, K.Z., Jeffreis, J.J., Martin, B.A. (1998). *Clinical Handbook of Psychotropic Drugs*, 8th rev. ed. Copyright 1998 by Hogrefe & Huber Publishers, Seattle, Toronto, Bern, Göttingen. Reprinted with permission.

[215]

ADVERSE EFFECTS AND THEIR MANAGEMENT

EXTRAPYRAMIDAL SIDE EFFECTS

The extrapyramidal side effects (EPS) caused by antipsychotics are a result of D2 blockade in the nigrostriatal system and are more common with the high potency agents. They include acute dystonias, akathisia, pseudoparkinsonism, pisa syndrome, and rabbit syndrome.

Acute dystonic reactions are involuntary muscle contractions that typically occur within the first week of initiating antipsychotic therapy. Symptoms are episodic and recurrent, lasting minutes to hours. They frequently involve muscles of the mouth, jaw, face, and neck. The tongue may swell causing swallowing difficulties. There may be trismus (lock-jaw) or opisthotonus (neck spasms with neck hyperextension). An oculogyric crisis is a painful dystonic reaction of the extraocular muscles presenting with a fixed gaze. Acute dystonic reactions may be very frightening and uncomfortable or even painful but are not usually dangerous. However, muscular dystonias may be so severe as to cause joint dislocations. The only life-threatening dystonic reactions are laryngeal and diaphragmatic dystonia that can result in respiratory compromise.

Young males are at highest risk for developing acute dystonic reactions, and they occur more commonly with high potency antipsychotics than low potency ones. Hypocalcemia has also been associated with the development of dystonic reactions and may be a risk factor.

Treatment with an anticholinergic or antihistaminergic agent or a benzodiazepine is effective. Parenteral administration is preferred due to the rapid onset of action; intravenous administration is preferable to intramuscular. Antidotes include benztropine (Cogentin) 1–2 mg, biperiden (Akineton) 2 mg, diphenhydramine (Benadryl) 50 mg, or lorazepam (Ativan) 1–2 mg. If there is no effect in 20 minutes, a repeat injection is indicated: Shorter intervals are acceptable in the case of laryngeal or diaphragmatic dystonia.

Following immediate relief, one of these agents should be started in a regular oral dosing regimen at the lowest possible dose to prevent future occurrences. Treatment may be tapered and discontinued within a few weeks since dystonias rarely occur after the initial period. Prophylaxis against dystonia may be started concomitantly with the antipsychotic in patients at high risk for dystonia (i.e., young men on haloperidol) for two weeks.

Akathisia is an intense subjective feeling of internal restlessness and a compulsion to be in motion. Patients frequently appear restless, pace endlessly, fidget, and are unable to sit or lie still. Patients describe this feeling as a need to keep moving or feeling like "jumping out of my skin" and appear to be in subjective distress. Akathisia is more common with high potency agents and usually occurs early in the course of antipsychotic treatment (within 10 days), although it may emerge after several months. This side effect may wane but is chronic in some patients. It may be confused with psychotic agitation but may be differentiated by the feeling of distress it causes the patient.

Treatment involves decreasing the antipsychotic dose if possible or switching to a lower potency agent. Unfortunately, akathisia does not respond as well to the antiparkinsonian drugs (see next section) as do the other extrapyramidal side effects. Beta-blockers such as propranolol (Inderal) are safe and effective for akathisia in doses of 10–40 mg tid. Benzodiazepines may also be effective. High caffeine intake and low iron may be associated with akathisia; if iron levels are low, supplementation may be beneficial.

Antipsychotic-induced parkinsonism resembles idiopathic Parkinson's disease and is characterized by bradykinesia, rigidity, and tremor. These side effects usually emerge after several weeks to months of treatment and are more common in women and the elderly. The most prominent sign of drug-induced parkinsonism is bradykinesia (slowness of motion). Patients adopt a flexed, stooped posture, walk with a wide-based, festinating gait with small rapid steps, have difficulty initiating movement, and turn on a small radius. They frequently have masked facies and decreased eye blinking. These signs may be easily confused with depression or with the negative symptoms of schizophrenia.

Rigidity is an increase in muscle tone that is detected by passive manipulation of the joints. To examine for rigidity, also known as "cogwheeling" in this population, have the patient sit quietly and passively while the clinician moves the arm. With thumb on the biceps tendon at the elbow, the clinician grasps the hand and manipulates the wrist and elbow while feeling for rigidity or cogwheeling. To accentuate this finding, have the patient move the contralateral hand in a repetitive alternating motion (as if screwing in a light bulb); this enhances the cogwheel rigidity and increases the sensitivity of the exam.

The tremor is a rhythmic oscillation of four to eight cycles per second. It typically involves the hands and has a characteristic "pill-rolling" appearance. It may also affect other body parts and is worse at rest. In drug-induced parkinsonism, the tremor is usually bilateral and occurs later in the course of treatment, whereas in Parkinson's disease, tremor is an early sign and is initially unilateral.

The pharmacological aim of treatment of EPS is to decrease dopamine blockade in the nigrostriatal pathway by either directly decreasing dopamine antagonism (decreasing antipsychotic dose or switching to a lower potency agent), potentiating dopamine transmission (adding dopamine agonists), or decreasing acetylcholine or histamine activity (adding antiparkinsonian agents). The agents with anticholinergic and antihistaminic properties are benztropine (Cogentin), diphenhydramine (Benadryl), and ethopropazine (Parsidol). Orphenadrine (Norflex) is only antihistaminic. Pure anticholinergic agents are biperiden (Akineton), procyclidine (Kemadrin), and trihexyphenidyl (Artane). The anticholinergic agents can produce cognitive side effects such as impairment of memory, time perception, and cognition. These agents also have the potential for abuse, particularly trihexyphenidyl (Artane). Amantadine (Symmetrel) is a dopamine agonist without anticholinergic properties and may be better tolerated by patients who are sensitive to anticholinergic effects. Because amantadine is a dopamine agonist, it has the potential to exacerbate psychosis. These agents are frequently dosed twice daily (Table 6–6).

Prophylaxis with antiparkinsonian agents is controversial. Concurrent administration of anticholinergics with antipsychotics during initiation of treatment significantly decreases the incidence of EPS.[75,76,77] Prophylaxis is most effective for dystonia in young male patients during the first four days of antipsychotic therapy, akathisia in females, and with high potency agents. However, anticholinergic prophylaxis is only partially effective against EPS. The disadvantage of prophylaxis is that patients are exposed to additional medications that may be unnecessary and have their own adverse effects and morbidity.

Extended prophylaxis with antiparkinsonian agents may be unnecessary.[78] After three months of treatment with an antiparkinsonian agent, it should be slowly tapered and stopped if possible. If EPS recur, the antiparkinsonian agent should be restarted with periodic attempts at reduction and discontinuation.[33]

The Pisa syndrome is also a late developing adverse effect and consists of leaning to one side. The "rabbit syndrome" is a repetitive tremor of the mouth resembling a rabbit's facial movements and develops usually after months of antipsychotic therapy. Both respond to antiparkinsonian drugs.

TARDIVE DYSKINESIA

Tardive dyskinesia (TD) is characterized by abnormal involuntary choreoathetoid movements of the face, mouth, tongue, extremities, or trunk. It usually begins with orobuccolingual movements such as lip smacking, puckering of the lips, tongue protrusion, cheek puffing, and chewing. An early sign is wormlike movements of the tongue. Other facial movements include grimacing, frowning, and blinking. These symptoms cause a variable degree of distress to the patient. In severe cases, the movements can result in profound functional impairment. TD may even interfere with breathing and swallowing. Symptoms are exacerbated by stress and disappear in sleep.

TABLE 6–6. ANTIPARKINSONIAN AGENTS

Antiparkinsonian Agent	Usual Dose	Therapeutic Effect					Adverse Effect
		Tremor	Rigidity	Dystonia	Akathisia		
Dopamine-releasing agent							
Amantadine (Symmetrel)	100 mg qd tid	+ +	+ +	+ +	+ +		Indigestion, nervous excitement, poor concentration, dizziness
Anticholinergic							
Benztropine (Cogentin)	1–2 mg qd tid	+ +	+ + +	+ + +	+ +		Dry mouth, blurred vision, urinary retention, constipation, delirium
Biperiden (Akineton)	2 mg qd	+ +	+ +	+ +	+ +		Same as benztropine, plus euphoria, increased tremor
Trihexyphenidyl (Artane)	5 mg qd	+ +	+ +	+ +	+ +		Dry mouth, blurred vision, GI distress, confusion/delirium, euphoria
Anticholinergic antihistamine							
diphenhydramine (Benadryl)	20–50 mg qid	+ +	+ +	+ +	+ + +		Somnolence, confusion
Benzodiazepines							
Clonazepam (Klonopin)	0.5–2 mg qd bid	–	+	+	+ + +		Drowsiness, lethargy
Lorazepam (Ativan)	1–2 mg qd qid	+	+	+ + +	+ + +		Drowsiness, lethargy
Beta-Blockers							
Propranolol (Inderal)	10–40 mg tid	+	–	–	+ + +		Monitor pulse and blood pressure; risk of rebound tachycardia with abrupt discontinuation

Adapted from Bezchlibnyk-Butler, K.Z., Jeffreis, J.J., Martin, B.A. (1998). *Clinical Handbook of Psychotropic Drugs*, 8th rev. ed. Copyright 1998 by Hogrefe & Huber Publishers, Seattle, Toronto, Bern, Göttingen. Reprinted with permission.

TD is a late side effect of chronic antipsychotic use, usually occurring after years of antipsychotic administration.[79] However, in some cases, it may begin after only three to six months of continuous antipsychotic exposure. Studies suggest that cumulative antipsychotic dose is linked to the development of TD. Approximately 20–30% of patients maintained on antipsychotic medication develop TD with an incidence rate estimated at 4% per year of patient exposure for at least the first five years.[80] Both high and low potency agents have been associated with TD. Clozapine has not been associated with TD and may, in fact, be an effective treatment. Antiparkinsonian agents may increase the risk for TD and aggravate symptoms. Patients with primary mood disorders seem to be at higher risk for developing TD than patients with schizophrenia. The elderly are also at higher risk for developing TD and are less likely to have complete resolution of symptoms with antipsychotic discontinuation.[81,82] There is also a significantly higher prevalence of TD accompanied by more severe symptoms in women.[83]

The pathophysiological mechanism for TD is not completely understood. A "dopamine excess" hypothesis has been proposed whereby chronic dopamine blockade in the nigrostriatal pathway results in up-regulation of postsynaptic dopamine receptors, leading to supersensitivity to dopamine. This proposed mechanism seems too simplistic and is not consistent with all the evidence. There is likely some contribution from other neurotransmitter systems including GABA, acetylcholine, and norepinephrine.

TD may appear or worsen when the antipsychotic dose is decreased and may actually improve in the short term when the dose is increased. Withdrawal dyskinesias may occur with a decrease or discontinuation of antipsychotic drug, but these are time-limited and resolve within days to weeks. TD is persistent and irreversible in some patients; however, evidence suggests that early detection and antipsychotic discontinuation may improve the movements of TD.[84,85]

Prevention of TD involves avoiding unnecessary exposure to antipsychotics by using the lowest effective doses to keep cumulative lifetime exposure to a minimum. When patients are exposed to maintenance antipsychotic treatment, early detection of abnormal movements is critical. This may be accomplished by routine biannual neurological examination or administration of a standardized examination and rating scale for TD, such as the Abnormal Involuntary Movement Scale (AIMS) shown in Figure 6–3.

When abnormal movements are detected, other extrapyramidal pathology should be ruled out such as Huntington's disease or Wilson's disease. See Table 6–7 for a differential diagnosis of TD.

Increasing the antipsychotic dose produces a temporary relief from TD but increases the chance of producing irreversible changes. Withdrawing the antipsychotic is the best treatment alternative from the standpoint of

TABLE 6–7. TARDIVE DYSKINESIA: DIFFERENTIAL DIAGNSOSIS

Dyskinesias on withdrawal from neuroleptic medication
Schizophrenic stereotypies and mannerisms
Spontaneous oral dyskinesias associated with aging (including Meige syndrome)*
Oral dyskinesias related to dental conditions or protheses**
Torsion dystonia
Idiopathic focal dystonia (oral mandibular dystonia, blepharospasm, spasmodic
  "habit spasms" [tics])
Huntington's disease***
Wilson's disease
Magnesium and other heavy metal
Fahr's syndrome or other disorders with calcification of the basal ganglia
Extrapyramidal syndromes following anoxia or encephalitis
Rheumatic (Sydenham's) chorea
Drug intoxications—L-dopa, amphetamines, anticholinergics, antidepressants,
  lithium, phenytoin
CNS complications of systemic metabolic disorders (e.g., hepatic or renal
  failure, hyperthyroidism, hypoparathyroidism, hypoglycemia, vasculitides)
Brain neoplasms (thalamic, basal ganglia)

*Meige syndrome is a disorder of middle age characterized by progressive oral, lingual, and buccal dystonia together with blepharospasm. The movements are indistinguishable from those of tardive dyskinesia, but patients with Meige syndrome need not have had antedating antipsychotic drug exposure, and Meige syndrome is a progressive disorder.
**Be sure to ask patients about the state of their mouth and teeth and whether they have any gum in their mouth when you are examining them for tardive dyskinesia.
***The abnormal movements of Huntington's disease are primarily chorea with little dystonia or athetosis. The movements are generalized, producing a "fidgety" appearance in the early stages. Although movements of tardive dyskinesia are more stereotyped and abnormal, the movements of Huntington's disease appear to be normal movements at an increased frequency. Patients with tardive dyskinesia have dyskinesias other than chorea. In general, patients with Huntington's disease have more trouble keeping their tongues out of their mouth, whereas tardive dyskinesia patients may have trouble keeping their tongues in their mouths.
From Gelenberg, A.J., Bassuk, E.L., Schoonover, S.C. (1991) *The Practitioner's Guide to Psychoactive Drugs*, 3rd ed. (p. 150). Copyright 1991 by Plenum Publishing Corp. Reprinted with permission.

TD. However, for patients with chronic schizophrenia, the risk of being off the antipsychotic is almost certain recurrence of a psychotic episode, which may have more dire consequences than the TD itself. When faced with this choice, patients and their families usually prefer to continue antipsychotic therapy. The antipsychotic should then be reduced to the lowest possible dose, anticipating that the TD will worsen temporarily.

Several strategies have been investigated to reduce the severity of the abnormal movements and to alleviate the discomfort. Benzodiazepines (i.e.,

text continues on page 226

ABNORMAL INVOLUNTARY MOVEMENT SCALE (AIMS)

Instructions: Complete Examination Procedure (reverse side) before making ratings.

Movement Ratings: Rate the highest severity observed.

Code:
0 = None
1 = Minimal, may be extreme normal
2 = Mild
3 = Moderate
4 = Severe

			(Circle One)			
Facial and Oral Movements:	1.	**Muscles of Facial Expression:** e.g., movements of forehead, eyebrows, periorbital area, cheeks; include frowning, blinking, smiling, grimacing	0	1	2	3	4
	2.	**Lips and Perioral Area:** e.g., puckering, pouting, smacking	0	1	2	3	4
	3.	**Jaw:** e.g., biting, clenching, chewing, mouth opening, lateral movement	0	1	2	3	4
	4.	**Tongue:** Rate only increase in movement both in and out of mouth NOT inability to sustain movement	0	1	2	3	4
Extremity Movements:	5.	**Upper:** (arms, wrists, hands, fingers): Include choreic movements, (i.e., rapid, objectively purposeless, irregular, spontaneous), athenoid movements (i.e., slow, irregular complex, serpentine). Do NOT include tremor (i.e., repetitive, regular, rhythmic)	0	1	2	3	4
	6.	**Lower (legs, knees, ankles, toes):** e.g., lateral knee movement, foot taping, heel dropping, foot squirming, inversion and eversion of foot	0	1	2	3	4

FIG. 6–3. Abnormal involuntary movement scale (AIMS). From Marsden, C. D., (1981). Br J Clin Pharm, 11:129–151. Copyright 1981 by Blackwell Science. Reprinted with permission.

		0	1	2	3	4
Trunk Movements:	7. Neck, shoulders hips: e.g., rocking, twisting, squirming, pelvic gyrations					
Global Judgements:	8. Severity of abnormal movements:			None, normal 0 / Minimal 1 / Mild 2 / Moderate 3 / Severe 4		
	9. Incapacitation due to abnormal movements:			None, normal 0 / Minimal 1 / Mild 2 / Moderate 3 / Severe 4		
	10. Patient's awareness of abnormal movements: Rate only patient's report	No awareness 0 / Aware, no distress 1 / Aware, mild distress 2 / Aware, moderate distress 3 / Aware, severe distress 4				
Dental Status:	11. Current problems with teeth and/or dentures:			No 0 / Yes 1		
	12. Does patient usually wear dentures?:			No 0 / Yes 1		

FIG. 6–3. Continued.

223

Either before or after completing the Examination Procedure observe the patient unobtrusively, at rest (e.g., in waiting room).

The chair to be used in this examination should be a hard, firm one without arms.

1. Ask the patient whether there is anything in his/her mouth. (i.e., gum, candy, etc.) and if there is, to remove it.

2. Ask patient about the current condition of his/her teeth. Ask patient if he/she wears dentures. Do teeth or dentures bother patient now?

3. Ask patient whether he/she notices any movements in mouth, face, hands, or feet. If yes, ask to describe and to what extent they currently bother patient or interfere with his/her activities.

4. Have patient sit in chair with hands on knees, legs slightly apart, and feet flat on floor. (Look at entire body for movements while in this position).

5. Ask patient to sit with hands hanging unsupported. If male, between legs, if female and wearing a dress, hanging over knees. (Observe hands and other body areas.)

6. Ask patient to protrude tongue. (Observe abnormalities of tongue movement.) Do this twice.

*7. Ask patient to tap thumb, with each finger, as rapidly as possible for 10-15 seconds; separately with right hand, then with left hand. (Observe facial and leg movements.)

8. Flex and extend patient's left and right arms (one at a time.) (Note any rigidity and rate on DOTES.)

9. Ask patient to stand up. (Observe in profile. Observe all body areas again, hips included.)

*10. Ask patient to extend both arms outstretched in front with palms down. (Observe trunk, legs, and mouth.)

*11. Have patient walk a few paces, turn, and walk back to chair. (Observe hands and gait.) Do this twice.

FIG. 6-3. Continued.

*Activated movements

Examiner's Comments: _____

_____

_____

_____

_____

_____

_____

_____

_____

_____

BACKER TO 2003-0000

FIG. 6–3. Continued.

clonazepam) may help some patients, possibly by increasing GABA-ergic activity. Stopping anticholinergic agents may help, although parkinsonian symptoms may worsen. Cholinergic agonists have been tried with disappointing results. High dose buspirone has been suggested. Switching to clozapine, an atypical antipsychotic, may actually improve the abnormal movements without increasing the long-term risk of irreversible TD that is inherent with increasing antipsychotic dose.

The hypothesized mechanism for TD is neurotoxic damage due to free radical formation. Vitamin E (alpha-tocopherol) is an antioxidant and has been postulated to protect membranes by its ability to decrease free radicals. Vitamin E has been studied in several well-controlled studies in patients with TD with mixed results.[86,87,88,89,90,91] The evidence suggests that vitamin E is effective in decreasing TD, especially in patients who have had it for five years or less.[91] Vitamin E may also have prophylactic benefit against TD, although this has not been systematically studied.

Patients should be informed about the risk of TD and give informed consent prior to starting antipsychotic therapy. They should also be reminded of the risk periodically during maintenance therapy.

TARDIVE DYSTONIA

Tardive dystonia appears late in antipsychotic therapy and may persist even after antipsychotic discontinuation. Tardive dystonia is less common than TD with a prevalence of 1–2%.[92] Tardive dystonia is characterized by slow, sustained involuntary twisting movements of the face (including blepharospasm), neck, extremities, or trunk. Anticholinergic agents are beneficial.

Temperature regulation in the hypothalamus may be impaired leaving patients more susceptible to hypothermia or hyperthermia. Transient temperature elevation occurs during the first three weeks of clozapine treatment in about half of the patients.

NEUROLEPTIC MALIGNANT SYNDROME

The neuroleptic malignant syndrome (NMS) is characterized by fever (often greater than 40°C), severe muscular rigidity, autonomic instability, and stupor. Physical exam is notable for tachycardia, tachypnea, hyperthermia, labile blood pressure, diaphoresis, and "lead-pipe" rigidity. Laboratory findings include leukocytosis, frequently with a left shift, markedly elevated serum creatine phosphokinase (CPK), and elevated hepatic transaminases and lactate dehydrogenase (LDH). It can lead to renal impairment and respiratory distress and is fatal in 20% of patients if untreated. It typically occurs within two weeks of initiating antipsychotic therapy, develops rapidly over 24–48 hours, and may last one to two weeks. It is more common with high potency agents with rapidly increased doses. Other risk factors include dehydration, agitation, and concurrent psychotropics, particularly lithium. Young males are most susceptible. The incidence of NMS is less than 1% of patients exposed to antipsychotics.[93]

The differential diagnosis includes malignant hyperthermia, psychomotor agitation, excited (lethal) catatonia, heat stroke, tetanus, viral encephalitis, and other infections.

Treatment involves immediate discontinuation of the offending antipsychotic agent and supportive measures in an intensive care unit including cooling blankets, ice packs, or ice-water enemas. Dopamine agonists such as dantrolene (Dantrium), bromocriptine, and amantadine reverse the dopamine antagonism that causes NMS.[33] Dantrolene is started at 2–3 mg/kg over 10–15 minutes with usual effective dose range of 0.8–10 mg/kg/day. Total dose should not exceed 10 mg/kg/day. Bromocriptine is dosed at 2.5–10 mg three times daily up to 60 mg/day. Dantrolene and bromocriptine may be given concomitantly at similar doses. Amantadine is given 200–400 mg/day divided twice daily. The mortality rate with treatment is about 10%.[94]

When a patient has a history of NMS, nonantipsychotic treatment strategies are preferable. If antipsychotics must be used, extreme caution should be exercised when initiating treatment. If the diagnosis of NMS is certain, the same antipsychotic should never be used again. A lower potency agent, preferably from a different family, should be tried. The new antipsychotic should not be started until at least two weeks after resolution of NMS symptoms, and titration should be slow and in a hospital setting.

Clozapine is a good alternative agent although a few cases of NMS have been reported.[95,96,97] Concomitant administration of benzodiazepines to decrease the antipsychotic dose along with bromocriptine for several weeks have been recommended when restarting an antipsychotic after NMS.[33]

Weight gain is another hypothalamus-mediated side effect that is more common with low potency drugs and results from a direct control of appetite. Molindone (Moban) has been associated with less weight gain than other antipsychotics.[98]

Sedation is common, particularly with initiation of antipsychotics or with dose increases. Tolerance usually develops. It is more common with the low potency agents and may be alleviated by giving the entire dose at bedtime.

SEIZURES

Antipsychotics, particularly the low potency agents, lower the seizure threshold and may precipitate seizures. This effect is dose-dependent and occurs more often with rapid dose increases. Patients at increased risk for developing seizures on antipsychotic therapy are those who already have seizure disorder or have other concomitant causes of decreased seizure threshold such as sedative-hypnotic or alcohol withdrawal or presence of another drug that also lowers the threshold. The risk of seizures with clozapine is 1–2% at doses less than 300 mg/day, 3–4% at 300–600 mg/day, and 5% on doses over 600 mg/day.

ANTICHOLINERGIC EFFECTS

The low potency agents are more likely to cause anticholinergic side effects than the high potency agents. Clozapine and thioridazine, in particular, are strongly anticholinergic. Central anticholinergic effects include confusion, impaired memory, and delirium. Peripheral anticholinergic effects include dry eyes, impaired visual accommodation, increased intraocular pressure, dry mouth, dry, warm flushing skin, drying of pulmonary secretions, tachycardia, constipation, urinary hesitancy, and delayed or retrograde ejaculation. Tolerance to these effects may develop over time, and anticholinergic rebound may be experienced with antipsychotic discontinuation. See Chapter 4 for a detailed discussion of anticholinergic side effects and their treatment.

Caution should be taken when using anticholinergic antiparkinsonian agents in patients who are on low potency antipsychotics since the anticholinergic effects may be additive between the two agents.

CARDIOVASCULAR EFFECTS

Orthostatic hypotension is also more common with the low potency agents, such as chlorpromazine and clozapine. It may be more pronounced in the elderly or in patients with preexisting orthostasis or dehydration. It is a dose-related phenomenon and is usually most prominent early in treatment. Because tolerance develops, beginning with low doses followed by slow titration may decrease the potential adverse effects. Supine and standing blood pressure should be monitored at the beginning of treatment, particularly with low potency agents. See Chapter 4 for a detailed discussion of treatment options.

Hypotension may occur with the initiation of clozapine or risperidone and with parenteral antipsychotic use. Epinephrine should not be used as it may lower blood pressure when used concomitantly with antipsychotics; phenylephrine should be used instead.

Cardiac conduction abnormalities may develop with antipsychotic therapy. Many antipsychotics are potentially cardiotoxic. Cardiac conduction effects range from benign changes in the electrocardiogram (inverted, flattened, or broadened T-waves), to conduction defects (prolongation of the QT and PR intervals and T-wave), depression of the ST segment, to cardiac arrhythmias including torsades de pointes. Again, the low potency agents tend to be more cardiotoxic. Coadministration of low potency antipsychotics and tricyclic antidepressants may produce additive cardiac effects and should be avoided or instituted cautiously.

HEMATOLOGICAL EFFECTS

Low potency agents may produce a transient leukopenia (WBC < $3500/mm^3$) or granulocytopenia (absolute neutrophil count [ANC] < $1500/mm^3$) due to toxicity to granulocyte stem cells. This phenomenon is of little clinical significance and only rarely leads to **agranulocytosis** (ANC < $500/mm^3$). The risk of agranulocytosis with chlorpromazine is about 1 in 3,000 or 4,000. Other possible hematological reactions to phenothiazines include thrombocytopenia, nonthrombocytopenic purpura, hemolytic anemia, and pancytopenia, necessitating a switch to an antipsychotic from a different chemical family.

Clozapine is associated with a 1% risk of agranulocytosis. The majority of cases develop within 5–25 weeks of initiation of therapy, almost all within 6 to 12 months. However, a few isolated cases of agranulocytosis have occurred after one year of treatment with clozapine. Because of the risk of agranulocytosis, weekly WBC counts must be obtained for 6 months and then every 2 weeks indefinitely while on clozapine. Early signs include sore throat, fever, oral ulcers, and weakness. Patients should be instructed to notify their physician immediately if they notice these or any other early signs of infection. Risk factors for development of agranulocytosis include female gender and increasing age.

If the WBC count falls below $5000/mm^3$, counts should be repeated three times per week. If WBC < 3500 and/or ANC < 1500, clozapine should be discontinued immediately. If WBC < 1000 or ANC < 500, the patient should be placed in reverse isolation. Clozapine should never be restarted in a patient whose ANC has been less than 500. WBC should be monitored weekly until counts return to normal.

Treatment of agranulocytosis involves reverse isolation to decrease the possibility of infection, aggressive treatment of any infection, and granulocyte colony stimulating factor. The mortality from agranulocytosis with infection is 40% and without infection is 15%.

HEPATIC EFFECTS

Some reports of cholestatic jaundice have been associated with low potency antipsychotic use, and the majority of reported cases have occurred in conjunction with chlorpromazine use. This is a hypersensitivity reaction and usually begins within weeks of initiating treatment. It is characterized by evidence of cholestasis (increased direct:indirect bilirubin ratio, increased alkaline phosphatase), elevated transaminases, absence of hepatomegaly, and eosinophilia. Discontinuing the medication produces complete recovery in a few weeks with the rare exception of the development of exanthematous biliary cirrhosis with a more chronic course that usually also eventually clears.

Since antipsychotics are metabolized in the liver by the cytochrome P450 system, hepatic impairment may result in decreased metabolism with increased accumulation of the antipsychotic compound and its active metabolites.

ENDOCRINE EFFECTS

Hyperprolactinemia may occur with antipsychotic administration due to decreased dopaminergic inhibition of prolactin release from the anterior pituitary. This may result in galactorrhea (more commonly in females but also rarely in males), gynecomastia in males and breast engorgement in females, amenorrhea (in women), and decreased libido (in both sexes). These side effects rarely require treatment, but they respond to dose reduction or switching to a different antipsychotic. Bromocriptine or amantadine may alleviate hyperprolactinemia and the associated symptoms.

Antipsychotics decrease testosterone levels that may also contribute to decreased libido. False-positive pregnancy tests have been reported.

Glucose-tolerance and insulin release may be altered by some antipsychotics, particularly the lower potency agents. Diabetes signs and symptoms may develop, and patients with diabetes may find their glucose more difficult to control.

DERMATOLOGICAL EFFECTS

An allergic rash may develop to an antipsychotic, usually between 2–10 weeks after initial exposure. Discontinuing the medication usually produces a complete recovery.

Low potency antipsychotics may increase photosensitivity and predispose to sunburn. Patients should be cautioned to use sunscreens containing PABA when they are exposed to sunlight to avoid burning. This reaction occurs most frequently with chlorpromazine and is less likely with higher potency agents.

Blue-gray skin discoloration may occur with prolonged use of low potency phenothiazines, particularly chlorpromazine. The skin changes occur on skin exposed to sunlight. These dermatological changes frequently occur with ocular pigmentary changes. There appears to be no clinical significance of this finding.

Seborrheic dermatitis may occur in conjunction with antipsychotic-induced parkinsonism.

OCULAR EFFECTS

The most serious potential ocular effect is pigmentary retinopathy that can occur with thioridazine (Mellaril) and results in visual impairment or even blindness. The risk of this adverse effect increases dramatically at doses greater than 800 mg/day and may be irreversible even after discontinuation of thioridazine. Therefore, daily doses of thioridazine should never exceed 800 mg/day.

Pigmentary changes may also occur in the lens, cornea, and conjunctiva with other low potency agents, evident only upon slit lamp examination. These changes are rarely of clinical importance and are reversible with drug discontinuation. This occurs particularly with long-term administration of chlorpromazine.

Increased intraocular pressure is an anticholinergic effect and may result in the precipitation of acute narrow-angle glaucoma in predisposed patients (see Chapter 4 on depression). Mydriasis may result in increased sensitivity to light. Impaired visual accommodation presents as blurry vision.

HYPERSALIVATION

Hypersalivation is a common side effect of clozapine, occurring in about one-third of patients. Patients may complain of drooling during the day and soaking their pillow at night. It may be so severe that discontinuation of the drug may be warranted. Anticholinergics may be helpful.

SEXUAL SIDE EFFECTS

Decreased libido is a common symptom of schizophrenia, but it is also a common side effect of antipsychotic therapy due to increased prolactin or decreased testosterone levels. Sexual function may also be impaired.[99] Delayed, altered, or inadequate orgasms may occur. Males may experience retrograde ejaculation. Switching to a higher potency agent or reducing the dose may be helpful. Bethanechol (Urecholine), yohimbine, cyproheptadine, or amantadine may be effective antidotes (see Chapter 4). Priapism may occur especially with thioridazine and chlorpromazine.

OVERDOSE/TOXICITY

The antipsychotic drugs have a high therapeutic index, meaning that there is a large difference between the therapeutic and the toxic dose. They are relatively safe in overdose; the most potentially dangerous ones are thioridazine and loxapine. The low potency agents may produce excess anticholinergic effects in overdose. Symptoms of toxicity include agitation, confusion, delirium, dystonic movements, EPS, seizures, hyperthermia, tachycardia, hypotension, arrhythmias, and cardiovascular collapse. Blood pressure abnormalities, particularly orthostatic hypotension, may be treated with alpha-adrenergic agents. Because of delayed gastric emptying, also an anticholinergic effect, suction and gastric lavage should be attempted even hours after the ingestion. Activated charcoal may also diminish absorption. The tricyclic compounds (the phenothiazines and loxapine) may produce arrhythmias. These should not be treated with Class 1A antiarrhythmics (quinidine, procainamide, and disopyramine) because of additive effects. Lidocaine is preferred as an antiarrhythmic. Dialysis is usually unsuccessful because of the high lipophilicity and strong protein and tissue binding of the antipsychotics, although lipoid dialysis may be beneficial.

ATYPICAL ANTIPSYCHOTICS

Since the introduction of chlorpromazine in the 1950s, many other antipsychotic agents have been synthesized and marketed. While there are many different agents with different chemical structures, they all have very similar pharmacological action with D2 blockade as the predominant feature. However, with more information about dopamine-receptor pharmacology and the interaction between dopamine and other neurotransmitter systems, the newer antipsychotics have been designed to affect other dopamine and serotonin receptor systems.

Clozapine, a D4 antagonist with a relatively high 5-HT2/DA ratio, was the first of the "atypical" antipsychotics available in the United States. Because of its effect at the D4 autoreceptor and lesser effect at D2, clozapine does not cause extrapyramidal side effects. It is also less likely to cause TD and may even alleviate TD symptoms. It has rarely been associated with NMS. Clozapine is effective in about 30% of patients who have been nonresponsive to multiple "typical" antipsychotics. Since the introduction of clozapine in the United States in 1990, many patients who were considered chronic "back-wards" patients have recovered enough to function in the community.

Risperidone was the next "atypical" antipsychotic and became available on the market in 1993. Risperidone has activity at serotonin 5-HT2 receptors and the 5-HT/DA ratio is also high. Its efficacy is similar to haloperidol and the other typical antipsychotics, but the incidence of EPS at therapeutic doses is much less. The typical effective dose range is 2–8 mg/day, and EPS increases above 8 mg/day. There is some evidence that it is more efficacious on the negative symptoms than typical antipsychotics but this finding is not consistent.

Olanzapine (Zyprexa) became available in the United States in 1996. The pharmacological profile is similar to clozapine with high affinities for 5-HT2A and M_1 muscarinic receptors but less affinity for adrenergic and D4 receptors than clozapine. Olanzapine is as effective as haloperidol in treating schizophrenia and may even be more effective against the negative symptoms while causing less EPS and akathisia. The usual dose range is 5–20 mg/day.

Quetiapine (Seroquel) became available in 1997. It is an atypical dibenzothiazepine with a pharmacological profile similar to clozapine with D2 and $5-HT_2$ antagonism. It is effective for positive and negative symptoms of psychosis and does not cause significant akathisia or EPS, and there is no need for routine blood monitoring. The usual dose range is 150–750 mg/day. Most common side effects are sedation, headache, and dizziness.

Other agents may soon be available including specific D1/D2 antagonists, partial D2 agonists, 5-HT antagonists, and mixed receptor antagonists.[100]

DISCONTINUATION/WITHDRAWAL REACTIONS

Discontinuation of antipsychotics may produce withdrawal symptoms. Physiological dependence does not develop, but post-synaptic receptor up-regulation with chronic antipsychotic exposure can result in an excess of dopaminergic function when the dopamine blockade of the antipsychotic is withdrawn. This may result in withdrawal dyskinesias or supersensitivity psychosis. Withdrawal dyskinesias typically resolve within a few weeks. Discontinuation of the low potency agents may cause cholinergic rebound including nausea, vomiting, increased sweating, sensations of heat or cold, insomnia, irritability, and headache.

Supersensitivity psychosis is analogous to TD in the mesolimbic system. Up-regulation and increased numbers of DA-receptors in the mesolimbic system as a consequence of prolonged antipsychotic treatment result in increased psychosis with a reduction or withdrawal of antipsychotic medication.[101,102] Patients with supersensitivity psychosis have other signs of dopamine receptor supersensitivity (i.e., TD), elevated prolactin levels, necessity of gradual increase in antipsychotic dose to maintain therapeutic response, and resolution of psychosis with increased antipsychotic dose. Patients with supersensitivity psychosis may become more psychotic after missing even a single dose. Finally, chronic antipsychotic treatment may induce relapse in some schizophrenics.[103]

Most important, antipsychotic discontinuation may lead to recurrent psychosis. While there is no definitive evidence supporting a gradual taper over abrupt discontinuation, anecdotal evidence and clinical experience suggest that gradual antipsychotic taper over at least several months is associated with less chance of recurrence. Recurrences may be less likely and if recurrent symptoms begin to emerge, quickly reinstituting a higher dose may prevent a full-blown episode. Pharmacologically, the gradual taper approach is rational, presumably giving DA-receptors time to down-regulate to avoid a supersensitivity state. Frequent visits and vigilant monitoring by family or friends can help prevent severe recurrences during antipsychotic drug withdrawal.

MONITORING

Routine laboratory monitoring for patients on antipsychotics is not necessary. Orthostatic blood pressures should be checked while titrating low potency agents, clozapine, and risperidone due to the possibility of hypotension.

Baseline and biannual examination for TD (AIMS exam) is prudent. Early signs of TD may be treated with dose reduction (if possible), vitamin E, or switching to clozapine.

Routine yearly liver function tests and complete blood count with differential is sufficient along with a yearly electrocardiogram for patients over age 30 or 40. All patients on pimozide and thioridazine should have a yearly electrocardiogram.

Patients on thioridazine, and possibly those on chlorpromazine, should have yearly ophthalmological examinations.

Female patients should have yearly breast exams and should be taught breast self-exam if possible.

Weekly white blood cell count with differential is necessary for patients on clozapine.

If patients develop signs of NMS (fever, rigidity, diaphoresis), white blood cell and creatinine phosphokinase should be monitored. Any signs of jaundice or pruritus should prompt liver function tests. Seizures or polydipsia should prompt electrolyte studies.

The presence of antipsychotic drugs may alter some laboratory tests. Falsely elevated serum transaminases, alkaline phosphatase, bilirubin, cholesterol, 17-hydroxysteroids, cerebrospinal fluid protein, urine diacetate, urine porphyrins, and urine bilinogen have been reported.[104] False-positive urinary phenylketonuria and pregnancy testing have also been reported. Inaccurate results of protein-bound iodine, radioactive iodine, and uric acid may also occur.

DRUG-DRUG INTERACTIONS

Because the antipsychotics are metabolized by the hepatic cytochrome P450 system, there are many potential drug interactions with other medications also metabolized by this system.[105] Genetic polymorphism in expression of these enzymes results in clinical heterogeneity with a small percentage of the population being poor metabolizers. There are also ethnic differences in cytochrome P450 2D6 activity with Asians generally having slower metabolism but fewer poor metabolizers. There seems to be no relationship between metabolic activity of cytochrome P450 2D6 or 1A2 and age.

Most antipsychotics are metabolized by cytochrome P450 2D6, and they act as competitive inhibitors of this enzyme. Antipsychotic administration can therefore result in increased levels of concomitantly administered TCAs, fluoxetine, paroxetine, venlafaxine, beta-blockers, type1C antiarrhythmics, dextromethorphan, and opiates. Haloperidol, fluphenazine, and thioridazine, in particular, are potent inhibitors of this enzyme. Metabolism of antipsychotics is inhibited by fluoxetine, paroxetine, sertraline, TCAs, and quinidine, as well as other drugs that are metabolized by this system, thus increasing antipsychotic levels. Haloperidol and clozapine are exceptions, because cytochrome P450 2D6 does not account for the majority of their metabolism.

Clozapine and haloperidol are primarily metabolized by cytochrome P450 1A2. This enzyme is inhibited by fluvoxamine and grapefruit juice. Concomitant fluvoxamine administration increases clozapine levels but has no effect on other antipsychotics. Cytochrome P450 1A2 is induced by smoking, charcoal-broiled foods, and cruciferous vegetables; these agents can decrease clozapine levels.

Concomitant administration of anticholinergic agents, such as **antiparkinsonian agents** and **TCAs**, with low potency antipsychotics may potentiate anticholinergic effects causing dry mouth, blurred vision, constipation, paralytic ileus, urinary retention, or delirium.

Coadministration of *propranolol* and antipsychotics may increase levels of both agents.

There have been reports of delirium and respiratory arrest when *benzodiazepines* are combined with clozapine.

Antacids and *cholestyramine* decrease oral absorption of antipsychotics and should be given at least one hour before or two hours after the antipsychotic.

Anticonvulsant levels need to be monitored when adding or adjusting antipsychotics. *Valproate* levels may increase with antipsychotics. *Carbamazepine* and *dilantin* may decrease antipsychotic levels due to induction of metabolism.

The antihistamines *terfenadine* and *astemizole* should be used with caution with mesoridazine, thioridazine, and pimozide due to potential QT prolongation and torsades de pointes.

Epinephrine and norepinephrine may cause paradoxical hypotension with antipsychotics. Phenylephrine is a safe substitute.

Smoking decreases plasma antipsychotic levels due to induction of metabolism. This drug interaction has clinical relevance because many patients with schizophrenia are heavy smokers. Patients stabilized on an antipsychotic dose in hospital where smoking may be limited or restricted may have a decline in antipsychotic level after discharge when they return to their usual smoking habits.

See Table 6–8 for a more complete listing of drug interactions.

DRUG-DISEASE INTERACTIONS

There are few absolute contraindications to antipsychotic drug use with comorbid medical conditions, but there are some relative contraindications and situations in which antipsychotics should be used with caution.

Autoimmune diseases are more prevalent in a subgroup of schizophrenia than in the general population, but there are no specific concerns with the use of antipsychotics in these patients. **Diabetes** may be more difficult to adequately control when the patient is on antipsychotics. Antipsychotics may cause hypoglycemia or hyperglycemia, glycosuria, and high or prolonged glucose tolerance tests, increased appetite, and weight gain, all of which interfere with diabetes management. Glucose should be monitored carefully and hypoglycemic medications may need to be adjusted.

Low potency agents, especially mesoridazine, thioridazine, and pimozide, should be used with caution in patients with **cardiac abnormalities** due to the potential of prolonging QT interval and torsades de pointes. **Hypotension** may be exacerbated by low potency agents and risperidone.

Narrow-angle glaucoma can be precipitated by anticholinergic effects of low potency agents and antiparkinsonian agents so these agents should not be used in patients who have uncorrected narrow angle glaucoma.

TABLE 6–8. DRUG INTERACTIONS

Class of Drug	Example	Interaction Effects
Adsorbent	Antacids, activated charcoal, cholestyramine, kaolinpectin	Oral absorption decreased significantly when used simultaneously; give at least 1 hour before or 2 hour after the neuroleptic
Anticholinergic	Antiparkinsonian drugs, antidepressants, antihistamines	Potentiate atropinelike effects causing dry mouth, blurred vision, constipation, etc.; may reduce inhibition of sweating and may lead to paralytic ileus; high doses can bring on a toxic psychosis; variable effects seen on metabolism and efficacy of neuroleptic
Anticonvulsant	Carbamazepine	Increased clearance and decreased neuroleptic plasma level (up to 60% with haloperidol)
	Phenytoin	Decreased neuroleptic plasma level due to induction of metabolism; reported with haloperidol, phenothiazines, and clozapine
	Valproic acid, valproate, divalproex	Increased neurotoxicity, sedation, and extrapyramidal side effects due to decreased clearance of valproic acid (by 14%)
Antidepressant		
Cyclic	Amitriptyline, trimipramine	Additive sedation, hypotension, and anticholinergic effects; increased serum level of either agent
SSRI	Fluoxetine, paroxetine	Increased plasma level of neuroleptic (20% increase with haloperidol); increased EPS and akathisia
Antihistamine	Terfenadine, astemizole	Potentiation of QT prolongation and torsades de pointes; caution with mesoridazine, thioridazine, pimozide, and fluspirilene
Antihypertensive	Methyldopa	Additive antihypertensive effect
	Guanethidine	Reversal of antihypertensive effect
	Propranolol	Increased plasma level of either drug
Anxiolytic		
Benzodiazepines	Clonazepam, lorazepam	Increased incidence of dizziness (collapse) and sedation when combined with clozapine; delirium and respiratory arrest reported
		Synergistic effect with neuroleptics; used to calm agitated patients
Busprione		May increase extrapyramidal reactions
Cimetidine		Increased haloperidol plasma level (by 26%)
		Inhibited metabolism of clozapine and thiothixene, with resultant increase in plasma level and adverse effects
CNS depressant	Antidepressants, hypnotics, antihistamines, alcohol, benzodiazepines	Increased CNS depression
Disulfiram		Alcohol may worsen EPS
		Decreased plasma level of perphenazine
Hypertensive	Epinephrine, norepinephrine	May result in paradoxical fall in blood pressure (due to alpha-adrenergic block produced by neuroleptics); phenylephrine is a safe substitute
Lithium		Increased neurotoxicity at therapeutic doses; may increase EPS; increased plasma level of molindone; possibly increased risk of agranulocytosis with clozapine
Rifampin		Decreased haloperidol plasma level due to induction of metabolism
Smoking		Decreased plasma level of neuroleptic due to induction of metabolism

Adapted from Bezchlibnyk-Butler, K.Z., Jeffreis, J.J., Martin, B.A. (1994). *Clinical Handbook of Psychotropic Drugs*, 8th rev. ed. Copyright 1998 by Hogrefe & Huber Publishers, Seattle, Toronto, Bern, Göttingen. Reprinted with permission.

Hyperprolactinemia, galactorrhea, and **amenorrhea** can occur with antipsychotic administration. Patients who have these as preexisting conditions likely will have exacerbations with antipsychotic use, particularly with high potency agents.

Leucopenia and **neutropenia** preclude a clozapine trial because of the risk of agranulocytosis. However, if a patient has been stable on clozapine for over a year and develops neutropenia from another known cause, clozapine may be continued safely.[106]

Seizure disorders may be exacerbated by antipsychotics by lowering the seizure threshold and interacting with anticonvulsants. High potency agents are less likely to alter the seizure threshold. Molindone appears to be the least likely to interfere with seizure threshold.

Idiopathic Parkinson's disease is exacerbated by antipsychotics. Clozapine is the best choice in these patients. Caution should be taken in Parkinson's patients with autonomic instability as clozapine can worsen orthostatic hypotension.

Most antipsychotics can cause weight gain that may be a particular problem in patients with **obesity**. Molindone is less likely to cause weight gain and may be a good choice in these patients.

CHOICE OF ANTIPSYCHOTIC/ADJUNCTIVE AGENT

SCHIZOPHRENIA SUBTYPE

There is no evidence from controlled clinical trials that symptom profile or schizophrenia subtype predicts response to a particular type of medication. There is anecdotal evidence, however, that monosymptomatic somatic delusions may preferentially respond to pimozide (Orap), but these data are not conclusive.[107]

Catatonic schizophrenia responds acutely to benzodiazepines and ECT. Maintenance treatment with antipsychotics alone may be sufficient or, if necessary, a benzodiazepine may be added.

COMORBID PSYCHIATRIC CONDITION

Depression comorbid with schizophrenia was discussed previously in the acute treatment section. Koreen et al. reports that depressive symptoms present with psychotic symptoms in 22–75% of schizophrenics during their first episode with almost complete resolution with resolution of the psychosis.[108] About 25–80% of schizophrenic patients experience post-psychotic depression after the acute episode has resolved.[70] Post-psychotic depression responds to tricyclic antidepressants with minimal risk of exacerbation of psychotic symptoms.[72] However, tricyclic antidepressants are not effective for negative symptoms or anergia, indicating that they specifically target depressive symptoms. SSRIs have not been adequately studied.

MANIA

Manic episodes can occur in the context of a schizoaffective disorder. Mood stabilizers used in primary bipolar disorder are also effective in treating schizophrenia with manic symptomatology. Lithium, carbamazepine, and valproate all have demonstrated efficacy for manic symptoms in schizophrenia.[41] Clozapine is also effective in treating mania of schizoaffective disorder.

SUBSTANCE ABUSE

Comorbid substance abuse complicates the treatment of schizophrenia.[109] About one-half of patients with schizophrenia or schizoaffective disorder suffer from a comorbid substance abuse disorder.[2] Preferred drugs among schizophrenics are alcohol, cannabis, stimulants, and hallucinogens. Because these drugs of abuse can cause psychotic symptoms, it is frequently difficult to differentiate whether the drug is producing or exacerbating the psychosis.

Substance use affects the course of schizophrenia. Alcohol use is associated with medication noncompliance.[110,111] Substance abuse correlates with difficulty complying with medications, social functional impairment (difficulty maintaining regular meals, managing finances, and maintaining stable housing), hostility, disorganized speech, and suicidal behavior.[112] Cocaine abuse is associated with paranoid subtype, depression, more hospitalizations, and increased risk of antipsychotic-induced dystonias.

Treatment should involve an integrated approach incorporating treatment for both the schizophrenia and the substance abuse in a general psychiatric setting. Appropriate pharmacotherapy for psychotic symptoms should include close attention to minimizing side effects to reduce antipsychotic-induced dysphoria or akathisia, which may spur substance abuse. The atypical antipsychotics, which have fewer of these side effects, may be promising. Agents specifically designed to prevent substance-abuse relapse may be beneficial, but there is no empirical support: examples include disulfiram and naltrexone for alcohol abuse and desipramine for cocaine abuse. Pharmacological therapy should be combined with nonconfrontational group therapy and self-help groups.

OBSESSIVE-COMPULSIVE SYMPTOMS

Obsessive compulsive symptoms are comorbid with schizophrenia in 20–25% of patients or may emerge with antipsychotic treatment, particularly with clozapine.[113,114] Clomipramine and fluoxetine have demonstrated efficacy for obsessive-compulsive symptoms in schizophrenia.[115,116,117] Coadministration of an SSRI with antipsychotics increases the levels of both agents.

SPECIAL POPULATIONS

CHILD AND ADOLESCENT

Only six antipsychotics are FDA approved for the treatment of psychosis in children: haloperidol, chlorprothixene, prochlorperazine, trifluoperazine, thioridazine, and chlorpromazine. High potency agents should be considered as first-line agents since children are exceedingly sensitive to the sedating and cognitive effects of the lower potency antipsychotics. We refer readers to Rosenberg et al. for a more detailed discussion of antipsychotic use in children and adolescents.[118]

PREGNANCY AND LACTATION

There are risks associated with the use of antipsychotic medications during pregnancy. There is concern about teratogenic effects of antipsychotics since they cross the placenta and are present in the fetus during development. However, babies of mothers with schizophrenia may have increased risk of congenital anomalies even without antipsychotic drug exposure. There have been no controlled studies of antipsychotics in pregnant women with schizophrenia and little retrospective uncontrolled data with most antipsychotics except chlorpromazine and haloperidol and then only in nonpsychotic women with hyperemesis gravidarum. The little data in this area have been reviewed extensively.[95,119]

Behavioral teratogenicity has been reported in animals, but there is no evidence for this in humans. There are case reports of morphological teratogenicity with various antipsychotics including chlorpromazine, haloperidol, trifluoperazine, and fluphenazine, but results of large studies do not support this.[120] Nevertheless, antipsychotic exposure during the first trimester, especially between weeks 4 and 10, should be avoided if possible. Keeping doses as low as possible to minimize exposure is also recommended. High potency agents are recommended because of fewer anticholinergic effects. Depot antipsychotics should be avoided due to the long half-life. Antiparkinsonian agents should be avoided during pregnancy due to morphological teratogenicity and neonatal withdrawal symptoms with anticholinergic agents and diphenhydramine. No antiparkinsonian agent is safer than any other. Low serum calcium, which may result from increased calcium need during pregnancy, combined with poor dietary habits and prenatal care in mothers with schizophrenia, may predispose to EPS. If NMS occurs during pregnancy, it may be more severe than usual. Bromocriptine is the safest antidote. Low potency agents that lower the seizure threshold predispose to eclampsia.

Withdrawal symptoms may occur in neonates exposed to antipsychotics in utero. Extrapyramidal side effects may persist for several months and include tremor, hyperactivity, motor restlessness, and abnormal movements. Anticholinergic effects include functional intestinal obstruction. Discontinuation of the antipsychotic at least 5–10 days before delivery is recommended to avoid withdrawal in the neonate.

Post-partum psychosis is very common in women with chronic psychotic illness. Therefore, antipsychotic medications should be restarted after delivery to prevent recurrence during the high-risk post-partum period.

Antipsychotics are secreted into breast milk, resulting in detectable levels of drug in nursing infants of lactating mothers who are exposed to these drugs.[119] The clinical significance of this small exposure is uncertain.

Physicians should counsel all female patients of reproductive age who are taking antipsychotics about the risks and benefits of continuing their psychotropic medication during pregnancy and should guide the patient in pregnancy planning. Although the use of any antipsychotic during pregnancy is not recommended, especially during the first trimester, the risk for the fetus of maternal psychosis must be weighed against the risk of possible teratogenesis or behavioral teratogenesis. Maternal psychosis may put the fetus in jeopardy by exposing it to poor nutrition, high-risk behavior, and possible death by suicide. If the patient's acute episodes are severe, the risk of recurrence may be greater than the possible risk of medication effects to the fetus, so the patient and fetus may be better off continuing the medication throughout the pregnancy, or at least restarting it at the beginning of the second trimester.

Psychotropics should be tapered prior to conception if possible, or at least as soon as the patient is aware of the pregnancy, if the decision to stop medication is made. At least, a trial off medication only during the first trimester may be tried. The treatment strategy during pregnancy may not be to achieve or maintain remission but simply to ameliorate the most threatening symptoms.

GERIATRICS

Elderly patients with schizophrenia include early-onset patients who have aged and late-onset patients who have developed the illness after age 45. Treatment is similar in both groups. In general, elderly patients require lower doses of antipsychotics than younger patients although women may require higher doses after menopause due to a drop in estrogen levels. The risk of relapse is the same as in younger patients, so maintenance antipsychotic therapy should be continued in late-life. However, the morbidity of antipsychotic therapy increases with age. Elderly patients are more susceptible to the EPS of high potency agents and to the anticholinergic effects of low potency agents. Midpotency agents such as perphenazine, or the atypical antipsychotics such as risperidone, olanzapine, or quetiapine, are often better tolerated by elderly patients. Also, the risk of TD increases with age. Elderly patients with only three months exposure to antipsychotics had a 16% rate of TD. The rate increases with duration of exposure to antipsychotics with 41% of elderly patients with greater than 10 years of exposure having TD, which is a relative risk of 4.1 compared with elderly patients not exposed to antipsychotics.[82]

Treatment recommendations for the use of antipsychotics in elderly patients have been compiled by Jeste et al. and Gregory and McKenna.[120,121] These include using the lowest possible doses, using midpotency agents as first-line choices, monitoring closely for EPS and anticholinergic side effects, and for emergence of TD.

REFERENCES

1. Kaplan, H.I., Sadock, B.J. (1995). (Eds.) *Compulsive Textbook of Psychiatry* (6th ed.). (Chapter 14). Baltimore: Williams & Wilkins.
2. Regier, D.A., Farmer, M.E., Rae, D.S., et al. (1990). Comorbidity of mental disorders with alcohol and other drug abuse: Results from the Epidemiologic Catchment Area (ECA) survey. *JAMA*, 264:2511–2518.
3. Loranger, A.W. (1984). Sex differences in age at onset of schizophrenia. *Arch Gen Psychiatry*, 41:157–161.
4. Seeman, M.V., Lang, M. (1990). The role of estrogens in schizophrenia gender differences. *Schizophr Bull*, 16(2):185–194.
5. Riecher-Rössler, A., Häfner, H. (1993). Schizophrenia and oestrogens—is there an association? *Eur Arch Psychiatry Clin Neurosci*, 242:323–328.
6. Flor-Henry, P. (1990). Influence of gender in schizophrenia as related to other psychopathological syndromes. *Schizophr Bull*, 16(2):211–227.
7. Andia, A.M., Zisook, S. (1991). Gender differences in schizophrenia: A literature review. *Annals Clin Psychiatry*, 3(4):333–340.
8. Shtasel, D.L., Gur, R.E., Gallacher, F., et al. (1992). Gender differences in the clinical expression of schizophrenia. *Schizophr Research*, 7:225–231.

9. Bartels, S.J., Teague, G.B., Drake, R.E., et al. (1993). Substance abuse in schizophrenia: Service utilization and costs. *J Nerv Ment Dis*, 181(4):227–232.

10. Wyatt, R.J., Heuter, I., Leary, M.C., et al. (1995). An economic evaluation of schizophrenia-1991. *Soc Psychiatry Psychiatr Epidemiol*, 30(5):196–205.

11. Rupp, A., Keith, S.J. (1993). The costs of schizophrenia: Assessing the burden. *Psychiatric Clin N Am*, 16(2):413–423.

12. Franks, D.D. (1987) The high cost of caring: Economic contributions of families to the care of the mentally ill. Unpublished PhD dissertation: Brandeis University.

13. Wyatt, R.J. (1991). Neuroleptics and the natural course of schizophrenia. *Schizophr Bull*, 17(2):325–351.

14. Johnstone, E.C., Geddes, J. (1994). How high is the relapse rate in schizophrenia? *Acta Psychiatr Scand*, 89(Suppl 382):6–10.

15. May, P.R.A., Tuma, A.H., Yale, C., et al. (1976). Schizophrenia—A follow-up study of results of treatment. II. Hospital stay over two to five years. *Arch Gen Psychiatry*, 33:431–506.

16. Hogarty, G.E. (1993). Prevention of relapse in chronic schizophrenic patients. *J Clin Psychiatry*, 54(Suppl 3):18–23.

17. Davis, J.M. (1985). Maintenance therapy and the natural course of schizophrenia. *J Clin Psychiatry*, 46(11):18–21.

18. Hogarty, G.E., Ulrich, R.F. (1977). Temporal effects of drug and placebo in delaying relapse in schizophrenic outpatients. *Arch Gen Psychiatry*, 34:297–301.

19. Schooler, N.R. (1986). The efficacy of antipsychotic drugs and family therapies in the maintenance treatment of schizophrenia. *J Clin Psychopharmacol*, 6:11S–19S.

20. Farr, R., Koegel, P., Burnam, A. (1986). A study of homelessness and mental illness in the skid row area of Los Angeles. In: Tessler, R.C., Dennis, D.L. A synthesis of NIMH-funded research concerning persons who are homeless and mentally ill. (1992). Rockville, MD: National Institute of Mental Health, (87M030467801D).

21. Bassuk, E.L. (1984). The homelessness problem. *Sci Am*, 251:40–45.

22. Black, D.W., Fisher, R. (1992). Mortality in DSM-IIIR schizophrenia. *Schizophr Res*, 7:109–116.

23. Roy, A. (1986). Depression, attempted suicide, and suicide in patients with chronic schizophrenia. *Psychiatric Clin N Am*, 9:193–206.

24. Caldwell, C.B., Gottesman, I.I. (1990). Schizophrenics kill themselves too: A review of risk factors for suicide. *Schizophr Bull*, 16:571–589.

25. Cheng, K.K., Leung, C.M., Lo, W.H., et al. (1990). Risk factors of suicide among schizophrenics. *Acta Psychiatr Scand*, 81(3):220–224.

26. Westermeyer, J.F., Harrow, M., Marengo, J.T. (1991). Risk for suicide in schizophrenia and other psychotic and nonpsychotic disorders. *J Nerv Ment Dis*, 179(5):259–266.

27. Keshavan, M.S., Ganguli, R. (1990). Biology of schizophrenia. In Pohl, R., Gershon, S. (Eds.), *The Biological Basis of Psychiatric Treatment* (Vol. 3, pp. 1–33). Basel: Karger.

28. Nasrallah, H.A. (1993). Neurodevelopmental pathogenesis of schizophrenia. *Psychiatric Clin N Am*, 16(2):269–280.

29. Buchsbaum, M.S. (1995). Positron emission tomography studies of abnormal glucose metabolism in schizophrenic illness. *Clin Neurosci*, 3:122–130.

30. Gur, R.E., Pearlson, G.D. (1993). Neuroimaging in schizophrenia research. *Schizophr Bull*, 19:337–353.

31. Davis, K.L., Kahn, R.S., Ko, G., et al. (1991). Dopamine in schizophrenia: A review and reconceptualization. *Am J Psychiatry*, 148:1474–1486.

32. Mednick, S.A., Huttunen, M.O., Machon, R.A. (1994). Prenatal influenza infections and adult schizophrenia. *Schizophr Bull*, 20:263–267.

33. Janicak, P.G., Davis, J.M., Preskorn, S.H., Ayd, F.J. (1993). *Principles and Practice of Psychopharmacology*. Baltimore: Williams & Wilkins.

34. Kane, J., Honigfeld, G., Singer, J., et al. (1988). Clozaril collaborative study group: Clozapine for the treatment of resistant schizophrenia: A double-blind comparison with chlorpromazine. *Arch Gen Psychiatry*, 45:789–796.

35. McEvoy, J.P. (1986). The neuroleptic threshold as a marker of minimum effective neuroleptic dose. *Compr Psychiatry*, 27:327–335.

36. McEvoy, J.P., Stiller, R.L., Farr, R. (1986). Plasma haloperidol levels drawn at neuroleptic threshold doses: A pilot study. *J Clin Psychopharmacol*, 6:133–138.

37. McEvoy, J.P., Hogarty, G.E., Steingard, S. (1991). Optimal dose of neuroleptic in acute schizophrenia. *Arch Gen Psychiatry*, 48:739–745.

38. Lieberman, J.A., Safferman, A.Z., Pollack, S., et al. (1994). Clinical effects of clozapine in chronic schizophrenia: Response to treatment and predictors of outcome. *Am J Psychiatry*, 151:1744–1752.

39. Dahl, S.G. (1986). Plasma level monitoring of antipsychotic drugs: Clinical utility. *Clin Pharmacokinet*, 11:36–61.

40. Darby, J.K., Pasta, D.J., Dabiri, L., et al. (1995). Haloperidol dose and blood level variability: Toxicity and interindividual and intraindividual variability in the nonresponder patient in the clinical practice setting. *J Clin Psychopharmacol*, 15:334–340.

41. Siris, S.G. (1993). Adjunctive medication in the maintenance treatment of schizophrenia and its conceptual implications. *Br J Psychiatry*, 163(Suppl 22):66–78.

42. Lingjaerde, O. (1991). Benzodiazepines in the treatment of schizophrenia: An updated survey. *Acta Psychiatr Scand*, 84(5):453–459.

43. Small, J.G., Kellams, J.J., Milstein, V., et al. (1975). A placebo-controlled study of lithium combined with neuroleptics in chronic schizophrenic patients. *Am J Psychiatry*, 132:1315–1317.

44. Growe, G.A., Crayton, J.W., Klass, D.B., et al. (1979). Lithium in chronic schizophrenia. *Am J Psychiatry*, 136:454–455.

45. Carman, J.S., Llewellyn, B.B., Wyatt, R.J. (1981). Lithium combined with neuroleptics in chronic schizophrenic and schizoaffective patients. *J Clin Psychiatry*, 42:124–128.

46. Simhandl, C., Meszaros, K. (1992). The use of carbamazepine in the treatment of schizophrenia and schizoaffective psychoses: A review. *J Psychiatry Neurosci*, 17(1):1–14.

47. Morgan, R., Cheadle, J. (1974). Maintenance treatment of chronic schizophrenia with neuroleptic drugs. *Acta Psychiatr Scand*, 50:78–85.

48. Davis, J.M., Andrivkactis, S. (1986). The natural course of schizophrenia and effective maintenance drug treatment. *J Clin Psychopharmacol*, 6:2S–10S.

49. Greenblatt, M., Soloman, M.H., Evans, A.S., Brooks, G.W. (Eds.) (1965). *Drug and Social Therapy in Chronic Schizophrenia*. Springfield, IL: Charles C. Thomas.

50. Prien, R.F., Levine, J., Switalski, R.W. (1971). Discontinuation of chemotherapy for chronic schizophrenics. *Hosp Comm Psychiatry*, 22:4–7.

51. Jolley, A.G., Hirsch, S.R., McRink, A., et al. (1989). Trial of brief intermittent neuroleptic prophylaxis for selected schizophrenic outpatients: Clinical outcome at one year. *Br Med J*, 298:985–990.

52. Jolley, A.0G., Hirsch, S.R., Morrison, E., et al. (1990). Trial of brief intermittent neuroleptic prophylaxis for selected schizophrenic outpatients: Clinical and social outcome at two years. *Br Med J*, 301(6756):837–842.

53. Herz, M.I., Glazer, W.M., Mostert, M.A., et al. (1990). Intermittent vs. maintenance medication in schizophrenia: Two year results. *Clin Neuropharmacol*, 13(Suppl 2):426–427.

54. Gaebel, W., Kopcke, W., Linden, M., et al. (1991). 2-year outcome of intermittent vs. maintenance neuroleptic treatment in schizophrenia. *Schizophr Res*, 4:288.

55. Carpenter, W.T., Hanlon, T.E., Heinrichs, D.W., et al. (1990). Continuous versus targeted medication in schizophrenic outpatients: Outcome results. *Am J Psychiatry*, 147(9):1138–1148.

56. Schooler, N.R. (1991). Maintenance medication for schizophrenia: Strategies for dose reduction. *Schizophr Bull*, 17(2):311–324.
57. Kane, J.M., Rifkin, A., Woerner, M., et al. (1983). Low-dose neuroleptic treatment of outpatient schizophrenics. I. Preliminary results for relapse rates. *Arch Gen Psychiatry*, 40:893–896.
58. Marder, S.R., Van Putten, T., Mintz, J., et al. (1987). Low- and conventional-dose maintenance therapy with fluphenazine decanoate. Two-year outcome. *Arch Gen Psychiatry*, 44:518–521.
59. Hogarty, G.E., McEvoy, J.P., Munetz, M., et al. (1988). Dose of fluphenazine, familial expressed emotion and outcome in schizophrenia. Results of a two-year controlled study. *Arch Gen Psychiatry*, 45:797–805.
60. Barnes, T.R., Curson, D.A. (1994). Long-term depot antipsychotics. A risk-benefit assessment. *Drug Safety*, 10(6):464–479.
61. Kissling, W., Moller, H.J., Walter, K., et al. (1985). Double-blind comparison of haloperidol decanoate and fluphenazine decanoate effectiveness, adverse effects, dosage and serum levels during a six months' treatment for relapse prevention. *Pharmacopsychiatry*, 18:240–245.
62. Wistedt, B., Persson, T., Heilbom, E. (1984). A clinical double-blind comparison between haloperidol decanoate and fluphenazine decanoate. *Curr Ther Res*, 35:804–814.
63. Chouinard, G., Annable, L., Campbell, W., et al. (1984). A double-blind, controlled clinical trial of haloperidol decanoate and fluphenazine decanoate in the maintenance treatment of schizophrenia. *Psychopharmacol Bull*, 20(1):108–109.
64. Burnett, P.L., Gallefly, C.A., Moyle, R. J., et al. (1993). Low-dose depot medication in schizophrenia. *Schizophr Bull*, 19:155–164.
65. Yadalam, K.G., Simpson, G.M. (1988). Changing from oral to depot fluphenazine. *J Clin Psychiatry*, 49:346–348.
66. Ereshefsky, L., Toney, G., Saklad, S.R., et al. (1993). A loading-dose strategy for converting from oral to depot haloperidol. *Hosp Comm Psychiatry*, 44(12):1155–1161.
67. Buchanan, A. (1992). A two-year prospective study of treatment compliance in patients with schizophrenia. *Psychol Med*, 22(3):787–797.
68. Hogarty, G.E., Goldberg, S.C., Schooler, N.R., et al. (1974). Drug and sociotherapy in the aftercare of schizophrenic patients. II. Two-year relapse rates. *Arch Gen Psychiatry*, 31:603–608.
69. Hogarty, G.E., Schooler, N.R., Ulrich, R., et al. (1979). Fluphenazine and social therapy in the aftercare of schizophrenic patients. Relapse analyses of a two-year controlled study of fluphenazine decanoate and fluphenazine hydrochloride. *Arch Gen Psychiatry*, 36:1283–1294.
70. DeLisi, L.E. (1980). *Depression in Schizophrenia*. Washington, DC: American Psychiatric Press.
71. Harrow, M., Yonan, C.A., Sands, J.R., et al. (1994). Depression in schizophrenia: Are neuroleptics, akinesia, or anhedonia involved? *Schizophr Bull*, 20(2):327–328.
72. Plasky, P. (1991). Antidepressant usage in schizophrenia. *Schizophr Bull*, 17(4):649–657.
73. Azorin, J.M. (1995). Long-term treatment of mood disorders in schizophrenia. *Acta Psychiatr Scand Supplementation*, 388:20–23.
74. Siris, S.G., Bermanzohn, P.C., Mason, S.E., et al. (1994). Maintenance imipramine therapy for secondary depression in schizophrenia: A controlled trial. *Arch Gen Psychiatry*, 51:109–115.
75. Hanlon, T.E., Schoenrich, C., Frenck, W., et al. (1966). Perphenazine benztropine mesylate treatment of newly admitted psychiatric patients. *Psychopharmacologia*, 9:328–339.
76. Chien, C.P., DiMascio, A., Cole, J.O. (1974). Antiparkinsonian agents and depot phenothiazine. *Am J Psychiatry*, 131:86–90.

77. Keepers, G.A., Clappison, V.J., Casey, D.E. (1983). Initial anticholinergic prophylaxis for neuroleptic-induced extrapyramidal syndromes. *Arch Gen Psychiatry*, 40:1113–1117.
78. Comaty, J.E., Janicak, P.G., Rajavatnam, J., et al. (1980). Is maintenance antiparkinsonian treatment necessary? *Psychopharmacol Bull*, 26:267–271.
79. Crane, G.E. (1968). Dyskinesia and neuroleptics. *Arch Gen Psychiatry*, 19:700–703.
80. Kane, J.M., Woerner, M., Borenstein, M., et al. (1985). Integrating incidence and prevalence of tardive dyskinesia. Read before the IVth World Congress of Biological Psychiatry. Philadelphia, September 8–13, 1985.
81. Jenike, M.A. (1983). Tardive dyskinesia: Special risk in the elderly. *J Am Ger Soc*, 31:71–73.
82. Sweet, R.A., Mulsant, B.H., Gupta, B., et al. (1995). Duration of neuroleptic treatment and prevalence of tardive dyskinesia in late life. *Arch Gen Psych*, 52:478–486.
83. Yassa, R., Jeste, D.V. (1992). Gender differences in tardive dyskinesia: A critical review of the literature. *Schizophr Bull*, 18(4):701–715.
84. Quitkin, F., Rifkin, A., Gochfeld, L., et al. (1977). Tardive dyskinesia: Are first signs reversible? *Am J Psychiatry*, 134:84–87.
85. Jeste, D.V., Potkin, S.G., Sinha, S., et al. (1979). Tardive dyskinesia—Reversible and persistent. *Arch Gen Psychiatry*, 36:585–590.
86. Lohr, J.B., Cadet, J.L., Lohr, M.A., et al. (1988). Vitamin E in the treatment of tardive dyskinesia: The possible involvement of free radical mechanisms. *Schizophr Bull*, 14:291–296.
87. Elkashef, A.M., Ruskin, P.E., Bacher, N., et al. (1990). Vitamin E in the treatment of tardive dyskinesia. *Am J Psychiatry*, 147:505–506.
88. Adler, L.A., Peselow, E., Rotrosen, J., et al. (1993). Vitamin E treatment of tardive dyskinesia. *Am J Psychiatry*, 150:1405–1407.
89. Egan, M.T., Hyde, T.M., Albers, G.W., et al. (1992). Treatment of tardive dyskinesia with Vitamin E. *Am J Psychiatry*, 149:773–777.
90. Shriqui, C.L., Bradwejn, J., Annable, L., et al. (1992). Vitamin E in the treatment of tardive dyskinesia: A double-blind placebo controlled study. *Am J Psychiatry*, 149:391–393.
91. Lohr, J.B., Caligiuri, M.P. (1996). A double-blind placebo-controlled study of vitamin E treatment of tardive dyskinesia. *J Clin Psychiatry*, 57:167–173.
92. Yassa, R., Nair, V., Dimitry, R. (1986). Prevalence of tardive dyskinesia. *Acta Psychiatr Scand*, 73:629–633.
93. Keck, P.E., McElroy, S.L., Pope, H.G. (1991). Epidemiology of NMS. *J Clin Psychiatry*, 21:148–151.
94. Sakkas, P., Davis, J.M., Hau, J., et al. (1991). Pharmacotherapy of NMS. *Psychiatr Ann*, 21:157–164.
95. Miller, D.D., Sharafuddin, M.J.A., Kathol, R.G. (1991). A case of clozapine-induced NMS. *J Clin Psychiatry*, 52:99–101.
96. Anderson, E.S., Powers, P.S. (1991). NMS associated with clozapine use. *J Clin Psychiatry*, 52:102–104.
97. DasGupta, K., Young, A. (1991). Clozapine-induced NMS. *J Clin Psychiatry*, 52:105–107.
98. Owen, R.R., Cole, J.O. (1989). Molindone hydrochloride: A review of laboratory and clinical findings. *J Clin Psychopharmacol*, 9:268–276.
99. Aizenberg, D., Zemishlany, Z., Dortman-Etrog, P., et al. (1995). Sexual dysfunction in male schizophrenic patients. *J Clin Psychiatry*, 56(4):137–141.
100. Fleischhacker, W.W. (1995). New drugs for the treatment of schizophrenic patients. *Acta Psychiatr Scand*, 91(Suppl 388):24–30.
101. Chouinard, G., Jones, B.D., Annable, L. (1978). Neuroleptic-induced supersensitivity psychosis. *Am J Psychiatry*, 135:1409–1410.
102. Chouinard, G., Jones, B.D. (1980). Neuroleptic-induced supersensitivity psychosis: Clinical and pharmacologic characteristics. *Am J Psychiatry*, 137:16–21.

103. Kirkpatrick, B., Alphs, L., Buchanan, R.W. (1992). The concept of supersensitivity psychosis. *J Nerv Ment Dis*, 180(4):265–270.
104. Gelenberg, A.J., Bassuk, E.L., Schoonover, S.C. (1991). *The Practitioner's Guide to Psychoactive Drugs* (3rd ed.). New York: Plenum Medical Book Co.
105. Nemeroff, C.B., Devane, C.L., Pollock, B.G. (1996). Newer antidepressants and the cytochrome P450 system. *Am J Psychiatry*, 153:
106. Wesson, M. (1996). Continuing clozapine despite neutropenia. *Br J Psychiatry*, 168:217–220.
107. Opler, L.A., Feinberg, S.S. (1991). The role of pimozide in clinical psychiatry: A review. *J Clin Psychiatry*, 52:221–233.
108. Koreen, A.R., Siris, S.G., Chakos, M., et al. Depression in first-episode schizophrenia. *Am J Psychiatry*, 150:1643–1648.
109. Selzer, J.A., Lieberman, J.A. (1993). Schizophrenia and substance abuse. *Psychiatric Clin N Am*, 16(2):401–412.
110. Pristach, C., Smith, C. (1990). Medication compliance and substance abuse among schizophrenic patients. *Hosp Comm Psychiatry*, 41:1345–1348.
111. Drake, R.E., Osher, F.C., Wallach, M.A. (1989). Alcohol use and abuse in schizophrenia: A prospective community study. *J Nerv Ment Dis*, 177:408–414.
112. Drake, R.E., Wallach, M.A. (1989). Substance abuse among the chronic mentally ill. *Hosp Comm Psychiatry*, 40:1041–1046.
113. Berman (Zaharovits), I. Obsessive-compulsive symptoms in schizophrenia. APA Annual Meeting, New York, May 1990.
114. Baker, R.W., Chengappa, K.N., Baird, J.W., et al. (1992). Emergence of obsessive compulsive symptoms during treatment with clozapine. *J Clin Psychiatry*, 53(12):439–442.
115. Berman, I., Sapers, B.L., Chang, H.L.J., et al. (1995). Treatment of obsessive-compulsive symptoms in schizophrenic patients with clomipramine. *J Clin Psychopharmacol*, 15:206–210.
116. Goff, D.C., Brotman, A.W., Waites, M., et al. (1990). Trial of fluoxetine added to neuroleptics for treatment-resistant schizophrenic patients. *Am J Psychiatry*, 147:492–494.
117. Goldman, M.B., Janecek, H.M. (1990). Adjunctive fluoxetine improves global function in chronic schizophrenia. *J Neuropsychiatry Clin Neurosci*, 2:429–431.
118. Rosenberg, D.R., Holttum, J., Gershon, S. (1994). *Textbook of Pharmacotherapy for Child and Adolescent Psychiatric Disorders*. Philadelphia: Brunner/Mazel.
119. Wisner, K.L., Perel, J.M. (1988). Psychopharmacologic agents and electroconvulsive therapy during pregnancy and the puerperium. In Cohen, R.L. (Ed.). *Psychiatric Consultation in Childbirth Settings: Parent- and Child-Oriented Approaches* (pp. 165–206). New York: Plenum Medical Book Co.
120. Jeste, D.V., Lacro, J.P., Gilbert, P.L., et al. (1993). Treatment of late-life schizophrenia with neuroleptics. *Schizophr Bull*, 19(4):817–830.
121. Gregory, C., McKenna, P. (1994). Pharmacological management of schizophrenia in older patients. *Drugs and Aging*, 5(4):254–262.

ANXIETY DISORDERS

INTRODUCTION

The anxiety disorders, panic disorder (with and without agoraphobia), generalized anxiety disorder, obsessive-compulsive disorder, and post-traumatic stress disorder are among the most common psychiatric disorders, with a one-year prevalence of 4 to 8% of the general population.[1] The term *anxiety* may be defined as an excessive level of arousal and/or awareness that is associated with functional impairment. The different anxiety disorders, as outlined in this chapter, all exhibit both subjective and objective symptoms.

DIAGNOSTIC CRITERIA

The DSM-IV criteria for a panic attack, panic disorder without agoraphobia, panic disorder with agoraphobia, generalized anxiety disorder, obsessive-compulsive disorder (OCD), and post-traumatic stress disorder (PTSD) are presented in Tables 7–1 through 7–6.

TABLE 7–1. CRITERIA FOR PANIC ATTACK

Note: A panic attack is not a codable disorder. Code the specific diagnosis in which the panic attack occurs (e.g., panic disorder with agoraphobia).

A discrete period of intense fear or discomfort, in which four (or more) of the following symptoms developed abruptly and reached a peak within 10 minutes:

palpitations, pounding heart, or accelerated heart rate
sweating
trembling or shaking
sensations of shortness of breath or smothering
feeling of choking
chest pain or discomfort
nausea or abdominal distress
feeling dizzy, unsteady, lightheaded, or faint
derealization (feelings of unreality) or depersonalization (being detached from oneself)
fear of losing control or going crazy
fear of dying
paresthesias (numbness or tingling sensations)
chills or hot flushes

Adapted with permission from the *Diagnostic and Statistical Manual of Mental Disorders*, 4th ed. (p. 395). Copyright 1994 by American Psychiatric Association.

TABLE 7–2. CRITERIA FOR PANIC DISORDER WITHOUT AGORAPHOBIA

A. Both (1) and (2):

    (1) recurrent unexpected panic attacks
    (2) at least one of the attacks has been followed by one month (or more) of one (or more) of the following:

        (a) persistent concern about having additional attacks
        (b) worry about the implications of the attack or its consequences (e.g., losing control, having a heart attack, "going crazy")
        (c) a significant change in behavior related to the attacks

B. Absence of agoraphobia

C. The panic attacks are not due to the direct physiological effects of a substance (e.g., a drug of abuse, a medication) or a general medical condition (e.g., hyperthyroidism).

D. The panic attacks are not better accounted for by another mental disorder, such as social phobia (e.g., occurring on exposure to feared social situations). Specific phobia (e.g., on exposure to a specific phobic situation), obsessive-compulsive disorder (e.g., on exposure to dirt in someone with an obsession about contamination), post-traumatic stress disorder (e.g., in response to stimuli associated with a severe stressor), or separation anxiety disorder (e.g., in response to being away from home or close relatives).

Adapted with permission from the *Diagnostic and Statistical Manual of Mental Disorders*, 4th ed. (p. 402). Copyright 1994 by American Psychiatric Association.

TABLE 7-3. CRITERIA FOR PANIC DISORDER WITH AGORAPHOBIA

A. Both (1) and (2):

(1) recurrent unexpected panic attacks

(2) at least one of the attacks has been followed by one month (or more) of one (or more) of the following:

(a) persistent concern about having additional attacks

(b) worry about the implications of the attack or its consequences (e.g., losing control, having a heart attack, "going crazy")

(c) a significant change in behavior related to the attacks

B. The presence of agoraphobia

C. The panic attacks are not due to the direct physiological effects of a substance (e.g., a drug of abuse, a medication) or a general medical condition (e.g., hyperthyroidism).

D. The panic attacks are not better accounted for by another mental disorder, such as social phobia (e.g., occurring on exposure to feared social situations). Specific phobia (e.g., on exposure to a specific phobic situation), obsessive-compulsive disorder (e.g., on exposure to dirt in someone with an obsession about contamination), post-traumatic stress disorder (e.g., in response to stimuli associated with a severe stressor), or separation anxiety disorder (e.g., in response to being away from home or close relatives).

Adapted with permission from the *Diagnostic and Statistical Manual of Mental Disorders*, 4th ed. (pp. 402–403). Copyright 1994 by American Psychiatric Association.

CLINICAL FEATURES OF ANXIETY DISORDERS

PANIC DISORDER

Panic disorder (PD), with and without agoraphobia, has at its root the panic attack. A panic attack is a time-limited episode of both physiological symptoms (tachycardia, dyspnea, sweating, nausea) and psychic symptoms (fear of dying, fear of "going crazy"). Agoraphobia is a situational based anxiety/phobia that progresses to phobic avoidance. While panic disorder is characterized by the presence of panic attacks, one panic attack does not equal panic disorder. Panic disorder, if untreated, may progress to include agoraphobia. Agoraphobia also may be found in patients who have not experienced panic attacks, however.

GENERALIZED ANXIETY DISORDER

Generalized anxiety disorder (GAD) is a syndrome of excessive anxiety about life situations and is defined by the presence of anxiety or nervousness and of three or more associated symptoms including restlessness,

TABLE 7–4. CRITERIA FOR GENERALIZED ANXIETY DISORDER

A. Excessive anxiety and worry (apprehensive expectation), occurring more days than not for at least 6 months, about a number of events or activities (such as work or school performance).

B. The person finds it difficult to control the worry.

C. The anxiety and worry are associated with three (or more) of the following six symptoms (with at least some symptoms present for more days than not for the past six months). Note: Only one item is required in children.

restlessness or feeling keyed up or on edge
being easily fatigued
difficulty concentrating or mind going blank
irritability
muscle tension
sleep disturbance (difficulty falling or staying asleep, or restless, unsatisfying sleep)

D. The focus of the anxiety and worry is not confined to features of an Axis I disorder, e.g., the anxiety and worry is not about having a panic attack (as in panic disorder), being embarrassed in public (as in social phobia), being contaminated (as in obsessive-compulsive disorder), being away from home or close relatives (as in separation anxiety disorder), gaining weight (as in anorexia nervosa), having multiple physical complaints (as in somatization disorder), or having a serious illness (as in hypochondriasis), and the anxiety and worry do not occur exclusively during post-traumatic stress disorder.

E. The anxiety, worry, or physical symptoms cause clinically significant distress or impairment in social, occupational, or other important areas of functioning.

F. The disturbance is not due to the direct physiological effects of a substance (e.g., a drug of abuse, a medication) or a general medical condition (e.g., hyperthyroidism) and does not occur exclusively during a mood disorder, a psychotic disorder, or a pervasive developmental disorder.

Adapted with permission from the *Diagnostic and Statistical Manual of Mental Disorders*, 4th ed. (pp. 435–436). Copyright 1994 by American Psychiatric Association.

sleep disturbance, irritability, and diminished concentration, as given in Table 7–4. Symptoms must be present for a minimum of six months for the diagnosis to be made.

OBSESSIVE-COMPULSIVE DISORDER

Obsessive-compulsive disorder (OCD) is a disorder characterized by the presence of obsessions and compulsions. Obsessions are recurring thoughts that are intrusive in nature, cannot be suppressed by the patient,

text continues on page 255

TABLE 7–5. CRITERIA FOR OBSESSIVE-COMPULSIVE DISORDER

A. Either obsessions or compulsions:

Obsessions as defined by (1), (2), (3), and (4):

(1) recurrent and persistent thoughts, impulses, or images that are experienced, at some time during the disturbance, as intrusive and inappropriate and that cause marked anxiety or distress

(2) the thoughts, impulses, or images are not simply excessive worries about real-life problems

(3) the person attempts to ignore or suppress such thoughts, impulses, or images, or to neutralize them with some other thought or action

(4) the person recognizes that the obsessional thoughts, impulses, or images are a product of his or her own mind (not imposed from without as in thought insertion)

Compulsions as defined by (1) and (2):

(1) repetitive behaviors (e.g., hand washing, ordering, checking) or mental acts (e.g., praying, counting, repeating words silently) that the person feels driven to perform in response to an obsession, or according to rules that must be applied rigidly

(2) the behaviors or mental acts are aimed at preventing or reducing distress or preventing some dreaded event or situation; however, these behaviors or mental acts either are not connected in a realistic way with what they are designed to neutralize or prevent or are clearly excessive

B. At some point during the course of the disorder, the person has recognized that the obsessions or compulsions are excessive or unreasonable. Note: This does not apply to children.

C. The obsessions or compulsions cause marked distress, are time-consuming (take more than one hour a day), or significantly interfere with the person's normal routine, occupational (or academic) functioning, or usual social activities or relationships.

D. If another Axis I disorder is present, the content of the obsessions or compulsions is not restricted to it (e.g., preoccupation with food in the presence of an eating disorder; hair pulling in the presence of trichotillomania; concern with appearance in the presence of body dysmorphic disorder; preoccupation with drugs in the presence of a substance use disorder; preoccupation with having a serious illness in the presence of hypochondriasis; preoccupation with sexual urges or fantasies in the presence of a paraphilia; or guilty ruminations in the presence of major depressive disorder).

E. The disturbance is not due to the direct physiological effects of a substance (e.g., a drug of abuse, a medication) or a general medical condition.

Specify if:

With Poor Insight: if, for most of the time during the current episode, the person does not recognize that the obsessions and compulsions are excessive or unreasonable.

Adapted with permission from the *Diagnostic and Statistical Manual of Mental Disorders*, 4th ed. (pp. 422–423). Copyright 1994 by American Psychiatric Association.

TABLE 7–6. CRITERIA FOR POST-TRAUMATIC STRESS DISORDER

A. The person has been exposed to a traumatic event in which both of the following were present:
   (1) the person experienced, witnessed, or was confronted with an event or events that involved actual or threatened death or serious injury, or a threat to the physical integrity of self or others
   (2) the person's response involved intense fear, helplessness, or horror. Note: In children, this may be expressed instead by disorganized or agitated behaviors

B. The traumatic event is persistently reexperienced in one (or more) of the following ways:
   (1) recurrent and intrusive distressing recollections of the event, including images, thoughts, or perceptions. Note: In young children, repetitive play may occur in which themes or aspects of the trauma are expressed
   (2) recurrent distressing dreams of the event. Note: In children, there may be frightening dreams without recognizable content
   (3) acting or feeling as if the traumatic event were recurring (includes a sense of reliving the experience, illusions, hallucinations, and dissociative flashback episodes, including those that occur on awakening or when intoxicated). Note: In young children, trauma-specific reenactment may occur
   (4) intense psychological distress at exposure to internal or external cues that symbolize or resemble an aspect of the traumatic event
   (5) physiological reactivity on exposure to internal or external cues that symbolize or resemble an aspect of the traumatic event

C. Persistent avoidance of stimuli associated with the trauma and numbing of general responsiveness (not present before the trauma), as indicated by three (or more) of the following:
   (1) efforts to avoid thoughts, feelings, or conversations associated with the trauma
   (2) efforts to avoid activities, places, or people that arouse recollections of the trauma
   (3) inability to recall an important aspect of the trauma
   (4) markedly diminished interest or participation in significant activities
   (5) feeling of detachment or estrangement from others
   (6) restricted range of affect (e.g., unable to have loving feelings)
   (7) sense of a foreshortened future (e.g., does not expect to have a career, marriage, children, or a normal life span)

D. Persistent symptoms of increased arousal (not present before the trauma), as indicated by two (or more) of the following:
   (1) difficulty falling or staying asleep
   (2) irritability or outbursts of anger
   (3) difficulty concentrating
   (4) hypervigilance
   (5) exaggerated startle response

E. Duration of the disturbance (symptoms in Criteria B, C, and D) is more than one month

F. The disturbance causes clinically significant distress or impairment in social, occupational, or other important areas of functioning.

Specify if:
   Acute: if duration of symptoms is less than three months
   Chronic: if duration of symptoms is three months or more

Specify if:
   With Delayed Onset: if onset of symptoms is at least six months after the stressor

Adapted with permission from the *Diagnostic and Statistical Manual of Mental Disorders*, 4th ed. (pp. 427–429). Copyright 1994 by American Psychiatric Association.

254

and cause anxiety or distress. Compulsions are repetitive behaviors or mental processes (washing, counting, etc.) that are performed in an attempt to suppress obsessions.

OCD has a lifetime prevalence rate of 2–3% in the United States and it affects men and women equally.[2] It is a clinical syndrome characterized by the presence of obsessive thoughts. These obsessions frequently involve fear of harmful events and may invoke compulsive rituals in an attempt to avoid "harm." While both the obsessions and compulsions may be seen as irrational by the OCD patient, he or she is eventually unable to resist them and they may interfere with his or her performance at home or at work. Comorbid symptoms of depression or anxiety may also appear.

POST-TRAUMATIC STRESS DISORDER

Post-traumatic stress disorder (PTSD) is a syndrome that may develop after exposure to a traumatic event outside the realm of normal human experience (i.e., an act of violence, a natural disaster, a trauma) over which the person has no control. The resulting symptom complex, as can be seen in Table 7–6, includes both anxiety symptoms (i.e., hyperarousal and hypervigilance) and affective symptoms (diminished affect, sense of detachment, belief in a foreshortened future).

DIFFERENTIAL DIAGNOSIS

Anxiety may be a symptom of medical illness as well as psychiatric illness, and common medical causes of anxiety must be ruled out before diagnosing a primary anxiety disorder. Cardiovascular, neurological, respiratory, hematological, and endocrine disorders can all manifest anxiety symptoms.

Angina pectoris or acute myocardial infarction frequently presents with chest pain. While it is common for sufferers of panic attacks to present to an emergency room complaining of chest pain, an electrocardiogram, history, and physical examination should be performed to rule out the above two conditions. Palpitations and dyspnea may also be presenting symptoms of an arrhythmia or congestive heart failure, as well as a panic attack.

Neurological and respiratory conditions that may present with symptoms mimicking panic include seizure, vertigo, tremor, asthma, chronic obstructive pulmonary disease, and an acute pulmonary embolism. Clues pointing to these nonfunctional diagnoses would be found on an initial physical examination.

Less commonly, anemia and endocrine abnormalities (hyper- or hypothyroidism, hyperparathyroidism, or pheochromocytoma) may present with anxiety symptoms. A final consideration in the differential diagnosis of anxiety symptoms is substance intoxication and withdrawal. Intoxication with illicit substances, like marijuana and cocaine to name only two, may present in part with symptoms of generalized anxiety or a panic attack.

NATURAL COURSE

PANIC DISORDER WITH OR WITHOUT AGORAPHOBIA

Panic disorder, with and without agoraphobia, is a chronic, recurrent disorder for which many patients require chronic pharmacotherapy. Pollock et al. followed 59 patients for a mean duration of 1.5 years who had completed an acute treatment program with either alprazolam, clonazepam, or placebo.[3] Of these, 78% remained on medication at the same mean dosage as during acute treatment. The authors noted that while overall symptom improvement was maintained, it had diminished slightly from that at the end of the acute treatment phase. Rickels et al. studied 123 benzodiazepine-dependent patients enrolled in a discontinuation study at follow-up of 2.7 to 5 years.[4] Forty-eight patients had completed the study. Of them, 78% were free of benzodiazepine use, and 35% still reported moderate-to-marked anxiety symptoms. The authors then argued that the high number of patients who were benzodiazepine-free but with continued symptomatology suggests these chronic symptoms were due to a chronic illness, rather than drug dependence.

One factor that distinguishes panic disorder from the other anxiety disorders is its robust placebo response. Dager et al. found that 27% of panic disorder patients in a 40-week, blinded study were placebo responders as defined by approximately a 42% decrease in ratings on symptom scales.[5] This response was noted at one week of placebo therapy, persisted throughout the 40 weeks, and was present one month after taper of the placebo at the end of the study. Dager et al. confirmed this early and robust response to placebo in a 32-week, double-blind trial with 138 PD patients with alprazolam.[6] They found that, overall, the subgroup of panic disorder patients with agoraphobia had the smallest placebo response when the groups were tapered over one month and that the alprazolam-treated group had a greater increase in anxiety symptoms than the placebo group. These findings illustrate a profound placebo response with this disorder that may be in part responsible for successful treatment with any pharmacological agent.

The discontinuation of therapy, particularly benzodiazepines, may play a role in the natural course of panic disorder by producing a withdrawal syndrome consisting of symptoms of anxiety, sleep disturbance, and disturbances of perception. Fyer et al. performed a discontinuation trial on 17 patients with PD with or without agoraphobia.[7] The patients were initially treated acutely for 13 weeks with alprazolam (mean dosage 5.25 mg/day) and then underwent a controlled taper of 10% of drug dose every three days. During the taper, 15 of the 17 patients experienced a recurrent or increased number of panic attacks and 9 of the 15 experienced withdrawal symptoms, most commonly malaise, weakness, insomnia, tachycardia, lightheadedness, and dizziness. Burrows et al. reported that discontinuation effects appear to be present regardless of benzodiazepine half-life, but that withdrawal of shorter half-life drugs is associated with a shorter time to onset of withdrawal symptoms than the longer half-life drugs.[8] While withdrawal symptoms occur commonly after discontinuation of benzodiazepines, they are more frequent after discontinuation of shorter acting drugs than longer acting drugs.[9]

Does a comorbid depressive illness alter the course of panic disorder? Nagy et al. found that treatment outcome with an initial course of imipramine/behavioral therapy at one to five years was unaffected by the presence of an initial diagnosis of major depression at the beginning of the study.[10] Noyes et al., however, found comorbid depression in 22% of their sample and reports of depressive symptoms in another 14%.[11] These episodes were more likely to occur in patients not receiving a tricyclic antidepressant. Depression may also develop as part of the course of the primary disorder, a so-called secondary depression, and has been reported in approximately 50% of PD with or without agoraphobic patients.[12,13]

GENERALIZED ANXIETY DISORDER

Details of the natural course of generalized anxiety disorder have yet to be fully described. Cloninger et al. reported a female:male ratio of 6:4, an age of onset of 20–35 years, and a familial clustering of cases.[14] Rickles et al. examined 131 patients with anxiety and 63% were found to relapse within one year of completing a treatment trial or dropping out.[15] Noyes et al. examined "anxiety neurosis" and stated that a longer duration of illness may predispose to a poorer outcome.[16] It is unclear what percentage of these "anxiety" or "anxiety neurosis" patients had GAD.

Mancusco et al. reported on 16-month follow-up data on 44 GAD patients who had initially completed a medication trial.[17] Fully 50% of them still fulfilled DSM-III-R criteria for GAD. Various Axis I comorbid diagnoses were present: dysthymia (11%), major depression (7%), and social phobia (7%). Ongoing GAD symptoms were more likely be associated with a comorbid Axis II disorder. The authors concluded by noting that 50% of GAD patients did not follow a chronic course.

OBSESSIVE-COMPULSIVE DISORDER

One unique factor in the course of OCD may be a very low placebo response. Mavissakalian et al. examined 30 patients treated in a single-blinded fashion with placebo for two weeks and then a subset of those patients (12) for an additional 10 weeks and found no improvement in both patient and clinician-rated symptoms of OCD.[18] Montgomery et al. also reported a very low placebo response rate (5.2%) in OCD.[19]

Psychiatric comorbidity or comorbid substance abuse may decrease the effectiveness of treatment for OCD. Baer et al. found that the diagnosis of schizotypal, borderline, or avoidant personality disorders, as well as the total number of DSM-III axis II diagnoses (greater than one), were predictive of poorer response to treatment.[20]

POST-TRAUMATIC STRESS DISORDER

Data are not currently available on the natural history of post-traumatic stress disorder but it appears clinically to be a chronic, lifelong condition.

ACUTE AND CONTINUATION PHARMACOLOGICAL TREATMENT

Schatzberg and Ballenger provided guidelines for the acute treatment of panic disorder which are given in Table 7–7.[21] They also noted that a delineation between primary and secondary panic needs to be made. If a patient's symptoms are in fact due to an underlying disorder (medical

TABLE 7–7. ACUTE THERAPY: GUIDELINES

Treat acutely if any one of the following is present:

Recent severe or frequent panic attacks or generalized anxiety
Clear morbidity:

    attacks have limited functioning at work or socially
    demoralization or suicidal ideation
    avoidant behavior or alcohol usage

Secondary comorbid disorders. e.g., alcohol abuse, major depression
Consider treating if significant family history of suicide or alcohol
    abuse is present.

Adapted from Schatzberg, A.F., Ballenger, J.C. (1991). Assessment and treatment of panic disorder. *J Clin Psychiatry*, 52(2 suppl): 26–30. Copyright 1991 by Plenum Publishing Corp. Reprinted with permission.

disease, alcoholism, or substance abuse), the primary condition needs to be treated and that one panic attack or a history of a remote series of panic attacks may be indications for observation rather than immediate treatment.

Charney et al. examined the comparative efficacy of imipramine, alprazolam, and trazodone in 74 PD patients in an eight-week, double-blind trial.[22] The authors found that while imipramine (maximum dosage 300 mg/day) and alprazolam (maximum dosage 8 mg/day), but not trazodone, were highly effective in decreasing symptoms of PD, the alprazolam group experienced decreasing symptoms during the first week while the imipramine group required four weeks of treatment until a treatment effect was seen. The data suggest that, as in affective illness, an appropriate trial of four to six weeks of a tricyclic is needed before declaring a treatment failure.

Ballenger et al. found in an eight-week trial of alprazolam versus placebo in 525 PD patients with agoraphobia that alprazolam (5 to 6 mg/day) decreased anxiety, decreased panic attacks (situational and spontaneous), decreased avoidance behavior, and decreased disability from panic symptoms after one week.[23] After four weeks, 82% of the alprazolam group experienced moderate improvement in anxiety symptoms, compared with 43% of the placebo group. After four weeks, 50% of the alprazolam group were without panic attacks, compared with 28% of the placebo group.

Panic disorder, panic attacks, and phobic symptoms did not respond to propranolol (median dose 240 mg/day) in an acute treatment trial comparing it with diazepam that was superior in efficacy.[24]

MAINTENANCE PHARMACOLOGIC TREATMENT

PANIC DISORDER WITH OR WITHOUT AGORAPHOBIA

Curtis et al. studied 181 patients with PD in a six-month, double-blind maintenance phase after an eight-week acute treatment phase (to which they responded) comparing alprazolam 6–7 mg/day, imipramine 150–175 mg/day, and placebo.[25] They found that twice as many acute treatment patients as placebo patients maintained or improved in symptom level, indicating a sustained efficacy of drugs and no evidence of tolerance.

Nagy et al. examined the long-term outcome of treatment in 28 patients with DSM-III diagnosed agoraphobia with panic attacks who received a four-month combined treatment of imipramine and behavioral therapy and were then discharged from treatment on imipramine therapy alone (mean dosage 74 mg/day).[10] The period of follow-up was between one to five years. They found that although only one-half of the patients remained on imipramine, the frequency of panic attacks and the symptoms of anxiety were reduced in all the patients. The authors concluded that the clinical improvement seen after a four-month combined treatment program was maintained for between one to five years, regardless of whether imipramine therapy was continued. The authors also emphasized the need for double-blind, controlled trials to further define the role of maintenance treatment of agoraphobia with panic disorder.

Lelliott et al. reported the results of a five-year follow-up study of 40 outpatients with agoraphobia.[26] All the patients had initially received exposure homework assignments and a combination of either imipramine (up to 200 mg/day) or placebo, plus ongoing exposure or relaxation therapy. Medication treatment was discontinued after six-and-a-half months. During the five-year follow-up, 58% of patients had required further medication treatment for agoraphobia and 25% remained on medications at the five-year point (benzodiazepines, tricyclic antidepressants, both or low-dose phenothiazines). The authors noted that those patients who were highly symptomatic at the end of the initial trial period were more likely to be symptomatic at five years and that those with a higher level of psychosocial functioning at the beginning of the trial were less symptomatic at five years. The authors, however, noted that a higher number of spontaneous panic attacks did not predict a poorer outcome.

Noyes et al. studied 107 patients with panic disorder who were treated openly with a tricyclic antidepressant and various psychotherapeutic interventions.[11] One-third of the group also received a benzodiazepine. After one to four years of follow-up, 63% of the patients continued on the tricyclic antidepressant and one-half of the subgroup receiving benzodiazepines at the onset of the study had discontinued them.

Schweizer et al. noted that although imipramine and alprazolam appear equally efficacious in treatment of PD, alprazolam has a greater degree of patient compliance.[27]

Schatzberg and Ballenger summarized the guidelines of a 1990 symposium on the acute and maintenance pharmacological treatment of panic disorder.[21] Their decision tree is shown in Figure 7–1. They emphasized that an acute treatment response over several months may be strengthened by continued treatment for several additional months (i.e., four to six months total) as too early discontinuation of therapy may lead to relapse. The authors provided indications for the need for maintenance treatment (shown below in Table 7–8) and noted that if active treatment has not been adequately effective, a dosage increase or an alternative agent should be tried. The long-term risks of the various drug therapies for PD are given in Table 7–9.

DURATION OF TREATMENT

Clinically, greater than 50% of PD patients require treatment for 6 to 8 months, while an additional 40% may need 12 months of treatment;

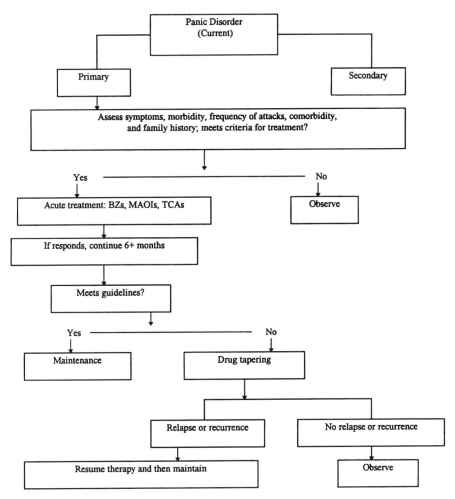

FIG. 7–1. Decision Tree: Assessment and treatment of panic disorder. From Schatzberg, A.F., Ballenger, J.C. (1991). Assessment and treatment of panic disorder. J. Clin Psychiatry, 52 (2 suppl.): 26–30. Copyright 1991 by Plenum Publishing Corp. Reprinted with permission.

20–40% may require chronic treatment. The authors also noted that definitive studies of treatment duration in PD have yet to be performed.

FAILURE RATE

As can be seen from the data reviewed above, the failure rate of pharmacological treatment is very low. In more severe cases, the intensity and frequency of panic attacks may be reduced, if not eliminated.

TABLE 7–8. MAINTENANCE THERAPY: GUIDELINES

Institute and continue maintenance therapy if the acute treatment was well tolerated and if any of the following are or were present:

Long duration of illness: severe and frequent attacks
Recent panic attacks while on medication
Secondary psychopathology, particularly if still present
Continued avoidant or other maladaptive behavior

Adapted from Schatzberg, A.F., Ballenger, J.C. (1991). Assessment and treatment of panic disorder. *J Clin Psychiatry*, 52(2 suppl): 26–30. Copyright 1991 by Plenum Publishing Corp. Reprinted with permission.

TABLE 7–9. LONG-TERM RISKS OF MAINTENANCE AND DISCONTINUATION OF DRUG TREATMENT

Monoamine oxidase inhibitors: weight gain, hypertensive crises, hyperpyrexic reactions, rebound mania
Tricyclic antidepressants: weight gain, rebound cholinergic symptoms on withdrawal, rebound mania, increased blood pressure
Benzodiazepines: cognitive impairment, ataxia (elderly), dependence, withdrawal

Adapted from Schatzberg, A.F., Ballenger, J.C. (1991). Assessment and treatment of panic disorder. *J Clin Psychiatry*, 52(2 suppl): 26–30. Copyright 1991 by Plenum Publishing Corp. Reprinted with permission.

FACTORS AFFECTING COMPLIANCE

Not surprisingly, the acceptability of the side-effect profile of the various pharmacological agents used is the major factor in medication treatment compliance. Benzodiazepines, as discussed below, have a less distressing side-effect profile than tricyclic antidepressants.

PREDICTORS OF RESPONSE/POOR OUTCOME

Pollack et al. reported that the presence of dysthymia and the presence of "less distress" on initial symptom rating was predictive of a favorable response to treatment.[3] They also found that the total duration of panic disorder, the presence of agoraphobia, and comorbid social phobia were predictors of poor outcome.[3] Pecknold noted that a prior use of benzodiazepines predicted difficulty upon treatment discontinuation.[28] Basoglu et al. summarized predictors of a poor outcome: longer duration of illness, older age, history of depression, and severity of phobias.[29] The authors also

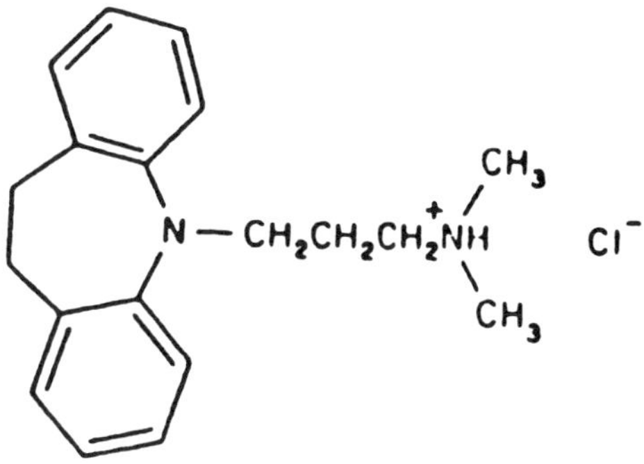

FIG. 7–2. Chemical structure of imipramine.

noted that treatment expectancy, pre-treatment morbidities (anxiety or depression), sex of patient, and referral source were not predictive of outcome.

TRICYCLIC ANTIDEPRESSANTS

Imipramine is the tricyclic antidepressant most studied and used clinically in panic disorder (Figure 7–2). Details of its usage are discussed fully in Chapter 4 on depression.

BENZODIAZEPINES

Alprazolam and clonazepam are the two most commonly used benzodiazepines in the treatment of anxiety (Figures 7–3 and 7–4). Tolerance, dependence, and rebound are three relevant pharmacological properties of benzodiazepines used in the maintenance treatment of anxiety disorders. *Tolerance is a decrease in the therapeutic response to a fixed dose of a drug over time.* With the advent of tolerance, larger and larger doses of a drug are required to achieve the original therapeutic effect. Tolerance does not appear to be a factor in PD treatment, as a slight decrease in the dosage requirement may be seen at the end of one year of treatment.[8] Rickles et al. enrolled 180 PD patients in a double-blind, continuous, 6 to 22 week trial of diazepam (15–40 mg/day) versus placebo and found that tolerance to the anxiolytic effects of the benzodiazepine did not occur.[30]

Dependence is a complex syndrome with both physical and psychological components. The DSM-IV diagnostic criteria for substance dependence are given in Table 7–10. Dependence on benzodiazepines may occur at

text continues on page 265

TABLE 7–10. CRITERIA FOR SUBSTANCE DEPENDENCE

A maladaptive pattern of substance use, leading to clinically significant impairment or distress, as manifested by three (or more) of the following, occurring at any time in the same 12-month period:

(1) tolerance, as defined by either of the following:

    (a) a need for markedly increased amounts of the substance to achieve intoxication or desired effect

    (b) markedly diminished effect with continued use of the same amount of the substance

(2) withdrawal, as manifested by either of the following:

    (a) the characteristic withdrawal syndrome for the substance (refer to Criteria A and B of the criteria sets for withdrawal from the specific substances)

    (b) the same (or a closely related) substance is taken to relieve or avoid withdrawal symptoms

(3) the substance is often taken in larger amounts or over a longer period than was intended

(4) there is a persistent desire or unsuccessful efforts to cut down or control substance use

(5) a great deal of time is spent in activities necessary to obtain the substance (e.g., visiting multiple doctors or driving long distances), use the substance (e.g., chain-smoking), or recover from its effects

(6) important social, occupational, or recreational activities are given up or reduced because of substance use

(7) the substance use is continued despite knowledge of having a persistent or recurrent physical or psychological problem that is likely to have been caused or exacerbated by the substance (e.g., current cocaine use despite recognition of cocaine-induced depression, or continued drinking despite recognition that an ulcer was made worse by alcohol consumption)

Specify if:

    With Physiological Dependence: evidence of tolerance or withdrawal (i.e., either Item 1 or 2 is present)

    Without Physiological Dependence: no evidence of tolerance or withdrawal (i.e., neither Item 1 nor 2 is present)

Course specifiers (see text for definitions):

    Early Full Remission
    Early Partial Remission
    Sustained Full Remission
    Sustained Partial Remission
    On Agonist Therapy
    In a Controlled Environment

clinical or supraclinical dosages or in conjunction with alcohol or opioid abuse.[31]

Rebound or withdrawal symptoms are those that occur when a drug is discontinued or when its serum concentration decreases. The most common symptoms of benzodiazepine withdrawal are rebound anxiety and insomnia, both of which are more common with the shorter half-life agents (alprazolam and lorazepam). Withdrawal seizures may also occur with abrupt discontinuation of short half-life agents, even at therapeutic doses. Withdrawal symptoms usually resolve within 4 to 12 weeks.

Uhlenhuth et al. took an opposing view following their review of a large data set regarding long-term benzodiazepine use.[32] They reported that while dependence may occur with regular use of clinically appropriate dosages, the risks are low when compared with the large numbers of patients taking benzodiazepines overall.

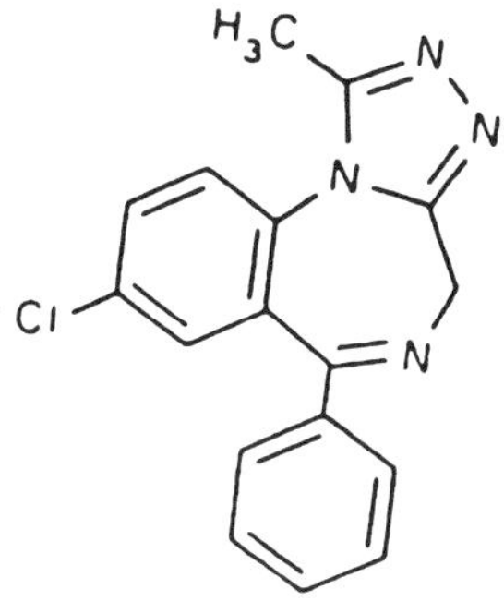

FIG. 7–3. Chemical structure of alprazolam.

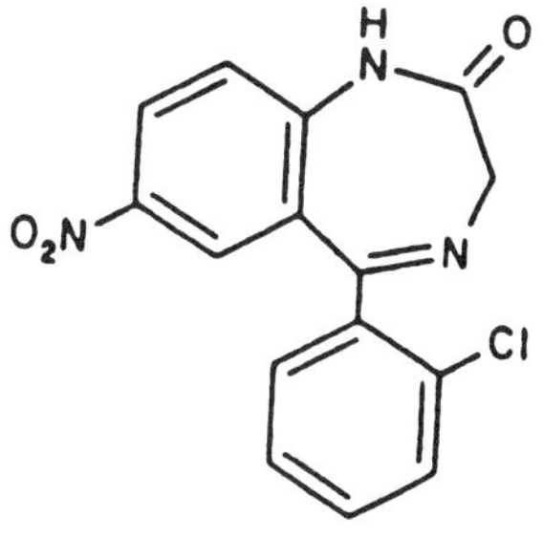

FIG. 7–4. Chemical structure of clonazepam.

DOSING/MONITORING THERAPY

The usual adult dosages of benzodiazepines are given in Table 7–11. Monitoring of benzodiazepine therapy is largely clinical as serum concentrations are not commonly obtained.

MANAGEMENT OF ADVERSE DRUG REACTIONS

Sedation is the most common side effect of benzodiazepine therapy and is seen most commonly at the initiation of treatment. It may be severe enough to limit a patient's driving or other functioning and the patient should be warned of this. While not usually prone to cause respiratory depression when used alone, the combination of benzodiazepines and other central nervous system depressants such as alcohol and barbiturates, may induce respiratory depression and even death. Therefore, the use of alcohol with benzodiazepines must be strongly discouraged. The sedative effects of benzodiazepines tend to diminish over time as tolerance to the drug develops. Less commonly, benzodiazepines may produce dizziness or ataxia in a patient and, if severe, may warrant discontinuation of the drug.

The presence of acute or chronic hepatic or renal dysfunction may increase the severity of benzodiazepine side effects by limiting the metabolism of the drugs. With the exception of lorazepam and oxazepam, the metabolism of the benzodiazepines occurs in the liver and involves some active metabolites that remain active in the central nervous system. Lorazepam and oxazepam are excreted unmetabolized through the kidneys, making them more favorable for use in the elderly, who possess a degree of age-related decline in hepatic function, and in patients with liver disease.

MANAGEMENT OF DRUG-DRUG INTERACTIONS

Commonly encountered interactions of benzodiazepines with other agents are given in Table 7–12. The best method for management of these interactions is to avoid concomitant use of benzodiazepines with these agents.

BETA-BLOCKERS

As discussed, the data for the use of propranolol in acute treatment are unfavorable. No studies exist on maintenance treatment. Clinically, propranolol or atenolol may be of use in situational anxiety, i.e., situations

text continues on page 268

TABLE 7–11. BENZODIAZEPINE DOSAGES

Drug	Approximate Dose Equivalents	Dosage Forms	Benzodiazepines Rate of Absorption	Major Active Metabolites	Average Half-Life of Metabolites (hrs)	Short or Long Acting	Usual Adult Dosage Range (mg per day)
Alprazolam (Xanax)	0.5	0.25, 0.5, 1, 2 mg tablets	Medium	α-Hydroxyalprazolam, 4-hydroxyalprazolam	12	Short	0.5–6
Clonazepam (Klonopin)	0.25	0.5, 1, 2 mg tablets	Rapid	None	34	Long	0.5–10
Diazepam (Valium)	5	2, 5, 10 mg tablets; 15 mg capsules (extended release); 5 mg/mt. parenteral; 5 mg/5 mt., 5 mg/mt. solution	Rapid	Desmethyldiazepam, oxazepam	100	Long	2–60
Lorazepam (Ativan)	1	0.5, 1, 2 mg tablets; 2 mg/mt. parenteral	Medium	None	15	Short	2–6

Adapted from Rosenberg, D.R., Holttum, J., Gershon, S. (1994). *Textbook of Pharmacotherapy for Child and Adolescent Psychiatric Disorders* (pp. 60–61). Philadelphia: Brunner/Mazel. Reprinted with permission.

TABLE 7-12. INTERACTIONS OF BENZODIAZEPINES WITH OTHER DRUGS

Decreased Absorption
Antacids

Increase CNS Depression
Antihistamines
Barbiturates and similarly acting drugs
Cyclic antidepressants
Ethanol

Increase Benzodiazepine Levels (Compete for microsomal enzymes; probably little or no effect on lorazepam, oxazepam, temazepam)
Cimetidine
Disulfiram
Erythromycin
Estrogens
Fluoxetine
Isoniazid

Adapted from Arana, G.W., Hyman, S.E. (1991). *Handbook of Psychiatric Drug Therapy*, 2nd ed. (p. 159). Copyright 1991 by Lippincott-Raven Publishers. Reprinted with permission.

in which the patient knows in advance that physiological symptoms (i.e., tachycardia, diaphoresis) may occur. For example, a person who becomes tachycardic when having to give a speech may use a beta-blocker to prevent the physiological symptoms of anxiety. In those cases, if relative contraindications to beta-blockade are not present (i.e., diabetes, asthma, bradycardia), a small dosage of either drug prior to the stressful situation will be helpful. Of note, beta-blockade will only remove the physiological manifestations of anxiety, not the psychic manifestations. Currently, these drugs appear to have no use in the treatment of panic disorder.

SEROTONIN SPECIFIC RE-UPTAKE INHIBITORS

No data are available currently regarding the use of these agents in PD. Clinically, they have been of benefit to some patients with PD. No one agent in this class appears to have a greater benefit than the others.

MONOAMINE OXIDASE INHIBITORS

While the MAOIs are effective agents in the treatment of affective and anxiety symptomatology in some patients, their side-effect profile precludes their use as first- or second-line therapy. While their side-effect profile is discussed fully in Chapter 4 on depression, a few comments are pertinent here. The tyramine-induced hypertensive/hyperpyrexic reactions may appear *at any time during the course of therapy.* Additional side effects of weight gain, orthostasis, and insomnia may not abate with prolonged use of the drugs. The use of MAOIs in panic disorder is likely to be restricted to a group of patients who have failed several other agents and who are able to maintain close follow-up with their physician. In addition, Sheehan et al. noted that the therapeutic effect of these agents in PD requires four to eight weeks of treatment until a decrease in anxiety symptoms is noted.[33]

BUPROPION

Bupropion has been found to be ineffective in decreasing both the frequency and the severity of symptoms in one study of PD patients with phobias.[34]

GENERALIZED ANXIETY DISORDER

MAINTENANCE PHARMACOLOGIC TREATMENT

Rickels et al. reported the results of an eight-week, double-blind, placebo-controlled study comparing imipramine, trazodone, and diazepam in 230 patients with GAD who were without other psychiatric morbidity.[35] Diazepam (mean dosage 26 mg/day) was most effective in reducing symptoms in the first two weeks, but at weeks 3 through 8, imipramine (mean dosage 143 mg/day) was superior to diazepam. At eight weeks, 73% of patients had moderate-to-marked improvement on imipramine, compared with 69% on trazodone (mean dosage 225 mg/day), 66% on diazepam, and 47% on placebo. Side effects were highest in the imipramine and trazodone group, and no impairment of cognitive functions was found across the treatment groups. Trazodone may have a role in the treatment of GAD, although not in PD, if other pharmacological treatments have failed.[22]

DURATION OF MAINTENANCE TREATMENT/FAILURE RATE

The duration of maintenance treatment for GAD is unclear due in part to a lack of experimental studies designed to answer that question. However, clinical experience demonstrates that after a six-month acute treatment period, a slow medication taper may be attempted. Fifty percent of GAD patients appear to follow a chronic course of illness, although the severity of their symptoms may be somewhat reduced.[17]

FACTORS AFFECTING COMPLIANCE/POOR OUTCOME

As discussed, the side-effect profile of the various pharmacological agents used is the major factor in medication treatment compliance, and benzodiazepines have a less distressing side effect profile than tricyclic antidepressants. A longer duration of illness, the presence of substance abuse, or the presence of an Axis III disorder are predictive of a poor response to drug treatment for GAD.[16]

TRICYCLIC ANTIDEPRESSANTS

Imipramine is the tricyclic antidepressant most used in GAD as evidenced by this literature review and its beneficial clinical experience. Details of its use are discussed in Chapter 4 on depression.

SEROTONIN SPECIFIC RE-UPTAKE INHIBITORS

No data are available currently on the use of SSRIs in GAD.

BENZODIAZEPINES

The use of benzodiazepines in GAD may be reserved for a second- or third-line treatment as the data regarding the use of imipramine and buspirone, as reviewed herein, are quite promising. Either of these agents should be tried as initial treatment strategies before turning to benzodiazepines.

BETA-BLOCKERS

Beta-blockers appear unlikely to have a role in the treatment of GAD. As discussed in the previous section, they remove only the physiological symptoms of anxiety, not the subjective feeling.

BUSPIRONE

Buspirone is a nonbenzodiazepine anxiolytic agent that acts as an agonist at pre- and post-synaptic 5-hydroxytryptamine receptors. Feighner et al. performed a 12-month, open-label trial to evaluate the effect of

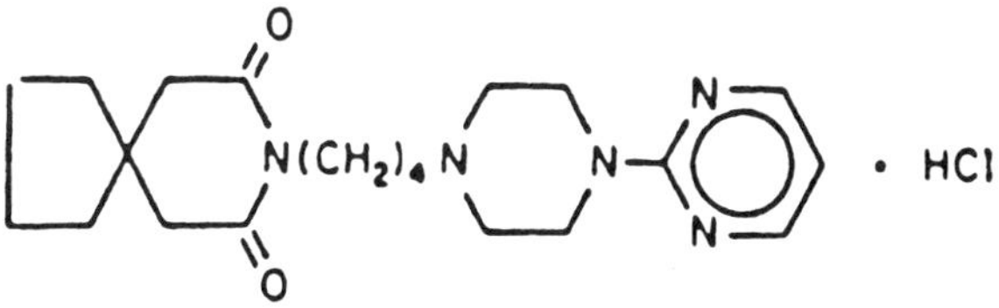

FIG. 7–5. Chemical structure of buspirone.

buspirone in GAD.[36] Seven hundred GAD patients, the majority with symptom duration of three months or greater, received buspirone 5 to 60 mg/day
(with the majority of patients receiving 15 to 20 mg/day). At three- and
six-month ratings, a mean decrease in anxiety symptoms was reported of
42.2% and 59.8%, respectively. Physicians who examined the patients after
six months documented improvement in 72%, half of whom had experienced
severe anxiety symptoms at study entry. The authors concluded that buspirone is an effective drug for GAD, with an optimum effective dose range
of 15 to 30 mg/day. Dell Chiaie et al. treated 44 GAD patients with lorazepam
(3 to 5 mg/day) for five weeks then randomized them in a double-blind fashion to either buspirone (15 mg/day) or placebo for six weeks while tapering
off the lorazepam over the first two weeks.[37] Patients were then followed
for two weeks after the end of the active trial, during which they received
placebo. The authors found that buspirone and lorazepam were of equal
efficacy in decreasing GAD symptoms and were clearly superior to placebo.
No rebound or increase in anxiety symptoms was seen in the buspirone
patients within the two weeks of placebo treatment at the end of the study
(Figure 7–5).

DOSING

Patients are usually started on 5 mg three times per day and increased
by 5 mg every two to three days to a final dose of 15 to 30 mg/day.
This increase may need to be done more slowly in elderly patients. Of note,
clinical experience now dictates that a person has not failed therapy with
this drug until he or she has been on 30 mg/day for a minimum of four
weeks.

MONITORING THERAPY

Monitoring of buspirone therapy is best accomplished by monitoring
the clinical course of the anxiety symptoms.

MANAGEMENT OF ADVERSE DRUG REACTIONS ON THERAPY

The side effects of buspirone therapy are drowsiness, dizziness, headache, nausea, and fatigue. If side effects do not appear within the first two months of treatment, they tend not to arise later and, overall, are better tolerated than the side effects of benzodiazepines.[36]

MANAGEMENT OF DRUG-DRUG INTERACTIONS

There is not much known about the interactions of buspirone with other psychotropics or other medications. Due to its activity as a serotoninergic agonist, the potential for an adverse interaction with an MAOI exists and these two agents should not be used together nor should an MAOI be started without a several week wash-out period after buspirone discontinuation. Clinically, concomitant use of buspirone with haloperidol may increase its serum concentration.

OBSESSIVE-COMPULSIVE DISORDER

MAINTENANCE PHARMACOLOGIC TREATMENT

The literature concerning the maintenance treatment of OCD deals primarily with clomipramine, a TCA, and SSRIs and is reviewed below. Prospective data on the duration of maintenance treatment in OCD are lacking. Clinically, however, it appears that the illness is chronic in nature and requires long-term treatment. As reported by Pato et al.[38], however, patients on long-term therapy may successfully tolerate a reduced dosage of medication as discussed below.

FAILURE RATE

Response of OCD to drug treatment is characterized not only by the presence or absence of a response, but also by the degree of response. Response rates are discussed in the sections on the individual agents.

FACTORS AFFECTING COMPLIANCE

Compliance is, as discussed, related directly to the side-effect profile of the agent chosen and is discussed elsewhere in the appropriate section.

PREDICTORS OF RESPONSE/POOR OUTCOME

Improvement at the end of acute treatment is the best predictor of response to maintenance treatment as was found in a six-year follow-up of patients receiving clomipramine.[39] Severity of symptoms pretreatment, the presence of comorbid tics, psychiatric comorbidity, or substance abuse appear to be predictive of a poorer response to drug treatment.

TRICYCLIC ANTIDEPRESSANTS

Clomipramine, a nonspecific serotonin re-uptake inhibitor, is the tricyclic antidepressant of first choice in the treatment of OCD (Figure 7–6). It differs from the other TCAs in its high degree of serotonergic re-uptake blockade. While its original use was for the treatment of affective disturbances, antiobessional effects occur in patients who lack concomitant affective symptoms[40] and these appear to be separate from the antidepressant effects.[41]

Clomipramine has been the subject of a series of double-blind, placebo-controlled studies and has demonstrated its beneficial effect on OCD and depressive symptoms. DeVeaugh-Geiss et al. reported the results of two placebo-controlled, 10-week, double-blind studies of 384 OCD patients with duration of illness greater than one to two years and found a 40 to 45% mean improvement in the clomipramine group (with a maximum dosage of 300 mg/day), but only a 4 to 5% mean improvement with placebo.[42] Jenike et al. found that at the end of 10 weeks of clomipramine versus placebo, the clomipramine group's scores on rating scales were statistically much improved, while the placebo group was unchanged.[43] Finally, a large study of 575 patients comparing clomipramine with placebo for 10 weeks

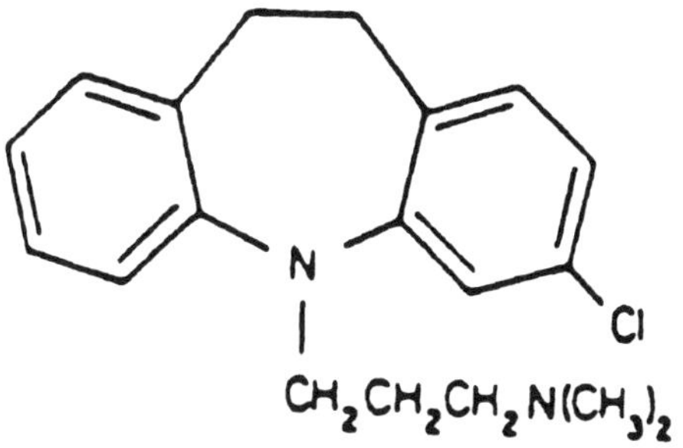

FIG. 7–6. Chemical structure of clomipramine.

demonstrated a 40% reduction in OCD symptoms in the clomipramine group (with a maximum dose of 300 mg/day), compared with a 5% reduction in the placebo group.[42] Clomipramine has also been found to be equally efficacious to phenelzine in a 12-week double-blind trial.[44]

Pato et al. performed a clomipramine dosage reduction study in 10 patients with OCD who had previously relapsed when clomipramine was discontinued.[38] All 10 patients tolerated a 40% decrease in clomipramine dosage (from 270 mg/day to 165 mg/day, mean dosages) without a statistically significant change in symptom rating scales. This study suggests that clomipramine dose in maintenance treatment may be decreased by up to 40% without changes in symptom level. This decrease may be attempted in the event of side effects with clomipramine treatment, prior to changing to a different agent.

DOSING

The usual adult dosage range for clomipramine is 150–250 mg/day, although as discussed, some OCD patients may require up to 300 mg/day. Adults may be started on 75 mg/day, for the first few days as a divided dose then as a single, hour of sleep dose. The dose may then be increased by 75 mg/week up to 300 mg/day. An OCD patient should be given at least a four-week trial at 300 mg/day, if possible, before he or she is called a nonresponder to clomipramine. Please see Chapter 4 for more general information on dosing tricyclic antidepressants.

MONITORING THERAPY

While the topic of plasma levels is discussed more fully in Chapter 4, the role of plasma clomipramine levels in OCD is discussed here. Mavissakalian et al. examined the correlation between treatment response versus the plasma levels of clomipramine and N-desmethylclomipramine, its major metabolite, in 33 patients with OCD in a 10-week study.[45] They found that a higher plasma clomipramine level (i.e., greater than 200 ng/ml) correlated in a statistically significant fashion with symptom diminution, while there was no correlation with the plasma level of N-desmethylclomipramine. The authors went on to report that the lower the N-desmethyl-clomipramine/clomipramine ratio, the more robust the clinical response. The authors postulated that slower demethylation of clomipramine may be responsible for a greater clinical response. They also noted that clomipramine is a potent serotonin reuptake blocker while N-desmethyl-clomipramine is a potent noradrenaline reuptake blocker.

MANAGEMENT OF ADVERSE DRUG
REACTIONS ON THERAPY

Clomipramine's side-effect profile of sedation, dry mouth, blurred vision, tremor, and sexual dysfunction is typical of the tricyclic antidepressant class and may contribute in large part to its poor tolerance by patients. Management of these side effects is discussed more fully in Chapter 4.

Clomipramine differs from the remainder of the tricyclics in its greater effect on lowering the seizure threshold. The onset of seizures appears to be dose related: 10/472 (2.1%) patients had seizures at doses greater than 300 mg/day compared with 12/2514 (0.48%) patients receiving 250 or less mg/day.[40]

MANAGEMENT OF DRUG-DRUG INTERACTIONS

Please see Chapter 4 for a discussion of drug-drug interactions of tricyclic antidepressants and their management.

SELECTIVE SEROTONIN REUPTAKE INHIBITORS

As a class of antidepressants, the SSRIs have failed to show homogeneity in their efficacy for OCD treatment. Fluoxetine has been shown to be effective in treating OCD. A large, multicenter study involving 355 patients in a double-blind, placebo-controlled, 13-week design demonstrated statistically significant effects of fluoxetine in doses of 20, 40, and 60 mg/day versus placebo.[46] The trend of greatest efficacy with the 60 mg/day dose was also reported. The most commonly reported side effects of fluoxetine were headache, nausea, insomnia, rhinitis, anorexia, dry mouth, somnolence, nervousness, tremor, and diarrhea. It is significant to note that it was not until week 5 of the study that a statistically significant improvement in OCD symptoms appeared in each of the fluoxetine study groups. This phenomenon of a slow and gradual therapeutic effect of fluoxetine in OCD, as well as the need for relatively higher fluoxetine doses than in affective illness, has been well described.[47] An earlier placebo-controlled, double-blind study involving 51 OCD patients, however, reported equal efficacy in dosages of 20, 40, or 60 mg/day.[48]

The experimental data regarding the effectiveness of sertraline in the treatment of OCD are mixed. Jenike et al. reported no improvement in OCD symptoms compared with placebo in a small 10-week double-blind study and felt this lack of effect may be due to an insufficient dosage (200 mg/day), too small a sample size (10 drug, 9 placebo), or to a unique pharmacological profile of sertraline.[49] Chouinard, however, reported positive results of three double-blind, placebo-controlled studies of sertraline. The first was an eight-week study of a fixed dose of 200 mg/day and demonstrated statistically significant improvement in three of the four rating scales used.[50] The other two studies were fixed dose studies of 8 and 12 weeks duration, using a maximum dose of 200 mg/day, and demonstrated efficacy at each of the dosages studied (50, 100, or 200 mg/day).[51]

Fluvoxamine has demonstrated equal efficacy to clomipramine in the treatment of OCD. Freeman et al. studied 66 outpatients with OCD randomized in a double-blind fashion to either fluvoxamine (100–250 mg/day) or clomipramine (100–250 mg/day) for 10 weeks.[52] They noted equal reduction in OCD symptoms in both drug groups and found that while fluvoxamine produced more insomnia and headache, clomipramine produced more anticholinergic effects and sexual dysfunction. Details of the use of SSRIs are discussed in Chapter 4.

MISCELLANEOUS AGENTS

Buspirone may have a minor role in the treatment of OCD as an adjuvant agent, but the data are mixed. Pigott reported the results of a double-blind study in which approximately 25% of OCD patients treated with buspirone experienced an additional 25% reduction in their OCD symptoms.[53] Grady and McDougle, however, reported that adjuvant treatment with buspirone conferred no additional benefit to OCD treatment.[54,55]

Trazodone was noted by Pigott et al. to lack any substantial antiobsessive effects in a 10-week, double-blind, placebo-controlled study.[56] Pigott et al. also studied the augmentation of clomipramine therapy with either lithium carbonate or triiodothyronine in an eight-week, double-blind, crossover study.[57] They found that, although the use of either drug as augmentation failed to decrease OCD symptoms by greater than 25%, the subset of subjects who received lithium carbonate experienced a greater than 25% decrease in their scores on depression indices.

Hewlett et al. compared clomipramine, clonazepam, and clonidine in a series of six-week trials, as well as a six-week trial of diphenhydramine as a control, in a double-blind, multiple crossover study and found that 40% of patients who failed clomipramine treatment (average dosage 239 mg/day) experienced a clinically significant improvement in symptoms with clonazepam (average dosage 6.85 mg/day).[58] The clonazepam response was the most pronounced of all the groups during the first three weeks of the study. No clinical benefit was noted in the clonidine group. The authors concluded that clonazepam may be a useful alternative treatment for OCD.

Finally, McDougle et al. examined haloperidol as an adjunct in OCD patients who had failed fluvoxamine monotherapy.[59] They found that 11 of 17 patients given haloperidol as an adjuvant to fluvoxamine experienced a reduction in severity of OCD symptoms whereas none of the 17 patients who received placebo in addition to fluvoxamine did. The authors also noted that the presence of a comorbid chronic tic disorder predicted a positive response to adjuvant haloperidol therapy.

MAINTENANCE TREATMENT OF POST-TRAUMATIC STRESS DISORDER

Maintenance pharmacotherapy for PTSD has yet to be a subject of prospective double-blind study and one must rely largely on clinical experience for treatment guidelines. Lipper et al. performed a small, open five-week study in 10 patients with PTSD (combat-induced) and noted a moderate or greater improvement in symptom rating scales in seven patients with carbamazepine.[60] Risse et al. reported a series of eight PTSD patients (combat-induced) who experienced severe withdrawal symptoms following a gradual taper of alprazolam therapy.[61]

When the clinician is faced with a choice of drug treatment for a PTSD patient, the appropriate choice might be based upon the predominant symptom cluster present, i.e., affective or anxiety. Depressed mood, anhedonia, sleep disturbance, hopelessness, and anergia may improve with antidepressant therapy. Irritability in PTSD, in our experience, has been quite responsive to SSRI treatment. Predominant symptoms of anxiety may require anxiolytic drug therapy. Benzodiazepine therapy should be reserved as a second- or third-line treatment in PTSD patients as these agents are difficult to discontinue in this population once they are started.[61]

SPECIAL POPULATIONS

PREGNANCY/LACTATION

The use of tricyclic antidepressants in pregnancy and lactation are discussed fully in Chapter 4. Maternal use of benzodiazepines is associated with risks to the fetus. Benzodiazepines easily cross the placenta to the fetal circulation that is ill-equipped to metabolize them, leading to increased concentrations that may persist up to several weeks after delivery. Symptoms of benzodiazepine toxicity in neonates include a poor suck, hypotonia, and global nervous system depression. While benzodiazepines alone carry minimal risk of teratogenicity, their chronic use combined with alcohol or other drugs may increase teratogenicity or other perinatal morbidity. Benzodiazepines are also secreted in breast milk, making their continued use a contraindication to breastfeeding.[62]

TREATMENT OF ELDERLY

The use of tricyclic antidepressants in the elderly is discussed fully in Chapter 4. Benzodiazepine use in the elderly is associated with an increased sensitivity to the side effects of drowsiness, confusion, and ataxia. This sensitivity results from a decreased volume of drug distribution, a decreased rate of metabolism (possibly both hepatic and renal), and increased sensitivity of GABA receptors. The use of these drugs in the elderly requires weighing the risk:benefit ratio before beginning treatment.

While there are no data available currently on the use of buspirone in the elderly, clinical experience has shown the drug to be quite effective and well tolerated in elderly patients with GAD-like symptoms.

TREATMENT OF ADOLESCENTS

What is known regarding the maintenance treatment of the anxiety disorders in adolescence? Data are available currently only on the treatment of OCD in adolescence. Flament et al. confirmed the effectiveness of clomipramine (mean dosage 141 mg/day) in 19 children with severe OCD in a 10-week, double-blind trial.[63] Symptom improvement was noted both by the patients and the examiners and was not found to have a correlation with serum concentrations. Leonard et al. reported the results of a maintenance treatment in which 26 children and adolescents with OCD treated with clomipramine (mean dosage 134.7 mg/day) for 4 to 32 months were switched in a double-blind fashion to either desipramine or clomipramine for two months and then returned to clomipramine for an additional two months.[64] Eighty-nine percent of the desipramine group experienced an increase in symptoms, compared with 18% of the clomipramine group. DeVeaugh-Geiss et al. described a 37% decrease in OCD symptoms with clomipramine, compared with an 8% decrease with placebo, in 27 children and adolescents in an eight-week, double-blind trial and noted continued effectiveness of clomipramine in the following one year of open treatment.[65] Riddle et al. reported a statistically significant decrease in OCD symptoms in 14 children and adolescents treated with fluoxetine (20 mg/day) in a placebo-controlled, double-blind fashion.[66]

REFERENCES

1. Weissman, M.M., Leaf, P.J., Holzer, C.E., Merikangas, K.R. (1985) The epidemiology of anxiety disorders: A highlight of recent evidence. *Psychopharmacol Bull*, 21:538–541.
2. Karno, M., Golding, J.M., Sorenson, S.B., et al. (1988) The epidemiology of obsessive-compulsive disorder in five US communities. *Arch Gen Psychiatry*, 45:1094–1099.
3. Pollock, M., Otto, M.W., Tesar, G.E., et al. (1993) Long-term outcome after acute treatment with clonazepam and alprazolam for panic disorder. *J Clin Psychopharmacol*, 13:257–263.
4. Rickels, K., Case, W.G., Schweizer, E., et al. (1991) Long-term benzodiazepine users three years after participation in a discontinuation program. *Am J Psychiatry*, 148(6):757–761.
5. Dager, S.R., Kahn, A., Cowley, D., et al. (1990) Characteristics of placebo response during long-term treatment of panic disorder. *Psychopharmacol Bull*, 26(3):273–278.
6. Dager, S.R., Roy-Byrne, P., Hendrickson, H., et al. (1992) Long-term outcome of panic states during double-blind treatment and after withdrawal of alprazolam and placebo. *Annals Clin Psychiatry*, 4(4):251–258.
7. Fyer, A.J., Liebowitz, M.R., Gorman, J.M., et al. (1987) Discontinuation of alprazolam treatment in panic patients. *Am J Psychiatry*, 144(3):303–308.
8. Burrows, G.D., Norman, T.R., Judd, F.K., et al. (1990) Short-acting versus long-acting benzodiazepines: Discontinuation effects in panic disorders. *J Psychiatric Research*, 24(Suppl 2): 65–72.
9. Noyes, R., Jr., Garvey, M.J., Cook, B., et al. (1991) Controlled discontinuation of benzodiazepine treatment for patients with panic disorder. *Am J Psychiatry*, 148(4):517–523.
10. Nagy, L.M., Krystal, J.H., Charney, D.S., et al. (1993) Long-term outcome of panic disorder after short-term imipramine and behavioral group treatment: 2.9-year naturalistic follow-up study. *J Clin Psychopharmcol*, 13(1):16–24.
11. Noyes, R., Jr., Garvey, M.J., Cook, B.L. (1989) Follow-up study of patients with panic disorder and agoraphobia with panic attacks treated with tricyclic antidepressants. *J Affect Dis*, 16:249–257.
12. Lesser, I.M., Rubin, R.T., Pecknold, J.C., et al. (1988) Secondary depression in panic disorder and agoraphobia: I. Frequency, severity, and response to treatment. *Arch Gen Psychiatry* 45:437–443.
13. Noyes, R., Jr. (1988) The natural history of anxiety disorders. In Roth, M., Noyes, R., Burrows, G.D. (Eds.) *Handbook of Anxiety* (pp. 115–334). New York: Elsevier.
14. Cloninger, C.R., Martin, E.L., Clayton, P. (1981) A blind follow up and family study of anxiety neurosis: Preliminary analyses of the St. Louis 500. In Klein, D.F., Rabkin, J.G. (Eds.). *Anxiety—New Research and Changing Concepts*. (pp. 69–79). New York: Raven Press.
15. Rickels, K., Case, W.G., Downing, R., et al. (1986) One year follow-up of anxious subjects treated with diazepam. *J Clin Psychopharmacol*, 6:32–36.
16. Noyes, R., Jr., Clancy J., Hoenk, P.R., et al. (1980) The prognosis of anxiety neurosis. *Arch Gen Psychiatry*, 37:173–178.
17. Mancuso, D.M., Townsend, M.H., Mercante, D.E. (1993) Long-term follow-up of generalized anxiety disorder. *Comprehensive Psychiatry*, 34(6):441–446.
18. Mavissakalian, M.R., Jones, B., Olson, S. (1990) Absence of placebo response in obsessive-compulsive disorder. *J Nerv Ment Disease*, 178(4):268–270.
19. Montgomery, S.A. (1980) Clomipramine in obsessional neurosis: A placebo-controlled trial. *Pharmacol Med*, 1:189–192.
20. Baer, L., Jenike, M.A., Black, D.W., et al. (1992) Effect of axis II diagnosis on treatment outcome with clomipramine in 55 patients with obsessive-compulsive disorder. *Arch Gen Psychiatry*, 49(11):862–866.

21. Schatzberg, A.F., Ballenger, J.C. (1991) Decisions for the clinician in the treatment of panic disorder: When to treat, which treatment to use, and how long to treat. *J Clin Psychiatry*, 52(Suppl 2):26–31.
22. Charney, D.S., Woods, S.W., Goodman, W.K., et al. (1986) Drug treatment of panic disorder: The comparative efficacy of imipramine, alprazolam and trazodone. *J Clin Psychiatry*, 47(12):580–586.
23. Ballenger, J.C., Burrows, G.D., Dupont, R.L., Jr., et al. (1988) Alprazolam in panic disorder and agoraphobia: Results from a multicenter trial, I. Efficacy in short-term treatment. *Arch Gen Psychiatry*, 45:413–422.
24. Noyes, R., Jr., Anderson, D.J., Clancy, J., et al. (1984) Diazepam and propranolol in panic disorders and agoraphobia. *Arch Gen Psychiatry*, 41(3):287–292.
25. Curtis, G.C., Massana, J., Udina, C., et al. (1993) Maintenance drug therapy of panic disorder. *J Psychiatric Res*, 27(Suppl 1):127–142.
26. Lelliott, P.T., Marks, I.M., Monterio, W.O. (1987) Agoraphobia five years after imipramine and exposure: Outcome and predictors. *J Nerv Ment Disease*, 175(10):599–605.
27. Schweizer, E., Rickels, K., Weiss, S., Zavodnick, S. (1993) Maintenance drug treatment of panic disorder: I: Results of a prospective placebo-controlled comparison of alprazolam and imipramine. *Arch Gen Psychiatry*, 50:51–60.
28. Pecknold, J.C. (1993) Discontinuation reactions to alprazolam in panic disorders. *J Psychiatric Res*, 27(Suppl 1):155–170.
29. Basoglu, M., Marks, I.M., Swinson, R.P., et al. (1994) Pre-treatment predictors of treatment outcome in panic disorder and agoraphobia treated with alprazolam and exposure. *J Affect Dis*, 30(2):123–132.
30. Rickels, K., Case, W.G., Downing, R.W., et al. (1983) Long-term diazepam therapy and clinical outcome. *JAMA*, 250(6):767–771.
31. Laux G., Puryear, D.A. (1984) Benzodiazepines: Misuse, abuse and dependency. *Am Fam Physician*, 30:139–147.
32. Uhlenhuth, E.H., DeWit, H., Balter, M.B., et al. (1988) Risks and benefits of long-term benzodiazepine use. *J Clin Psychopharmacol*, 8(3):161–162.
33. Sheehan, D.V., Ballenger, J., Jacobsen, G. (1980) Treatment of endogenous anxiety with phobic, hysterical and hypochondriacal symptoms. *Arch Gen Psychiatry*, 37:51–59.
34. Sheehan, D.V., Davidson, J., Manschreck, T., et al. (1983) Lack of efficacy of a new antidepressant (Bupropion) in the treatment of panic disorder with phobias. *J Clin Psychopharmacol*, 3(1):28–31.
35. Rickels, K., Downing, R., Schweizer, E., et al. (1993) Antidepressants for the treatment of generalized anxiety disorder. *Arch Gen Psychiatry*, 50(11):884–895.
36. Feighner, J. (1987) Buspirone in the long-term treatment of generalized anxiety disorder. *J Clin Psychiatry*, 48(Suppl 12):3–6.
37. Delle Chiaie, R., Pancheri, P., Casacchia, M. (1995) Assessment of the efficacy of buspirone in patients affected by generalized anxiety disorder, shifting to buspirone from prior treatment with lorazepam: A placebo-controlled, double-blind study. *J Clin Psychopharmcol*, 15(1):12–19.
38. Pato, M.T., Hill, J.L., Murphy, D.L. (1990) A clomipramine dosage reduction study in the course of long-term treatment of obsessive-compulsive disorder patients. *Psychopharmacol Bull*, 26(2):211–214.
39. O'Sullivan, G., Noshirvani, H., Marks, I., et al. (1991) Six-year follow-up after exposure and clomipramine therapy for obsessive-compulsive disorder. *J Clin Psychiatry*, 52(4):150–155.
40. Katz, R.J., DeVeaugh-Geiss, J. (1990) The antiobsessional effects of clomipramine do not require concomitant affective disorder. *Psychiatry Res*, 31(2):121–129.
41. Mavissakalian, M., Turner, S.M., Michelson, L., et al. (1985) Tricyclic antidepressants in obsessive-compulsive disorder: Antiobsessional or antidepressant agents? *Am J Psychiatry*, 142:572–576.

42. DeVeaugh-Geiss, J., Landau, P., Katz, R. (1989) Preliminary results from a multicenter trial of clomipramine-obsessive-compulsive disorder. *Psychopharmocol Bull*, 25(2):36–40.
43. Jenike, M.A., Baer, L., Summergrad, P., et al. (1989) Obsessive-compulsive disorder: A double-blind, placebo controlled trial of clomipramine in 27 patients. *Am J Psychiatry*, 146:1328–1330.
44. Vallejo, J., Olivares, J., Manos, T., et al. (1992) Clomipramine versus phenelzine in obsessive compulsive disorder. A controlled trial. *Br J Psychiatry*, 161:665–670.
45. Mavissakalian, M.R., Jones, B., Olson, S. (1990) Clomipramine in obsessive-compulsive disorder: Clinical response and plasma levels. *J Clin Psychopharmacol*, 10(4):261–268.
46. Tollefson, G.D., Rampey, A.H., Jr., Potvin, J.H., et al. (1994) A multicenter investigation of fixed-dose fluoxetine in the treatment of obsessive-compulsive disorder. *Arch Gen Psychiatry*, 51(7):559–567.
47. Wood, A., Tollefson, G.D., Birkett, M. (1993) Pharmacotherapy of obsessive compulsive disorder-Experience with fluoxetine. *Int Clin Psychopharmacol*, 8(4):301–306.
48. Dominguez, R.A. (1992) Serotonergic antidepressants and their efficacy in obsessive compulsive disorder. *J Clin Psychiatry*, 53 (Suppl): 56–59.
49. Jenike, M.A., Baer, L., Summergrad, P. (1990) Sertraline in obsessive compulsive disorder: A double-blind comparison with placebo. *Am J Psychiatry*, 147(7):923–928.
50. Chouinard, G., Goodman, W., Greist, J., et al. (1990) Results of a double-blind placebo controlled trial of a new serotonin uptake inhibitor, sertraline, in the treatment of obsessive-compulsive disorder. *Psychopharmacol Bull*, 26(3):279–284.
51. Chouinard, G. (1992) Sertraline in the treatment of obsessive compulsive disorder: Two double-blind, placebo-controlled studies. *Int Clin Psychopharmacol*, 7(Suppl 2):37–41.
52. Freeman, C.P., Trimble, M.R., Deakin, J.F., et al. (1994) Fluvoxamine versus clomipramine in the treatment of obsessive compulsive disorder: A multicenter, randomized double-blind, parallel group comparison. *J Clin Psychiatry*, 55(7):301–305.
53. Pigott, T.A., L'Heureux, F., Rubenstein, C.S., et al. (1992) A double-blind, placebo-controlled study of trazodone in patients with obsessive-compulsive disorder. *J Clin Psychopharmacol*, 12(3):156–162.
54. Grady, T.A., Pigott, T.A., L'Heureux, F., Hill, J.L., et al. (1993) Double-blind study of adjuvant buspirone for fluoxetine treated patients with obsessive-compulsive disorder. *Am J Psychiatry*, 150(5):819–821.
55. McDougle, C.J., Goodman, W.K., Leckman, J.F., et al. (1993) Limited therapeutic effect of addition of buspirone in fluvoxamine-refractory obsessive-compulsive disorder. *Am J Psychiatry*, 150(4):647–649.
56. Pigott, T.A., L'Heureux, F., Hill, J.L., et al. (1992) A double-blind study of adjuvant buspirone hydrochloride in clomipramine-treated patients with obsessive-compulsive disorders. *J Clin Psychopharmacol*, 12(1):11–18.
57. Pigott, T.A., Pato, M.T., L'Heureux, F., et al. (1991) A controlled comparison of adjuvant lithium carbonate or thyroid hormone in clomipramine-treated patients with obsessive-compulsive disorder. *J Clin Psychopharmacol*, 11(4):242–248.
58. Hewlett, W.A., Vinogrodov, S., Agras, W.S. (1992) Clomipramine, clonazepam and clonidine treatment of obsessive-compulsive disorder. *J Clin Psychopharmacol*, 12(6):420–430.
59. McDougle, C.J., Goodman, W.K., Leckman, J.F., et al. (1994) Haloperidol addition in fluvoxamine-refractory obsessive-compulsive disorder. A double-blind, placebo-controlled study in patients with and without tics. *Arch Gen Psychiatry*, 51(4):302–308.
60. Lipper, S., Davidson, J.R.T., Grady, T.A., et al. (1986) Preliminary study of carbamazepine in post-traumatic stress disorder. *Psychosomatics*, 27(12):849–854.
61. Risse, S.C., Whitters, A., Burke, J., et al (1990) Severe withdrawal symptoms after discontinuation of alprazolam in eight patients with combat induced post-traumatic stress disorder. *J Clin Psychiatry*, 51(5):206–209.

62. Ashton, H. (1995) Toxicity and adverse consequences of benzodiazepine use. *Psychiatric Annals*, 25(3):158–165.

63. Flament, M.F., Rapoport, J.L., Berg, C.J., et al. (1985) Clomipramine treatment of childhood obsessive-compulsive disorder: A double-blind controlled study. *Arch Gen Psychiatry*, 42:977–983.

64. Leonard H.L., Swedo, S.E., Lenane, M.C., et al. (1991) A double-blind desipramine substitution during long-term clomipramine treatment in children and adolescents with obsessive compulsive disorder. *Arch Gen Psychiatry*, 48(10):922–927.

65. DeVeaugh-Geiss, J., Moroz, G., Biederman, J., et al. (1992) Clomipramine hydrochloride in childhood and adolescent obsessive-compulsive disorder—A multicenter trial. *J Am Acad Child Adolesc Psychiatry*, 31(1):45–49.

66. Riddle, M.A., Scahill, L., King, R.A., et al. (1992) Double-blind, crossover trial of fluoxetine and placebo in children and adolescents with obsessive-compulsive disorder. *J Am Acad Child Adolesc Psychiatry*, 31(6):1062–1069.

SEIZURE DISORDERS

INTRODUCTION

The link between epilepsy and behavioral disorders has long been recognized. There has been considerable literature published in the past 30 years to remind us of the interaction between seizure disorders and psychopathology, particularly psychosis. A seizure is a paroxysmal cerebral neuronal firing with or without perceptual or motor alterations or altered consciousness. Epilepsy is a disorder characterized by recurrent seizures.

CLASSIFICATION

The International Classification of Epileptic Seizures (ICES) is listed in Table 8–1.[1] Mesial temporal lobe focus seizures are characterized by rising epigastric discomfort, nausea, autonomic signs, pallor, flushing, pupillary dilatation, fear, panic, and olfactory hallucinations. Lateral temporal lobe seizures are characterized by auditory and visual hallucinations and language dysfunction. Frontal lobe seizure manifestations include motor automatisms, rapid generalization, and minimal post-ictal confusion. Focal seizures may be simple (without affecting consciousness) or complex (with impaired consciousness). Generalized seizures may present as tonic-clonic,

text continues on page 285

TABLE 8–1. INTERNATIONAL CLASSIFICATION OF EPILEPSIES AND EPILEPTIC SYNDROMES

1	Localization-related (focal, local, partial) epilepsies and syndromes
1.1	Idiopathic (with age-related onset)

- Benign childhood epilepsy with centrotemporal spike
- Childhood epilepsy with occipital paroxysms
- Primary reading epilepsy

1.2	Symptomatic

- Chronic progressive epilepsia partialis continua of childhood (Kojewnikow's syndrome)
- Syndromes characterized by seizures with specific modes of precipitation
- Temporal lobes epilepsies
- Frontal lobe epilepsies
- Parietal lobe epilepsies
- Occipital lobe epilepsies

1.3	Cryptogenic
2	Generalized epilepsies and syndromes
2.1	Idiopathic (with age-related onset—listed in order of age)

- Benign neonatal familial convulsions
- Benign neonatal convulsions
- Benign myoclonic epilepsy in infancy
- Childhood absence epilepsy (pyknolepsy)
- Juvenile absence epilepsy
- Juvenile myoclonic epilepsy (impulsive petit mal)
- Epilepsy with grand mal (GTCS) seizures on awakening
- Other generalized idiopathic epilepsies not defined above
- Epilepsies with seizures precipitated by specific modes of activation

2.2	Cryptogenic or symptomatic (in order of age)

- West syndrome (infantile spasms, Blitz-Nick-Salaam Krampfe)
- Lennox-Gastaut syndrome
- Epilepsy with myoclonic-astatic seizures
- Epilepsy with myoclonic absences

2.3	Symptomatic
2.3.1	Nonspecific etiology

- Early myoclonic encephalopathy
- Early infantile epileptic encephalopathy with suppression burst
- Other symptomatic generalized epilepsies not defined above

2.3.2	Specific syndromes

- Epileptic seizures may complicate many disease states. Under this heading are included diseases in which seizures are a presenting or predominant feature

3	Epilepsies and syndromes undetermined whether focal or generalized
3.1	With both generalized and focal seizures

- Neonatal seizures

(Contd.)

TABLE 8–1. (Continued)

- Severe myoclonic epilepsy in infancy
- Epilepsy with continuous spike-waves during slow wave sleep
- Acquired epileptic aphasia (Landau-Kleffner syndrome)
- Other undetermined epilepsies not defined above

3.2 Without unequivocal generalized or focal features. All cases with generalized tonic–clonic seizures in which clinical and EEG findings do not permit classification as clearly generalized or localization related, such as in many cases of sleep–grand mal (GTCS) considered not to have unequivocal generalized or focal features

4 Special syndromes

4.1 Situation-related seizures (Gelegenheitsanfalle)

- Febrile convulsions
- Isolated seizures or isolated status epilepticus
- Seizures occurring only when there is an acute metabolic or toxic event due to factors such as alcohol, drugs, eclampsia, nonketotic hyperglycemia

From Proposal for Revised Classification of Epilepsies and Epileptic Syndromes. (1989). *Epilepsia*, 30(4). Copyright 1989 by Lippincott-Raven Publishers. Reprinted with permission.

tonic, clonic, absence, or myoclonic. In generalized seizures, the epileptiform activity begins bilaterally and is associated with impaired consciousness.

Temporal lobe epilepsy (TLE) is an example of a complex partial seizure with a temporal lobe focus. TLE is no longer used in the official classification scheme but is used in this chapter to refer to focal seizures with a temporal lobe focus. TLE is the seizure type most frequently associated with neuropsychiatric manifestations and psychopathology, so these seizures are described in greater detail in a later section.

EPIDEMIOLOGY

The incidence of epilepsy is 20–70/100,000 per year and is age dependent with the highest incidence in early childhood and then increasing with age in the elderly.[2] Point prevalence is 3–5/1000 and lifetime prevalence is 3.5%. This 10-fold difference suggests that epilepsy is not a lifetime disorder in the majority of patients.[2] Focal seizures account for about 70% of epilepsy. Primary generalized seizures account for approximately 30% of epilepsy, and less than 5% are absence or myoclonic.[2]

PROGNOSIS

The risk of recurrence after a first seizure is 27–84% depending on the length of follow-up.[2] The prevailing view of epilepsy as a chronic disorder in the vast majority of patients is not substantiated.

Most patients go into one-year remission with treatment. The treatment recommendation is to withdraw antiepileptic drugs (AEDs) after two years seizure free. The relapse rate after two years seizure free is 12–72% and decreases to 11–53% after three years seizure free.[2] However, as many as 25% of patients have intractable seizures despite optimal anticonvulsant medication.[3] This group suffers primarily from complex partial seizures.

There is some controversy over whether adequate treatment, thus preventing more seizures, improves the long-term outcome. It is possible that with improved treatment over recent years, the natural course of epilepsy has improved and been transformed into a less severe and less chronic disorder.

ETIOLOGY

The biochemical abnormalities associated with epilepsy have been proposed to be either a deficit of inhibitory neurotransmission or an excess of excitatory neurotransmission. The primary inhibitory neurotransmitter in the brain is GABA and there is evidence that there are alterations in GABA-A receptors and glutamic acid decarboxylase (GAD), the enzyme that synthesizes GABA. The primary excitatory neurotransmitters are the amino acids glutamate and aspartate. These bind to the NMDA receptor that is a glutamate-mediated calcium channel. Excess excitatory amino acid neurotransmission may be the mechanism underlying TLE since there is evidence of NMDA receptor changes in the parahippocampal gyrus in this condition.

Epilepsy is often associated with other forms of cerebral pathology especially perinatal anoxia that can damage the hippocampus, encephalitis, closed head injury, brain trauma, stroke, and cerebral masses such as tumors or infections.

DIAGNOSIS

The diagnosis of epilepsy is made on the basis of a clinical history of seizures, a neurological examination, and electroencephalographic evidence of paroxysmal epileptiform activity. Structural brain imaging such as magnetic resonance imaging (MRI) may be useful to assess concomitant structural pathology. Functional brain imaging, such as single photon emission computed tomography and positron emission tomography, may demonstrate hypermetabolism at the seizure focus. Neuropsychological testing is useful to determine concomitant cognitive or personality impairment and to help optimize educational and rehabilitation efforts.

TREATMENT

Treatment of seizures is primarily with AEDs that increase the seizure threshold thereby decreasing the frequency and severity of seizures. About 75% of patients are adequately controlled with monotherapy while an additional 15% require a second agent. Table 8–2 lists the first- and second-line agents for each of the common seizures types.

For the 5–10% of patients who are treatment refractory, surgical excision of the seizure focus is an option. Most refractory patients have temporal

TABLE 8–2. ANTIEPILEPTIC DRUGS BY SEIZURE TYPE

Seizure Type	First-Line Agent	Second-Line Agent
General idopathic epilepsies	VPA	
Primary generalized		
tonic-clonic	VPA	CBZ, PHT
absence	ESM	VPA, VPA, ESM
myoclonic	VPA	ESM, MSM
Secondary epilepsies (symptomatic)		
West syndrome (infantile spasms)	ACTH, cortosteroids	VPA, VGB
Lennox-Gastaut syndrome	VPA	CBZ, PHT, PB, CZP, BZD, FBM combinations
Localization-related epilepsies and epileptic syndromes (focal, local, and partial)	CBZ, PHT	PB, VPA
Idiopathic benign childhood epilepsy with centrotemporal spikes	CBZ	PHT, PB, PRM
Symptomatic epilepsies		
secondary generalized tonic–clonic seizures	CBZ, PB, PHT, PRM, VPA	
partial seizures	CBZ, VPA, PHT	PB, PRM

VPA = valproate, CBZ = carbamazepine, PHT = phenytoin, ESM = ethosuximide, MSM = methsuximide, VGB = vigabatrin, PB = phenobarbital, CZP = clonazepam, BZD = benzodiazepines, FBM = felbamate, PRM = primidone. Adapted from Mattson, R.H. (1995). Efficacy and adverse effects of established and new antiepileptic drugs. *Epilepsia*, 36(suppl 2):S13–S26. Copyright 1995 by Lippincott-Raven Publishers. Reprinted with permission.

lobe foci so temporal lobectomy is the most common surgical procedure for intractable epilepsy.

NEUROPSYCHIATRIC MANIFESTATIONS

ASSOCIATION BETWEEN SEIZURE AND PSYCHOPATHOLOGY

There is a higher rate of psychopathology in epilepsy patients than in the general population, although the rate is approximately equal to that in other chronic illnesses.[3] Also, patients with epilepsy are overrepresented in psychiatric hospitals, and about 10% of these patients have schizophrenia, suggesting that there is a strong link between epilepsy and psychosis.[3] Factors associated with psychopathology in epilepsy include anatomical location of seizure focus, ictal firing, kindling, other cerebral pathology, psychosocial aspects associated with having a chronic illness, developmental effects, and factors associated with treatment such as folate deficiency, alterations in monoamine neurotransmitter metabolism, and endocrine effects.[3,4] Psychopathology is more predominant in TLE than in generalized epilepsy.[3] Much of this chapter focuses on TLE.

LIMBIC SYSTEM

Papez first described the limbic system and recognized its role in regulating behavior and emotion.[5] The limbic system includes the amygdala, hippocampus, parahippocampal gyrus, limbic forebrain (nucleus accumbens, ventral striatum), hypothalamus, thalamus, and midbrain tegmentum. The circuit mediates emotional expression and affective modulation and is thought to be involved in some types of epilepsy, particularly TLE.

NEUROPATHOLOGY IN TLE

Pathological changes in parts of the limbic system have been seen in TLE. The most notable change is sclerosis of mesial temporal structures, especially the hippocampus. This change can be a result of anoxia during an early developmental period such as perinatal complications, febrile seizures, or encephalitis. Mesial temporal tumors may also be seen in TLE.

NEUROPSYCHIATRIC MANIFESTATIONS OF TLE

TLE is associated with behavioral disorders including psychosis. In fact, the psychosis seen in TLE is almost indistinguishable from schizophrenia. Slater et al. in their five part series on the schizophrenia-like psychoses of epilepsy suggest that the same underlying anatomical abnormality is responsible for the development of both epilepsy and schizophrenia.[7] Subsequent studies have identified this as neuroanatomical disarray in the mesial temporal lobe.[8]

PSYCHOSOCIAL FACTORS

The stress of having a chronic, paroxysmal disorder with a constant threat of an unexpected seizure may contribute to maladjustment and psychopathology.[5] In addition, the social and functional restrictions imposed on individuals suffering from epilepsy may lead to dependency.

LOCATION OF SEIZURE FOCUS

Laterality of seizure focus effects psychopathology. Left hemisphere foci are associated with psychotic symptoms and thought disorder, while right hemisphere foci tend to have a greater association with affective symptoms.[9]

RELATIONSHIP OF NEUROPSYCHIATRIC MANIFESTATIONS TO TIMING OF SEIZURE

Neuropsychiatric symptoms may occur at different times in relation to the ictus. Symptoms may occur during the preictal prodrome or aura period, during the ictal period, post-ictally, or interictally.

TEMPORAL LOBE SYMPTOMS

TLE is the seizure type most commonly associated with neuropsychiatric manifestations. Simple partial temporal lobe seizures begin with olfactory hallucinations and may have psychic symptomatology such as flashbacks and deja vu. Temporal lobe absence seizures have a 10–30 second loss of consciousness accompanied by minor motor automatism such as masticatory movements, buttoning or speech automatisms, drop attacks, staring spells, post-ictal perplexity, and disorientation. Other temporal lobe phenomena include auditory buzz or hum, complex verbalization, aphasia, illusions, tactile distortions, olfactory and gustatory phenomena, flashbacks, deja vu, jamais vu, depersonalization, and derealization.

PSYCHOSIS

There is some controversy as to whether epilepsy is associated with a high rate of psychosis. The incidence of psychosis in epilepsy is 2–9%

in neurology and general medicine clinics but is much higher (21–60%) in specialized psychiatry clinics.[2] Some studies demonstrate that there is no greater incidence of psychosis in epilepsy than in the general population.[8] However, psychosis in epilepsy is four to seven times more likely to occur in TLE than in primary generalized epilepsy.[5] Comparing complex partial seizures with and without psychosis, patients with psychosis have significantly more neurological signs, spike patterns on electroencephalogram (EEG), history of brain damage, and absence of family histories of seizure disorder,[5] and more psychosocial problems.[5] Comparing psychotic patients with complex partial seizure and with generalized epilepsy, patients with complex partial seizures are more treatment refractory, require higher AED doses, are more likely to be treated with polypharmacy, have more seizures, and have evidence of associated organic brain syndrome.[5]

There is no universally accepted classification system for epilepsy plus psychosis. Conventionally, psychotic syndromes are classified by their temporal relationship to the ictus.

PRE-ICTAL

Pre-ictal phenomena are divided into the prodrome, which may last for days prior to the seizure, and the aura, which usually lasts only seconds immediately before the seizure. Altered insight and reality testing, psychosis, and thought disorder have been described during the prodromal period in some patients. The aura may consist of hallucinations (olfactory, auditory, visual, or visceral) or other psychic phenomena.

PERI-ICTAL

Simple focal status epilepticus may present with complex hallucinations, thought disorder, and affective symptoms. Complex focal status epilepticus may be continuous or cyclic and may be marked by prolonged confusional states and "psychotic behavior."[2] These two states may resemble an acute psychotic episode of schizophrenia with psychomotor automatisms, misinterpretations, forced thinking, hallucinations, flashbacks, depersonalization, derealization, and paranoia. Generalized nonconvulsive status is in some cases characterized by altered consciousness, disorientation, apathy, delusions, and hallucinations.

What has been described as peri-ictal psychosis with an altered level of consciousness and disorientation is probably better categorized as delirium. It usually presents with undirected, nonspecific aggression, especially when the patient is restrained.

POST-ICTAL

Post-ictal psychosis accounts for about 25% of psychosis in epilepsy. It may be precipitated by a series of tonic-clonic seizures, especially of complex focal origin, and usually follows a lucid period of several days after the seizure. Common symptoms include paranoid delusions, altered mood state, fluctuating level of consciousness, disorientation, and confusion. This state resembles delirium, and the EEG demonstrates increased epileptiform and slow wave activity. This state resolves spontaneously within days to weeks and rarely proceeds to a chronic state.

INTER-ICTAL

Inter-ictal psychosis accounts for about 10–30% of epileptic psychoses and most closely resembles schizophrenia. Several studies have demonstrated that the phenomenology of psychosis of epilepsy is not significantly different from schizophrenia.[2,10] However, some differences have been reported. Psychosis of epilepsy is characterized by delusions of mystical or religious content, less well-organized delusions, predominant visual rather than auditory hallucinations, no formal thought disorder or catatonia, rare negative symptoms, normal affect, and a worse long-term outcome.[2,11]

POST-TEMPORAL LOBECTOMY

Temporal lobectomy does not improve psychosis even when it does treat the seizures effectively. In fact, psychosis can occur de novo after temporal lobectomy in some patients.

RISK FACTORS FOR PSYCHOSIS IN EPILEPSY

Some risk factors have been identified (but these are controversial because they are based on uncontrolled retrospective studies)[7] including prevalence of head trauma, history of encephalitis, temporal lobe seizures, and cortical atrophy. Psychosis is associated with early adolescent onset of seizures. There is a mean of 14 years between onset of seizures and onset of psychosis,[7] possibly supporting the hypothesis that kindling contributes to the development of schizophrenic psychosis in epilepsy. TLE accounts for 76% of the cases of psychosis in epilepsy in uncontrolled studies, which is approximately the prevalence of epilepsy which is TLE.[2] There is considerable evidence for a predominance of dominant hemisphere mesial temporal foci in patients who develop psychosis.[12] TLE with a dominant hemisphere focus is associated with thought disorder while a nondominant hemisphere focus is associated with affective symptomatology.[13] In controlled studies, the rates of psychosis in TLE and in generalized seizures are the same. Psychosis in generalized seizures is more mild, confusional, and shorter lasting with no paranoia or hallucinations and prominent affective symptoms. On the other hand, the psychosis in TLE is marked by Schneiderian first rank symptoms and chronicity, similar to schizophrenia.

There appears to be an inverse relationship between psychosis and seizures, with psychosis worsening when seizures are under better control in many, but not all, cases.

ACUTE TREATMENT

Antipsychotics are effective in treating psychosis in epilepsy, but there are a few additional concerns when using these medications in patients with epilepsy that do not apply to other patient populations. Antipsychotics lower the seizure threshold, thus potentially exacerbating the underlying seizure disorder. The phenothiazines (chlorpromazine) have the greatest effect on seizure threshold while pimozide has the least. Antipsychotics also increase serum levels of the AEDs. When using antipsychotics, serum levels of AEDs must be monitored carefully during initiation and titration. The AED dose may be decreased in anticipation of this effect if the level is already at the upper limit of normal range or there are some signs of neurotoxicity. AEDs decrease the levels of antipsychotics, so higher doses of antipsychotics may be needed for therapeutic effect. Phenobarbital and multiple AEDs should be avoided if possible when using antipsychotics.

While there are no published studies of maintenance treatment of psychosis in epilepsy, lifelong treatment with antipsychotics is recommended. Often a balance must be struck between control of seizures and control of psychosis. AED levels should be monitored with any change in antipsychotic dose.

DEPRESSION

There is an association between epilepsy and depression although there have not been any good studies comparing the rate of depressive disorders in epilepsy with the general population. The rate of suicide in epilepsy is about five times the general population.[2] Mania, however, is rarely associated with epilepsy.

Etiological factors contributing to depression in epilepsy range from psychosocial to biological factors.[2] The following two variables may be related to the development of depression although there is little evidence: the social stigma and stress of having a chronic episodic illness with externally imposed restrictions on functioning (for example, driving, working in certain jobs), and some of the AEDs, particularly phenobarbital. The use of carbamazepine is the least associated with depression. Some of the medications can also lead to folate deficiency thus indirectly affecting the metabolism of many neurotransmitters involved in affective regulation. Temporal lobe (limbic system) pathology may also be directly related to depression. There is a higher rate of depression after temporal lobectomy. Left temporal lobe seizure foci are more highly associated with depression while right temporal lobe seizure foci are associated with hypomania (this is a similar lateralization as seen in post-stroke depression).[2]

PRODROMAL

Depressed or irritable mood may last several days during the prodromal period and is relieved by the seizure.

PERI-ICTAL/INTER-ICTAL

Depression is relatively rare in the peri-ictal period, but when it does occur, it tends to last longer than other emotional symptoms. A syndrome consistent with major depressive disorder may occur during the inter-ictal period in some patients. Depression in epileptics is associated with more dysthymia, fewer "neurotic traits," and more agitation and anxiety than in nonepileptics.[2] It may also be associated with certain personality traits that are described in the next section.

ACUTE TREATMENT

The first step in treating depression is to optimize seizure control, preferably with the fewest number of medications possible. If the patient is on phenobarbital or vigabatrin, both of which may exacerbate or contribute to depression, these should be discontinued and replaced with carbamazepine if possible.

Antidepressant use in epilepsy has been reported in several acute treatment studies.[14] Robertson and Trimble report a double-blind, placebo-controlled trial of nomifensine and amitriptyline that demonstrated nomifensine significantly more effective than amitriptyline in treating depression in epilepsy.[15] Some antidepressants, especially the TCAs, decrease the seizure threshold. The SSRIs have little effect on seizure threshold. Antidepressants increase serum levels of AEDs, so AED levels must be monitored closely during antidepressant dose titration. AEDs decrease antidepressant levels, so higher doses than usual of antidepressants may be needed. The maintenance treatment of depression in epilepsy has not been studied.

PERSONALITY CHANGE

The *epileptic character* has long been recognized as a discrete entity and occurs in 7–21% of epileptics.[2] However, there is some controversy over the nature and etiology of the personality changes. Psychosocial factors relating to living with a chronic illness that usually begins during adolescence before coping skills or personality is completely developed, may interfere with normal cognitive and personality development. Long-term AED exposure may also lead to personality changes. The characteristic personality may be directly related to the underlying pathology of the seizures (namely head injury that may have predated the onset of seizures), the brain pathology associated with the seizure focus, or a result of recurrent seizures. The psychiatric manifestations, including personality changes, appear to be more dependent on the location of the seizure focus, especially the anterior temporal lobe, than on psychosocial factors.

The character traits associated with epilepsy have been described variably by several different authors. Waxman and Geschwind identified hypergraphia, diminished sexuality, and preoccupation with philosophical and moral concerns as the hallmark features.[16] Bear and Fedio also included humorlessness, dependence, circumstantiality, and a heightened sense of personal destiny.[17] Perini differentiated personality styles by hemisphere of seizure focus; patients with left temporal lobe lesions are characteristically paranoid, depressed, guilt-ridden, aggressive, angry, and have a negative self-image, while patients with right hemisphere lesions have a more positive self-image and elation.[18]

ACUTE AND MAINTENANCE TREATMENT

While there is no demonstrated effective treatment for the personality changes associated with epilepsy, some suggest that the AEDs, carbamazepine in particular, may help relieve these character traits. Rodin and Schmalz report that carbamazepine has a beneficial effect on the interictal personality syndrome, decreasing elation, philosophical interests, sense of destiny, hypergraphia, and normalizing sexual functioning.[19] While no maintenance studies have been done, long-term treatment is presumably necessary since personality changes are chronic, lifelong problems.

COGNITIVE IMPAIRMENT

Patients with epilepsy frequently have cognitive impairment. The etiology is likely multifactorial and may be related directly to the seizures or to the preexistent brain damage underlying the seizure disorder. Seizures also frequently result in additional head injury from trauma during seizures.

AEDs may also contribute to cognitive impairment. Phenytoin, primidone, and phenobarbital are the most likely culprits. These agents impair concentration and attention more than memory. Polypharmacy should be avoided when possible because of multiplicative effects on cognitive functioning. The AEDs associated with the least cognitive impairment are valproate, carbamazepine, and vigabatrin.

PSEUDOSEIZURES

The term pseudoseizures refers to nonepileptic attacks that may in some way resemble epileptic seizures. Clinically, the fits of pseudoseizures are usually distinguishable from real epileptic seizures, although some forms of frontal lobe and simple partial seizures may be difficult to differentiate. The EEG is diagnostic. In pseudoseizures, video EEG monitoring reveals no epileptiform discharge during the "seizures." After an epileptic seizure, prolactin levels rise dramatically and a prolactin level drawn 20 minutes after a seizure should be markedly elevated and then fall by 1 hour after the seizure. The prolactin rise is not seen in pseudoseizures.

The differential diagnosis of pseudoseizures includes anxiety disorder (generalized anxiety disorder or panic disorder), depressive disorders, schizophrenia, conversion disorder, somatization disorder, episodic dyscontrol disorder, and malingering. Some sleep disorders, including night terrors and REM behavior disorder, may also present with pseudoseizures. Vasovagal syncope and hypoglycemia also should be considered.

ACUTE AND MAINTENANCE TREATMENT

Appropriate treatment for the underlying psychiatric or medical disturbance is the treatment of choice for pseudoseizures. AEDs are not effective since there is no underlying seizure focus or electrical abnormality in the brain.

PSYCHIATRIC DISORDERS SECONDARY TO AEDs

All the AEDs are potentially neurotoxic, with some agents more likely to cause toxicity than others. Polypharmacy carries a higher risk of psychiatric and cognitive morbidity than monotherapy.

There is a higher association of depression with phenobarbital than with any other agent. Vigabatrin is also associated with depression, especially in patients who have a past history of depression. Carbamazepine appears to be the least likely to cause depression and in fact may decrease the rate of depression and act as a mood stabilizer.

Conduct disorder and ADHD in children have also been associated with the use of particular AEDs, most notably phenobarbital, clonazepam, and vigabatrin.[2]

Folate deficiency is caused by several of the AEDs, especially phenytoin and phenobarbital. Folate deficiency is associated with more severe psychopathology. However, folate replacement is not an adequate treatment for psychopathology.

REFERENCES

1. Commission on Classification and Terminology of the International League Against Epilepsy. (1989). Proposal for revised classification of epilepsies and epileptic syndromes. *Epilepsia*, 30(14):389–399.
2. Trimble, M.R., Ring, H.A., Schmitz, B. (1996). Neuropsychiatric aspects of epilepsy. In Fogel, B.S., Schiffer, R.B. (Eds.), *Neuropsychiatry* (pp. 771–803). Baltimore: Williams & Wilkins.
3. Sillanpa, M. (1993). Remission of seizures and predicters of intractability in long-term follow-up. *Epilepsia*, 34(5):930–936.
4. Hermann, B.P., Whitman, S. (1984). Behavioral and personality correlates of epilepsy: A review, methodological critique, and conceptual model. *Psychol Bull*, 95:451–497.
5. Neppe, V.M., Tucker, G.J. (1992). Neuropsychiatric aspects of seizure disorders. In Yudofsky, S.C., Hales, R.E., (Eds.), *The American Psychiatric Press Textbook of Neuropsychiatry* (pp. 397–425). Washington, DC: American Psychiatric Press.
6. Papez, J.W. (1937). A proposed mechanism of emotion. *Arch Neurol Psychiatry*, 38:725–733.
7. Slater, E., Beard, A.W., Glithero, E. (1963). The schizophrenia-like psychoses of epilepsy. *Br J Psychiatry*, 109:95–150.
8. Stevens, J.R. (1988). Epilepsy, psychosis and schizophrenia. *Schizophr Res*, 1:79–89.
9. Bear, D.M., Fedio, P. (1977). Quantitative analysis of interictal behavior in temporal lobe epilepsy. *Arch Neurol*, 34:454–467.
10. Perez, M.M., Trimble, M.R. (1980). Epileptic psychosis - diagnostic comparison with process schizophrenia. *Br J Psychiatry*, 137:245–249.
11. Oyebode, F., Davison, K. (1989). Epileptic schizophrenia: Clinical features and outcome. *Acta Psychiatr Scand*, 79:327–331.
12. Trimble, M.R. (1985). The psychoses of epilepsy and their treatment. *Clin Neurosci*, 8(3):211–220.
13. Kraft, A.M., Price, T.R.P., Peltier, D. (1984). Complex partial seizures and schizophrenia. *Compr Psychiatry*, 25:113–124.

14. Robertson, M.M. (1989). The organic contribution to depressive illness in patients with epilepsy. *J Epilepsy*, 2:189–320.
15. Robertson, M.M., Trimble, M.R. (1985). The treatment of depression in patients with epilepsy: A double-blind trial. *J Affect Disord*, 9:127–136.
16. Waxman, S.G., Geschwind, N. (1975). The interictal behavior syndromes of temperal lobe epilepsy. *Arch Gen Psychiatry*, 32:1580–1586.
17. Bear, D., Levin K., Blumer, D., et al. (1982). Interictal behavior in hospitalized temporal lobe epileptics: relationship to idiopathic psychiatric syndromes. *J Neurol Neurosurg Psychiatry*, 45:481–488.
18. Perini, G.I. (1986). Emotions and personality in complex partial seizures. *Psychother Psychosomatics*, 45:141–148.
19. Rodin, E., Schmalz, S., Twitty, G. (1984). What does the Bear-Fedio inventory measure? In Porter, R.J., Mattson, R.H., Ward, Jr., A.A., Dam, M. (Eds.), *The XVth Epilepsy International Symposium* (pp. 551–555). New York: Raven Press.

CHAPTER

9

PARKINSON'S DISEASE

INTRODUCTION

A movement disorder is a neurologic illness that features abnormal movements as major symptoms. Parkinson's disease (PD) is one of the most common and is characterized by progressive neurodegeneration of dopaminergic neurons in the substantia nigra. The disease triad consists of bradykinesia, rigidity, and tremor. Dopaminergic drugs are the mainstay of pharmacological treatment. Both PD and the medications used to treat it may promote psychiatric symptoms.

PSYCHIATRIC SEQUELAE OF PARKINSON'S DISEASE

Psychiatric symptoms in PD may result from either the primary illness or the side effects of the dopaminergic medications used as treatment. Depression, dementia, delirium, and psychosis are the most common psychiatric disorders, present in 10 to 50% of PD patients treated with levodopa.[1]

DEPRESSION

Depression in PD is characterized by "sadness without guilt."[2] Symptoms of sadness, irritability, dysphoria, and suicidal ideation are

299

prominent, while feelings of guilt and self-reproach are less so. Anxiety symptoms are more prominent in PD patients with depression, while psychotic depression and suicide are less prominent compared with MDD patients.[3]

Depression in PD is a common finding and carries with it moderate disability. Cummings reported that in 26 studies the mean prevalence of depression in PD was 40% (range 4–70%) and that approximately 54% of patients fulfilled criteria for a moderate-to-severe depressive episode. A family history of affective illness does not appear to predispose to depression in PD.[4]

The duration of untreated depressive symptoms in PD is unclear. Mayeux et al. noted remission of depressive symptoms in 1 of 14 PD patients with depression followed for $2\frac{1}{2}$ years.[5] Brown et al. noted in a group of PD patients followed for approximately $1\frac{1}{2}$ years that while 11% of depressive episodes remitted, approximately the same percentage of nondepressed patients went on to develop depressive symptoms.[2]

DEMENTIA

Dementia is common in many forms of neurodegenerative illness with an incidence that is generally related to the duration of illness. The prevalence of dementia in PD is unclear, as estimates have ranged from 0 to 81%.[6] Dementia in PD does not appear to be homogeneous either clinically or pathologically and its etiology is unclear.[7]

PSYCHOSIS

Psychotic symptoms include delusions, hallucinations, and delirium and are thought to be induced by dopaminomimetic drugs. Psychiatric disturbances are the third most common side effect of levdopa therapy[1] and may be induced by other antiparkinsonian agents as well (i.e., bromocriptine, pergolide, and selegiline). Musser and Akil reviewed the phenomenon of psychosis in PD and found prevalence rates ranged from 7.5 to 65%.[8] The clinical presentation of psychosis in PD has been well described by Greene et al. and ranges from a mild sleep disturbance with infrequent hypnagogic and hypnopompic hallucinations to florid psychotic symptoms.[9] Delusions are usually paranoid in nature, classically involving concerns of infidelity, and hallucinations are usually visual. Curiously, the PD patient may appear unconcerned about the delusions. Finally, PD patients with dementia are more likely to develop psychotic symptoms than nonndemented PD patients.[10]

PHARMACOTHERAPY OF DEPRESSION IN PD

The tricyclic antidepressants and buproprion have been investigated in PD patients with depression. Cummings summarized the results of four prospective double-blind studies of antidepressant use in PD patients with depression.[4] The results are summarized in Table 9–1. Collectively, they demonstrate approximately a 40 to 60% response rate as well as improvement in parkinsonian symptoms (tremor, rigidity, and akinesia) with two of the tricyclic antidepressants (imipramine and desipramine) presumably secondary to their anticholinergic effects. Intuitively, buproprion seems an appropriate agent for use in PD, given its dopaminergic effects, but it appeared somewhat less effective than the tricyclic agents.

The role of maintenance antidepressant therapy in PD depression has yet to be studied prospectively, so firm recommendations cannot be made currently. However, given that PD is a chronic, progressive neurodegenerative illness with a significant prevalence of depressive symptoms, it is likely that antidepressant therapy, once initiated, may need to be lifelong. While the SSRIs have yet to be studied prospectively in this patient population, clinical experience suggests a role for these agents in PD patients with depression.

Selegiline, a selective monoamine oxidase type B inhibitor that sometimes is used as a treatment in early PD, may have mild antidepressant properties, as might be expected given its membership in the MAOI class of drugs. However, dosages in PD are small (10 mg/day) and may be too low to achieve an antidepressant effect. In addition, at doses above 10 mg/day, the drug loses its selectivity and concern for hypertensive crisis and other MAOI side effects becomes an issue, requiring compliance with an MAOI diet and avoiding coadministration of other serotonergic agents (SSRIs, clomipramine).

Psychostimulants (methylphenidate, etc.) appear to have no antidepressant effects in PD depression. Cantello et al. reported that methylphenidate did not have antidepressant effects in PD patients with depression compared with either nondepressed controls or patients with primary depression.[11]

Electroconvulsive therapy has been used successfully to treat depressive symptoms in PD patients, but data are sparse and limited to case reports.[12] Its role in maintenance therapy is unclear at present, due to a lack of experimental data, but it may be used as a third- or fourth-line strategy.

PHARMACOTHERAPY OF DEMENTIA IN PD

Specific pharmacologic treatments for dementia in PD do not exist currently, either for acute or maintenance therapy use. General principles of the pharmacology of dementia are discussed in Chapter 11.

TABLE 9–1. FINDINGS OF DOUBLE-BLIND STUDIES OF ANTIDEPRESSANT TREATMENT FOR PATIENTS WITH PARKINSON'S DISEASE (PD) AND DEPRESSION

Study	Year	Agent	Dose (mg/day)	Number of Subjects	Patients Whose Depression Responded (%)	Positive Effect on PD (%)	Study Design
Strang (5)*	1965	Imipramine	150–200	20	60	Rigidity, 42; tremor, 28; akinesia, 54	Double-blind
Andersen et al. (78)	1980	Nortriptyline	150	22	—**	No effect	Double-blind crossover
Laitinen (79)	1969	Desipramine	100	39	50	Rigidity, 25; tremor, 15	Double-blind
Goetz et al. (80)	1984	Bupropion	450	20	42	30	Double-blind followed by open-label phase

*Reference numbers in table's source.

**Depression rating scale scores were significantly improved in the active treatment group.

Adapted from Cummings, J. L. (1992). Depression and Parkinson's disease: A review, *Am J Psychiatry*, 149(4):443–454. Copyright 1992 by American Psychiatric Press. Reprinted with permission.

PHARMACOTHERAPY OF PSYCHOSIS

Musser and Akil reviewed the pharmacologic options for the treatment of psychosis in PD.[8] While reducing antiparkinsonian drug dosages is usually effective in diminishing psychotic symptoms, it is not always clinically possible. Traditional antipsychotics, while effective in treating psychosis, are usually intolerable in the PD patient whose Parkinsonian symptoms worsen.

Clozapine is a promising agent for PD psychosis. While the majority of studies of clozapine in PD are open (one involved a double-blind, crossover design), the drug has shown promise in treating psychotic symptoms. The required dosage is low, under 25 mg/day, compared with the average starting dose of 300–400 mg/day in schizophrenic patients. Common side effects of clozapine treatment include sedation, weight gain, anticholinergic side effects, sialorrhea, and tachycardia. In addition, delirium may develop with clozapine treatment; but if the drug is continued at a low dose, it may resolve.[9] Agranulocytosis, a potential adverse effect of clozapine treatment, must be monitored in any treatment population and is discussed more fully in Chapter 6 on schizophrenia. It may be a greater risk in these patients, as the incidence of clozapine-induced agranulocytosis has been found to increase with age.[13] While clozapine is an effective agent in PD psychosis, the decision to initiate clozapine treatment should be made in conjunction with a psychiatrist skilled in its use. Other atypical antipsychotics may also be useful for the treatment of psychosis in PD.

Maintenance studies of psychosis in PD do not exist currently. Clinically, however, as with PD depression, the symptoms appear to be chronic and therefore may need lifelong treatment.

REFERENCES

1. Goodwin, F.K. (1971). Behavioral effects of l-dopa in man. *Semin Psychiatry*, 3:477–492.
2. Brown, R.G., MacCarthy, B., Gotham, A.M., et al. (1988). Depression and disability in Parkinson's disease: A follow-up study of 132 cases. *Psychol Med*, 18:49–55.
3. Henderson, R., Kurlan, R., Kersun, J.M., et al. (1992). Preliminary examination of the comorbidity of anxiety and depression in Parkinson's disease. *J Neuropsychiatry Clin Neurosci*, 4:257–264.
4. Cummings, J.L. (1992). Depression and Parkinson's disease: A review. *Am J Psychiatry*, 149:443–454.
5. Mayeux, R., Stern, Y., Sano, M., et al. (1988). The relationship of serotonin to depression in Parkinson's disease. *Mov Disord*, 3:237–244.
6. Boyd, J.L., Cruickshank, C.A., Kenn, C.W., et al. (1991). Cognitive impairment and dementia in Parkinson's disease: A controlled study. *Psychol Med*, 21:911–921.
7. Duyckaerts, C., Gaspar, P., Coosta, C., et al. (1993). Dementia in Parkinson's disease: Morphometric data. *Am J Neurol*, 60:447–455.

8. Musser, W.S., Akil, M. (1996). Clozapine as a treatment for psychosis in Parkinson's disease: A review. *J Neuropsychiatry Clin Neurosci*, 8:1–9.

9. Greene, P., Cote, L., Fahn, S. (1993). Treatment of drug-induced psychosis in Parkinson's disease with clozapine. *Adv Neurol*, 60:702–706.

10. Sacks, O.W., Kohl, M.S., Measeloff, C.R., et al. (1972). Effects of levodopa in Parkinson's patients with dementia. *Neurology*, 22:516–519.

11. Cantello, R., Aguggia, M., Gilli, M., et al. (1989). Major depression in Parkinson's disease and the mood response to intravenous methyphenidate: Possible role of the "hedonic" dopamine synapse. *J Neurol Neurosurg Psychiatry*, 52:724–731.

12. Asnis, G. (1977). Parkinson's disease, depression, and ECT: A review and a case. *Am J Psychiatry*, 134:2;191–195.

13. Alvir, J.M.J., Lieberman, J.A., Safferman, A.Z., et al. (1993). Clozapine-induced agranulocytosis: Incidence and risk factors in the United States. *N Engl J Med*, 329:162–167.

MULTIPLE SCLEROSIS

INTRODUCTION

Disorders of central nervous system (CNS) demyelination (loss or destruction of the myelin sheath that covers the nerve axon), of which multiple sclerosis is the prototypic example, may present with psychiatric symptoms at some point in their course. Multiple sclerosis (MS) is characterized by the formation of plaques, focal areas of demyelination of white matter tracts (axons) in either the brain and spinal cord. The nerve cell bodies (gray matter) are rarely affected. MS is a chronic disorder that may be characterized either by discrete episodes of relapses and remissions or by a slow progression of neurologic deficits (i.e., visual difficulties, spasticity, tremor, and urinary difficulties).

Psychiatric symptoms of an affective nature are a common development in MS and include depression, bipolar disorder, emotionalism, and euphoria. Indeed, psychiatric symptomatology may herald the onset of MS.[1] Cognitive dysfunction (i.e., memory impairment and intellectual decline) is also common in MS but is not reviewed here as pharmacologic treatments are lacking. Psychosis in the context of MS is rare.

PSYCHIATRIC SEQUELAE OF MULTIPLE SCLEROSIS

DEPRESSION

Depressive symptoms are quite common in MS, with a prevalence rate of 27 to 54%.[2] Depressive symptoms in MS include primarily irritability, anger, and anxiety without the more characteristic ruminations, apathy, or social withdrawal seen in a major depressive episode.[3] A higher prevalence and greater severity of depression is present in MS than in other medical or neurologic illnesses,[1] and there does not appear to be an increased incidence of depression in MS patients with a positive family history of primary affective illness.[2] The location of MS plaques is associated with depressive symptoms: Patients with brain plaques have a higher prevalence of depressive symptoms than those with plaques of the spinal cord.[4] As with affective symptoms in other neurological illnesses, depressive symptoms in MS appear to be underrecognized and remain untreated,[3] even though they appear amenable to biological therapies.

BIPOLAR DISORDER

A comorbidity between bipolar disorder and MS appears to exist. An epidemiological study identified 10 patients in one county of approximately 702,000 people with both bipolar disorder and MS.[5] The authors noted that this was twice the rate expected based on the prevalence rate for each of the two illnesses. Joffe et al.,[6] in a survey of 100 MS patients, found that 13% fulfilled research criteria for bipolar disorder and noted that the prevalence appeared to be 13 times higher than that of the general population. Kellner et al.[7] described two patients with treatment-resistant rapid cycling bipolar disorder who were subsequently found to have MS and postulated that the demyelinating illness contributed to the treatment-refractoriness of the affective disorder. Symptoms of mania may arise as a side effect of steroid therapy for MS and should resolve with discontinuation.

EMOTIONALISM

Disordered emotional expression in MS is manifest as pathologic laughter or tearfulness. That is, the MS patient may spontaneously laugh or cry without regard to external or internal stimuli. The prevalence rate of these symptoms is unknown.

EUPHORIA

Euphoria in MS is a neurologically mediated, sustained emotional state of outward cheerfulness, sometimes in complete opposition to the patient's internal state. MS patients with euphoria appear outwardly happy, even if they do not feel so internally. Patients with clinical depression may outwardly appear euphoric.[8] Rabins[9] reported the prevalence rate of euphoria to be 0 to 63%. The presence of euphoria is associated with a progressive course of MS and a greater degree of neurologic impairment.[4] The necessity of treatment of euphoria in MS is unclear.

PSYCHOSIS

Psychotic symptoms resulting from multiple sclerosis are rare,[10] but they may occasionally be seen clinically.

PHARMACOTHERAPY OF PSYCHIATRIC SYMPTOMS OF MULTIPLE SCLEROSIS

Despite the prevalence of affective symptoms in MS, a paucity of experimental data on treatment exists. There has been one double-blind study to date of antidepressant therapy in MS patients with major depression. Schiffer and Wineman[11] reported that desipramine produced significant improvement in depressive symptoms compared with placebo but that approximately one-third of the patients experienced side effects. Clinically, the SSRIs have been found to be effective in treating depressive symptoms in MS patients and are more easily tolerated. No studies exist on the longitudinal course of depression in these patients nor its response to treatment. Clinically, one may follow the guidelines described previously for primary major depression.

Bipolar illness from MS appears to be a rare entity. The role of lithium in treating bipolar disorder in MS is unclear, and the data are limited to case reports. Kemp et al.[12] describe a young female patient with an agitated depression who, when given steroid therapy for her MS, developed manic symptoms that were successfully treated with lithium carbonate 900–1200 mg/day (serum levels 0.6–1.0 mmEq/l). Peselow et al.[13] describe a patient with a nine-year history of mania who went on to develop multiple sclerosis during an episode of treatment-resistant mania that eventually responded to steroid therapy and lithium carbonate 1200 mg/day. The patient was successfully maintained on lithium for over one year without recurrence of mania.

Treatment studies for pathological laughter and tearfulness are limited to one double-blind study and several open studies. Schiffer et al.[14] performed a double-blind, placebo-controlled crossover design study of amitriptyline in 12 MS patients with pathologic laughter and weeping. Mean amitriptyline dosage was 57.8 mg/day. Eight of the 12 patients had statistically significant decreases in their affective symptoms (laughing and weeping) while concomitant measurements of mood were unchanged. The authors concluded that the effect of amitriptyline on emotionalism was separate from its antidepressant effects. Wolf et al.[15] reported a small open series of patients (one of whom carried the diagnosis of MS) whose "emotional incontinence" was relieved by levodopa. As in emotionalism from cerebrovascular disease,[16] the SSRIs may be an effective alternative to amitriptyline.

No data exist currently on the pharmacological treatment of euphoria in MS, although it is a benign symptom that usually does not require treatment.

REFERENCES

1. Whitlock, F.A., Siskind, M.M. (1980). Depression as a major symptom in multiple sclerosis. *J Neurol Neurosurg Psychiatry*, 43:861–865.
2. Beatty, W.W. (1993). Cognitive and emotional disturbances in multiple sclerosis. *Neurologic Clinics*, 11:1;189–204.
3. Minden, S.L., Orav, J., Reich, P. (1987). Depression in multiple sclerosis. *Gen Hosp Psychiatry*, 9:426–434.
4. Rabins, P.V., Brooks, D.R., O'Donnell, P., et al. (1986). Structural brain correlates of emotional disorder in multiple sclerosis. *Brain*, 109:585–597.
5. Schiffer, R.B., Wineman, N.M., Weitkamp, L.R. (1986). Association between bipolar affective disorder and multiple sclerosis. *Am J Psychiatry*, 143:94–95.
6. Joffe, R.T., Lippert, G.P., Gray, T.A., et al. (1987). Mood disorder and multiple sclerosis. *Arch Neurology*, 44:376–378.
7. Kellner, C.H., Davenport, Y., Post, R.M., et al. (1984). Rapidly cycling bipolar disorder and multiple sclerosis. *Am J Psychiatry*, 141:112–113.
8. Surridge, D. (1969). An investigation into some psychiatric aspects of multiple sclerosis. *Br J Psychiatry*, 1115:749–764.
9. Rabins, P.V. (1990) Euphoria in multiple sclerosis. In Rao, S.M. (Ed.), *Neurobehavioral Aspects of Multiple Sclerosis* (p. 180). New York: Oxford University Press.
10. Trimble, M.R., Grant, I. (1982). Psychiatric aspects of multiple sclerosis. In Benson, D.F., Bluner, D. (Eds.), *Psychiatric Aspects of Neurologic Disease*, Vol. 2 (pp. 279–299). New York: Grune and Stratton.
11. Schiffer, R.B., Wineman, N.M. (1987). Antidepressant pharmacotherapy of depression associated with multiple sclerosis: A double-blind placebo controlled trial. Presented at the Symposium on Mental Disorders, Cognitive Deficits, and their Treatment in Multiple Sclerosis. Odense: Denmark, December 1987.
12. Kemp, K., Lion, J.R., Magram, G. (1977). Lithium in the treatment of a manic patient with multiple sclerosis: A case report. *Dis Nerv Syst*, 38:210–211.
13. Peselow, E.D., Fieve, R.R., Deutsch, S.I., et al. (1981). Coexistent manic symptoms and multiple sclerosis. *Psychosomatics*, 22:824–825.

14. Schiffer, R.B., Herndon, R.M., Rudick, R.A. (1985). Treatment of pathologic laughing and weeping with amitriptyline. *N Engl J Med*, 312:1480–1482.
15. Wolf, J.K., Santana, H.B., Thorpy, M. (1979). Treatment of 'emotional incontinence' with levodopa. *Neurology*, 29:1435–1436.
16. Anderson, G., Vestergaard, K., Riis, J.O. (1993). Citalopram for post-stroke pathological injury. *Lancet*, 342:837–839.

CHAPTER

11

DEMENTIA

INTRODUCTION

Dementia refers to a heterogeneous group of degenerative disorders characterized by progressive global cognitive decline and usually accompanied by neuropsychiatric manifestations in both affective and behavioral realms. The cognitive deterioration of dementia has an insidious onset and a progressive course. It may affect memory, language, visuospatial construction, and executive functions such as abstraction, calculation, problem-solving, motor sequencing, planning, recognition, and praxis. The affective component of dementia is manifest as depression, mania, anxiety, emotional liability, or personality change. Apathy and abulia are also characteristic affective changes of dementia. In addition to the progressive cognitive decline and affective dysregulation, behavioral disturbances including psychosis, altered sleep-wake cycle, agitation, wandering, aggressivity, repetitive vocalizations, and resistance to care are common in dementia.

All these abnormalities contribute to progressive social and occupational functional impairment, eventually necessitating assistance with activities of daily living and close supervision. The majority of demented individuals receive long-term care from their families at home. However, as global functioning declines, many demented patients require institutionalization in long-term care facilities such as nursing homes. Dementia is a growing

311

health and social concern as the population ages and the number of affected individuals increases dramatically.

EPIDEMIOLOGY

Degenerative dementia is an age-dependent illness and the incidence increases with increasing age. Approximately 5–15% of individuals over the age of 65 suffer from dementia.[1] Above age 85, this figure jumps to 30%.[2] The prevalence of Alzheimer's disease is about 6% for individuals over age 65, 20% for those over age 80, and 45% for those over age 95.[3] Because the oldest age group (over age 85) is the fastest growing segment of the U.S. population, dementia is affecting a growing number of individuals, influencing health care and delivery needs in the elderly.

The most common causes of dementia are Alzheimer's disease (AD) and Lewy body disease (LBD). Cerebrovascular disease, i.e., multi-infarct dementia, is the next most common cause. These three causes alone or together account for about 90% of dementia cases. The remaining 10% are attributed to Parkinson's disease, Huntington's disease, frontal-temporal atrophy, and Creutzfeldt-Jakob disease.

DIAGNOSTIC CRITERIA

The DSM-IV criteria for dementia of the Alzheimer's type are listed in Table 11–1. Criteria A and B are the same for all dementias while the subsequent ones reflect other etiologies including vascular, HIV, head trauma, Parkinson's disease, Huntington's disease, Pick's disease, Creutzfeldt-Jakob disease, other medical conditions, substance induced, and mixed etiologies.

AD is a histologic diagnosis made only at brain biopsy or autopsy. However, specific criteria for possible and probable Alzheimer's disease have been enumerated by McKhann and are listed in Table 11–2.[4]

The primary degenerative cortical dementias include AD, LBD, the frontal-temporal atrophies including Pick's disease, frontal lobe degeneration of the Alzheimer's type, dementia lacking distinctive histological features, progressive subcortical gliosis, and focal lobar atrophies. Primary subcortical dementias include Parkinson's disease and Huntington's disease. Specific clinical criteria for the diagnosis of LBD are being developed.[5]

The secondary dementias are caused by a neurological, medical, or psychiatric illness. The nondegenerative dementias include vascular dementia, hydrocephalus, infectious diseases (neurosyphilis, Lyme disease, HIV, fungal and bacterial infections, Whipple's disease, Creutzfeldt-Jakob disease),

text continues on page 315

TABLE 11–1. DIAGNOSTIC CRITERIA FOR DEMENTIA OF THE ALZHEIMER'S TYPE

A. The development of multiple cognitive deficits manifested by both
   (1) memory impairment (impaired ability to learn new information or to recall previously learned information)
   (2) one (or more) of the following cognitive disturbances:
      (a) aphasia (language disturbance)
      (b) apraxia (impaired ability to carry out motor activities despite intact motor function
      (c) agnosia (failure to recognize or identify objects despite intact sensory function)
      (d) disturbance in executive functioning (i.e., planning, organizing, sequencing, abstracting)

B. The cognitive deficits in Criteria A1 and A2 each cause significant impairment in social or occupational functioning and represent a significant decline from a previous level of function.

C. The course is characterized by gradual onset and continuing cognitive decline.

D. The cognitive deficits in Criteria A1 and A2 are not due to any of the following:
   (1) other central nervous system conditions that cause progressive deficits in memory and cognition (e.g., cerebrovascular disease, Parkinson's disease, Huntington's disease, subdural hematoma, normal-pressure hydrocephalus, brain tumor)
   (2) systemic conditions that are known to cause dementia (e.g., hypothyroidism, vitamin B_{12} or folic acid deficiency, niacin deficiency, hypercalcemia, neurosyphilis, HIV infection)
   (3) substance-induced conditions

E. The deficits do not occur exclusively during the course of a delirium.

F. The disturbance is not better accounted for by another Axis I disorder (e.g., major depressive disorder, schizophrenia).

Code based on type of onset and predominant feature:

With Early Onset: if onset is at age 65 years or below
290.11 With Delirium: if delirium is superimposed on the dementia
290.12 With Delusions: if delusions are the predominant feature
290.13 With Depressed Mood: if depressed mood (including presentations that meet full symptom criteria for a major depressive episode) is the predominant feature. A separate diagnosis of mood disorder due to a general medical condition is not given.
290.10 Uncomplicated: if none of the above predominates in the current clinical presentation

With Late Onset: if onset is after age 65 years
290.3 With Delirium: if delirium is superimposed on the dementia
290.20 With Delusions: if delusions are the predominant feature
290.21 With Depressed Mood: if depressed mood (including presentations that meet full symptom criteria for a major depressive episode) is the predominant feature. A separate diagnosis of mood disorder due to a general medical condition is not given.
290.0 Uncomplicated: if none of the above predominates in the current clinical presentation

Specify if:
With Behavioral Disturbance
Coding note: Also code 331.0 Alzheimer's disease on Axis III.

Adapted with permission from the *Diagnostic and Statistical Manual of Mental Disorders*, 4th ed. (pp. 142–143). Copyright 1994 by American Psychiatric Association.

TABLE 11–2. CRITERIA FOR CLINICAL DIAGNOSIS OF ALZHEIMER'S DISEASE

I. The criteria for the clinical diagnosis of PROBABLE Alzheimer's disease include:

dementia established by clinical examination and documented by the Mini-Mental Test, Blessed Dementia Scale, or some similar examination, and confirmed by neuropsychological tests;
deficits in two or more areas of cognition;
progressive worsening of memory and other cognitive functions;
no disturbance of consciousness;
onset between ages 40 and 90, most often after age 65; and
absence of systemic disorders or other brain diseases that in and of themselves could account for the progressive deficits in memory and cognition.

II. The diagnosis of PROBABLE Alzheimer's disease is supported by:

progressive deterioration of specific cognitive functions such as language (aphasia), motor skills (apraxia), and perception (agnosia);
impaired activities of daily living and altered patterns of behavior;
family history of similar disorders, particularly if confirmed neuropathologically; and
laboratory results of:
normal lumbar puncture as evaluated by standard techniques,
normal pattern or nonspecific changes in EEG, such as increased slow-wave activity, and
evidence of cerebral atrophy on CT with progression documented by serial observation.

III. Other clinical features consistent with the diagnosis of PROBABLE Alzheimer's disease, after exclusion of causes of dementia other than Alzheimer's disease, include:

plateaus in the course of progression of the illness;
associated symptoms of depression, insomnia, incontinence, delusions, illusions, hallucinations, catastrophic verbal, emotional, or physical outbursts, sexual disorders, and weight loss;
other neurologic abnormalities in some patients, especially with more advanced disease and including motor signs such as increased muscle tone, myoclonus, or gait disorder;
seizures in advanced disease; and
CT normal for age.

IV. Features that make the diagnosis of PROBABLE Alzheimer's disease uncertain or unlikely include:

sudden, apoplectic onset;
focal neurologic findings such as hemiparesis, sensory loss, visual field deficits, and incoordination early in the course of the illness; and
seizures or gait disturbances at the onset or very early in the course of the illness.

V. Clinical diagnosis of POSSIBLE Alzheimer's disease:

may be made on the basis of the dementia syndrome, in the absence of other neurologic, psychiatric, or systemic disorders sufficient to cause dementia, and in the presence of variations in the onset, in the presentation, or in the clinical course;
may be made in the presence of a second systemic or brain disorder sufficient to produce dementia, which is not considered to be the cause of the dementia; and
should be used in research studies when a single, gradually progressive severe cognitive deficit is identified in the absence of other identifiable cause.

VI. Criteria for diagnosis of DEFINITE Alzheimer's disease are:

the clinical criteria for probable Alzheimer's disease and histopathologic evidence obtained from a biopsy or autopsy.

VII. Classification of Alzheimer's disease for research purposes should specify features that may differentiate subtypes of the disorder, such as:

familial occurrence;
onset before age of 65;
presence of trisomy-21; and
coexistence of other relevant conditions such as Parkinson's disease.

Adapted from McKhann, M.D., Drachman, D., Folstein, M., et al. (1984) Clinical diagnosis of Alzheimer's disease. *Neurology,* 34:940. Copyright 1984 by American Academy of Neurology. Reprinted with permission.

neoplasms, nutritional deficiencies (vitamin B_{12}, folate, niacin), endocrine abnormalities (hypothyroidism), vasculitis, metachromatic leukodystrophy, demyelinating diseases, metabolic abnormalities (hyponatremia), and toxic disorders (alcohol, heavy metals), and trauma. Some of these conditions are treatable and appropriate treatment may result in partial or complete resolution of dementia symptoms.

NEUROPSYCHIATRIC MANIFESTATIONS

Cognitive impairment is only one of the neuropsychiatric manifestations and is the symptom least amenable to treatment. Depressive and anxiety symptoms may be present relatively early in the course of dementia and respond well to pharmacological treatment. Mania is less common but also responds to medications. Psychosis usually presents later in the course of dementia and may be associated with behavioral disturbances. Disruptive behaviors are the most troublesome symptom of dementia and may be manifestations of other neuropsychiatric disturbances or of medical illness, and frequently bring patients to medical attention or prompt institutionalization.

PSYCHOSOCIAL/ENVIRONMENTAL INTERVENTIONS

Some of these neuropsychiatric manifestations respond to environmental manipulation that families or long-term care staff can easily learn. Creating a consistent environment with a structured routine and adequate but not excessive sensory stimulation can help eliminate confusion. Providing familiar personal objects such as pictures and mementos, as well as cues for orientation like calendars and clocks, can help patients' orientation. Communications should be clear and simple. Patients should be encouraged to be active participants in their care and in decision-making as much as possible. Supportive psychotherapy, interpersonal psychotherapy, reminiscence therapy, or grief therapy may be beneficial in individual cases. We refer readers to Mace and Rabins, Aronson, and Gruetzner for a further discussion of environmental, behavioral, and psychotherapeutic interventions.[6,7,8]

EVIDENCE FOR PSYCHOPHARMACOLOGICAL TREATMENT

The literature supporting psychopharmacological treatment of the neuropsychiatric manifestations of dementia is very limited although it has been extensively reviewed.[9,10,11,12,13] The majority of published reports are case reports and retrospective or open clinical series, many of which include patients with the diagnosis of "organic mental disorder," and nondementing illnesses. Many controlled studies of psychiatric disorders common in dementia specifically exclude patients with dementia.

Because the literature in this area is so limited, practitioners frequently extrapolate from studies in other populations and develop treatment strategies based on evidence in younger or nondemented patients. There is an inherent risk in this assumption, since the process of dementia alters the neurochemical and neuroanatomical substrates in the brain. In fact, treating all dementia as a homogeneous disorder is likely also incorrect because of the different etiologies of dementia.

POLYPHARMACY AND DRUG-DRUG INTERACTIONS

The average elderly patient takes 9.3 medications for an average of 9.6 medical conditions.[14] Therefore, polypharmacy and drug-drug interactions are important considerations when treating elderly demented patients who are on multiple medications and have multiple medical comorbidities. Drug-drug interactions of particular importance to the elderly are addressed in Chapters 4–7. Many psychotropic medications are metabolized by and inhibit the hepatic P450 isoenzyme system. Many other medications are also metabolized by this system and may enhance or inhibit metabolism of the psychotropic agent. Therefore, drug levels of psychotropics and other medications may change with the addition or discontinuation of another agent, possibly causing either toxicity or decreased efficacy of the medication. Physicians must be aware of and anticipate these potential interactions. Psychotropics that are highly protein bound also pose a problem because they may displace other highly protein bound drugs, increasing free levels and potentially causing toxicity. Drugs metabolized by the hepatic isoenzymes are presented in Chapter 4 on Depressive Disorders.

COGNITIVE IMPAIRMENT

There is no known effective treatment for arresting or reversing the cognitive deterioration of the degenerative dementias. However, there is some promise for slowing the progression of degeneration, at least temporarily, in Alzheimer's disease, although there is no evidence that currently available treatments alter the underlying disease process.

The pathophysiological mechanism of cognitive impairment in Alzheimer's dementia is loss of cholinergic neurons. Therefore, potential strategies to increase cholinergic function have been investigated. There are currently two agents available that have demonstrated efficacy in slowing the progression of cognitive decline in a subset of AD patients.

TACRINE

Tacrine, tetrahydroaminoacridine (THA), is a potent central cholinesterase inhibitor that also affects cholinergic functioning, acetylcholine receptors, monoamine neurotransmitter levels, MAO-A and -B activity, sodium and potassium ion channels, and cyclic AMP phosphodiesterase.[15,16] It has a palliative effect, especially in higher doses.[17] Tacrine is more effective in mild-to-moderately demented patients and is less effective in the severely demented. Improvements are small when measured on cognitive scales. These small cognitive improvements may have no clinical relevance, although in some cases even modest cognitive improvement may be associated with pronounced behavioral improvement, enough to allow a patient to be cared for at home longer and to postpone nursing home placement. Only about 33–50% of patients derive any benefit from tacrine treatment compared with 16–25% with placebo.[14]

However, a larger percentage of patients experience significant adverse effects that limit treatment, specifically hepatotoxicity and gastrointestinal symptoms. At the higher doses where tacrine is most effective, approximately 66% of patients have significant adverse reactions. In a large series, about 50% of patients had ALT elevations above the upper limit of normal (ULN), 25% had elevations three times the ULN, and 2% had elevations 20 times the ULN.[18] Most patients with hepatotoxicity were asymptomatic, and women were affected more frequently than men. Fully 90% of cases of hepatotoxicity occurred within the first 12 weeks of treatment. Transaminase elevations were reversible with discontinuation of the drug in all cases, and there have been no deaths reported. Upon rechallenge, 88% of patients were able to resume long-term treatment, most at the original dose.[18] GI side effects (nausea, vomiting, diarrhea, dyspepsia, and weight loss) are the other most common treatment-limiting side effects of tacrine, and 16% of patients withdrew from one study due to these complaints.[17]

Prophylactic effects do not extend indefinitely. In a 30-week study, improvement dropped off after 24 weeks of treatment.[17] Few long-term maintenance treatment studies of tacrine have been performed. Minthon et al. examined patients for 14 months and found both clinical and functional neuroimaging evidence that long-term tacrine treatment may delay the progression of cognitive impairment.[19] Clinically, 7 out of 9 patients on tacrine were unchanged or slightly improved while 8 of the 11 untreated patients had deteriorated or not improved. Regional cerebral blood flow (rCBF) studies showed increased rCBF in central-parietal regions with long-term tacrine treatment compared with the typical decrease in rCBF with time in untreated patients.[19]

Drug-drug interactions with tacrine include increased levels of theophylline, increased levels of tacrine with cimetidine, synergistic effect with cholinergic agents (bethanechol), succinylcholine and cholinesterase inhibitors, and antagonism of anticholinergic medications. Precaution should be used when administering tacrine to patients with "sick sinus syndrome" due to potential vagotonic effects, ulcer disease due to increased gastric acid secretion, liver disease, seizure disorder, and asthma.

Tacrine has a low oral bioavailability of 17%. Half-life is about two to four hours so dosing must be four times per day. Protein binding is 55%. It is hepatically metabolized by cytochrome P450 1A2, which it also inhibits. Tacrine (Cognex) is available in 10, 20, 30, and 40 mg tablets.

Tacrine should be initiated at 10 mg po qid and titrated gradually by 40 mg/day at six-week intervals with weekly monitoring of liver function tests (particularly ALT) for six weeks after each dose increase.[15] Once stable on a dose for at least six weeks, the patient's hepatic monitoring can be decreased to once every three months. The maximum dose is 160 mg/d. If ALT rises to greater than three times the ULN, tacrine should be discontinued with persistent weekly monitoring of the liver function tests for four weeks or until they normalize. Patients may be rechallenged with tacrine after ALT elevation resolves, especially if they were deriving some benefit from the drug. Patients should not be rechallenged with tacrine if they had jaundice with total bilirubin >3 mg/dL or ALT >10 times the ULN.

DONEPEZIL

Donepezil (Aricept) is the second FDA approved drug for use for cognitive impairment in Alzheimer's disease. It is also a cholinesterase inhibitor that has been shown to significantly improve memory and cognition compared with placebo at doses of 5 or 10 mg/day. Donepezil produces greater inhibition of acetylcholinesterase than tacrine which contributes to its better side effect profile. The most common side effects are nausea, diarrhea, and weight loss. Hepatotoxicity does not occur and routine monitoring of liver function is unnecessary.[20] Weight loss may be severe in some patients and necessitates routine monitoring of the patients weight. Patients should be initiated at 5 mg po, usually in the morning before breakfast unless nausea is a complaint, at which donepezil should be given with food. If the drug is well-tolerated, the dosage should be increased to 10 mg/day in a single dose after four to six weeks. Clinical use of donepezil is much more common given its ease of use and better side effect profile than tacrine.

OTHERS

Other drugs have also been studied but with disappointing and mixed results. Acetylcholine precursors, lecithin and choline, and muscarinic cholinergic agonists have been studied with negative results. Other agents such as NSAIDs, vitamin E, vasodilators, calcium-channel blockers, nootropics, NMDA antagonists, selegeline, neuropeptides, vitamin B_{12}, and opiate antagonists have been suggested to improve cognitive function, but there is still a paucity of convincing evidence for efficacy of any of these agents.

BEHAVIORAL DISTURBANCE

Behavioral disturbances occur in the majority of moderate to severely demented patients and are the major cause of institutionalization in this population. Common behaviors include agitation, aggressivity, assaultiveness, catastrophic reactions, suspiciousness, responding to hallucinations and delusions, disinhibition, sleep disturbances, restlessness, wandering, repetitive inappropriate vocalizations and screaming, and inappropriate sexual behavior.

The behavioral disturbances commonly seen in demented patients can be divided into several categories based on the type of disruptive behaviors and associated neuropsychiatric features. Treatment approaches vary by type of behavioral disturbance. Rosen et al. classify behavioral disturbances or agitation into the following six causes:

1. Pain or discomfort.
2. Delirium.
3. Depression.
4. Anxiety or distress.
5. Psychosis.
6. Caregiver burden.

Each category requires a different treatment approach.[12]

The diagnostic evaluation of agitated behavior in dementia should begin with a thorough medical evaluation to search for a treatable medical cause. Physical illnesses such as infection (commonly urinary tract infection or pneumonia), bone fracture, decubitus, and constipation with obstruction or ileus should be ruled out. Once a physical illness has been ruled out, the underlying psychopathology should be determined: delirium, depression, anxiety, or psychosis. These associated symptoms should be targeted appropriately first with behavioral interventions if indicated, and then with pharmacotherapy.

Caregiver burden is treated by providing support, community services, and respite to the caregiver and possibly placement of the patient.

When behavioral strategies are ineffective, pharmacological treatment should be employed. This literature has been extensively reviewed.[1,11,12,13,21,22,23] There are few adequately controlled prospective studies of behavioral disturbance in dementia, and there is little evidence supporting commonly employed treatment approaches. Behaviors that are most amenable to pharmacological interventions include restlessness, aggression, violence, and psychosis. Distressing repetitive behaviors, wandering, hoarding, stealing, clinging, inappropriate voiding, hypersexuality, and difficult personality traits are less responsive to pharmacological treatment.[21]

Pharmacological treatments and the evidence supporting their use are presented by category of behavioral disturbance and associated psychopathology. Some medications that have been suggested to be effective are listed in Table 11–3.

DEPRESSION

Depressive symptoms and depressive disorders are relatively common in dementia, especially early in the course of the illness. The estimated prevalence of comorbid depressive disorders in dementia ranges from 0–86% with most studies reporting an incidence of 10–20%.[24] Patients with comorbid depression are more cognitively impaired and disabled than nondepressed demented patients.[25] The presence of depression in dementia is associated with higher rates of institutionalization, mortality, and functional impairment.

Depression is more common in dementia than in the general population and more common in subcortical than cortical dementias. Depressive disorder affects approximately 10–20% of patients with Alzheimer's disease, 25% with vascular dementia, 40% with Huntington's disease, and 40% of patients with Parkinson's disease.[24,26,27,28]

The diagnosis of depression in dementia may be complicated. Patients may develop a depressed mood early in the course of the dementing illness as they are faced with numerous losses including diminished cognitive abilities, functioning, and resultant loss of independence. To meet criteria for a depressive disorder, the depressed mood must be a persistent state rather than merely a transitory symptom in response to a particular situation. Affective lability or emotional incontinence may be confused with depression. Patients with dementia, especially with right hemisphere dysfunction, may

TABLE 11–3. PHARMACOLOGIC TREATMENT FOR BEHAVIORAL
DISTURBANCES IN DEMENTIA

Medication	Special Considerations	Adverse Effects
Antidepressants		
SSRIs	Affective symptoms, irritability, apathy, amotivation, panic	Headache, dyspepsia, diarrhea, restlessness, akathisia, insomnia, lethargy
Trazodone	Affective behavioral disturbances	Sedation, orthostatic hypotences, excitement, priapism
Mood Stabilizers		
Lithium	Agitation, aggression, mania, episodic symptoms	Neurotoxicity at "therapeutic" levels
Carbamazepine	Agitation, affective symptoms, abnormal EEG	Neurotoxicity, ataxia, blood dyscrasias
Valproic acid	Agitation, affective symptoms, abnormal EEG	Sedation, confusion, ataxia, hepatitis, thrombocytopenia
Anxiolytics		
Benzodiazepines	Anxiety, apprehension, distress, hyperactivity, impulsivity	Worsening cognitive impairment, sedation, ataxia, disinhibition, delirium
Buspirone	Agitation, anxiety, depression, impulsivity	Headache, nausea, agitation, dyskinesia, dystonia
Beta-blockers	Agitation, aggression	Hypotension, bradycardia, psychosis, aggravation of diabetes, asthma and heart failure, depression
Antipsychotics	Agitation due to paranoia, hallucinations, delusions	Extrapyramidal side effects, anticholine effects, confusion, falls, tardive dyskinesia
Psychostimulants	Lack of response to other treatments	Agitation, hypertension, psychosis, confusion

lose the ability to express affect directly.[29] These patients may not necessarily endorse a depressed mood but instead may display irritability, negativism, emotional lability, anxiety, agitation, self-neglect, multiple somatic complaints, and cognitive impairment out of proportion to the extent of brain pathology. Other characteristic symptoms include the neurovegetative signs (insomnia, decreased appetite with weight loss, psychomotor retardation, anergia, decreased libido), hopelessness, chronic anger, social withdrawal, refusal to eat or take responsibility for their care, passive death wish, and psychotic features such as nihilism, morbid hallucinations, or delusions of death or suffering. Depression may also be accompanied by behavioral disturbances such as agitation, assaultive behavior, and screaming.

Cognitive impairment in patients with depression is associated with late onset major depressive disorder, manic symptoms, and poorer outcome.[30] This cognitive impairment is reversible and improves as the depression improves. This condition is called the dementia of depression.[31] While it is initially reversible, dementia of depression usually heralds the development of dementia within several years in the majority of patients.[32]

Few randomized, double-blind, placebo-controlled studies of the treatment of depression in the elderly have been reported. There is only one published study of acute treatment of depression in elderly demented patients, and there are no studies on maintenance treatment in this population. Reifler et al. reported a double-blind, placebo-controlled, randomized eight-week trial of imipramine in depressed and nondepressed patients with Alzheimer's disease.[33] There was significant improvement in all groups with no advantage of imipramine over placebo. However, the authors report significantly greater cognitive decline with imipramine. There was no significant cognitive improvement in the depressed demented patients with adequate treatment of the depression.

Nyth and Gottfries reported the results of a multicenter randomized, double-blind, placebo-controlled study of citalopram, an SSRI not currently available in the United States, in the treatment of "emotional disturbances" in Alzheimer's and vascular dementia.[34] The emotional disturbances were decreased motivation, emotional blunting, and anxiety, and patients were only mildly depressed. Citalopram produced significant improvement in depression, irritability, emotional bluntness, confusion, anxiety, fear, panic, and restlessness. This response was confined to the Alzheimer's dementia patients and was not seen in the vascular dementia patients.

Despite the lack of evidence supporting the use of antidepressants in the treatment of depressive disorders and depressive symptoms in dementia, treatment strategies are extrapolated from late life depression studies in nondemented patients. This may not be justified since the presence of dementia likely alters the pathophysiology of the depression. Nevertheless, treatment is guided by evidence from the nondemented elderly.

Predictors of response to antidepressants in patients with mixed dementia and depression include greater initial depressive symptoms, higher cognitive functioning, and moderate sleep disturbance.[35] Older patients may take longer to respond to antidepressants than younger patients, and an adequate trial in the elderly should probably be 12 weeks at therapeutic dose or level.

Choice of antidepressant is guided by side-effect profile. The better tolerated agents (SSRIs) should be tried first. Tertiary amine tricyclic antidepressants (TCAs) should be avoided due to the high anticholinergic burden.

SELECTIVE SEROTONIN REUPTAKE INHIBITORS (SSRIs)

The SSRIs have demonstrated efficacy in only one placebo-controlled acute study in late life depression.[36] In many comparison studies between SSRIs and TCAs, the SSRIs are as effective if not more effective than the TCAs and are much better tolerated and devoid of cognitive side effects.[37]

Fluoxetine's long half-life and active metabolite makes it a less desirable agent in the elderly, because if patients do have an adverse reaction, drug-drug interaction with another agent, or need to switch to a different agent, it takes much longer to wash out than the other SSRIs (four weeks compared with one week). Paroxetine is the most anticholinergic of the SSRIs and theoretically may have more negative effects on cognition. Fluvoxamine is metabolized by cytochrome P450 3A4 and may cause fatal ventricular arrhythmias with astemizole and terfenadine so patients taking these agents should avoid fluvoxamine. Sertraline has the fewest interactions with the P450 system and little cholinergic activity so it is a good first choice SSRI in the elderly.

The most common adverse effects with all the SSRIs are transient headache, GI upset, diarrhea, anxiety, restlessness, psychomotor agitation, insomnia, and lethargy. Notably, there are far fewer anticholinergic side effects than with the TCAs. Initial doses should be half those used in adults but should be increased to adequate doses; elderly patients may require the same doses as young healthy adults. For more information on the clinical use of SSRIs, see Chapter 4, Depressive Disorders.

TRICYCLIC ANTIDEPRESSANTS (TCAs)

TCAs have demonstrated efficacy in five placebo-controlled acute trials of amitriptyline and imipramine in late life depression in nondemented patients and in one maintenance trial of nortriptyline.[38,39] In the only reported study of depression in dementia, imipramine had no benefit over placebo.[33] The most significant adverse reactions are orthostatic hypotension, which is a risk factor for falls and hip fractures, cardiac conduction delays, and anticholinergic effects such as constipation, urinary retention, and cognitive impairment or delirium. The question of cognitive impairment with TCAs is a controversial one; Reifler et al. demonstrated increased cognitive impairment with imipramine (average dose 82 mg/day), while Reding et al. did not detect a cognitive change in a double-blind, placebo-controlled study of 17 Alzheimer's disease patients on 25–100 mg/day of amitriptyline.[33,40] Tertiary amines, which are more anticholinergic, are demethylated to secondary amines. This process is slowed in the elderly, leading to accumulation of the more toxic parent compound. Therefore, the secondary amines, nortriptyline and desipramine, are preferred in the elderly due to less anticholinergic activity.

Initial doses should be 10 mg nortriptyline or desipramine and a serum level and electrocardiogram should be checked every five to seven days before each dose increase. Elderly patients may require lower doses of TCAs to achieve therapeutic plasma levels, but they require the same plasma levels as younger patients for therapeutic effect. Therefore, it is important to push the dose to therapeutic levels as tolerated even in elderly patients. Target levels of nortriptyline are 50–150 ng/ml, the same as in adults. One common mistake is to fail to push the level to therapeutic range for fear of adverse effects. Common drug-drug interactions that affect the elderly are listed in Table 11–4.

MONOAMINE OXIDASE INHIBITORS (MAOIs)

The MAOI phenelzine has demonstrated efficacy in the acute treatment of depression in nondemented elderly patients in one acute controlled trial each and in one maintenance study in late life depression.[39,41] MAOIs may be especially effective for apathy and low motivation and in patients with anxiety accompanied by physical symptoms, atypical features (rejection sensitivity, mood reactivity), and intolerance or lack of response to the TCAs.[42,43] L-deprenyl, an MAO-B selective inhibitor at low doses, has been shown to decrease anxiety, depression, tension, and excitement and improve cognitive functioning in 17 AD patients with mild behavioral symptoms in a placebo-controlled study.[44]

MAOIs may produce more adverse effects in elderly patients than the TCAs.[41] These include sedation, activation, headache, paradoxical reactions, memory loss, confusion, ataxia, insomnia, mania, psychosis, orthostatic hypotension, anticholinergic side effects, sexual dysfunction, paresthesias, peripheral neuropathy, myoclonus, tremor, myalgias, and arthralgias. MAOIs are contraindicated in carcinoid and pheochromocytoma. Hypertensive crisis is no more common in the elderly than in younger patients but is potentially more devastating in elderly patients with fragile cerebrovasculature.[38] High tyramine foods and certain over-the-counter medications, especially sympathomimetics, should be avoided as these may precipitate hypertensive crisis. These restrictions pose the greatest danger for demented patients taking MAOIs, because they may forget the restrictions. Acute treatment for hypertensive crisis in younger patients is chlorpromazine, which should be avoided in the elderly secondary to risk of hypotension and anticholinergic side effects. Nifedipine 10 mg chewed and placed sublingual should be used acutely.[45] Potential drug interactions are listed in Table 11–4.

TABLE 11–4. SOME POTENTIAL HETEROCYCLIC ANTIDEPRESSANT INTERACTIONS

Medication	Interacting Medication	Interaction
Tricyclic antidepressants (TCAs)	Anticholinergic drugs	Additive anticholinergic effects
	Tranquilizers, sedatives, and low-potency neuroleptics	Increased sedation
	Low-potency neuroleptics and antihypertensive drugs	Increased orthostatic hypotension
	Antihypertensives (clonidine, guanethidine, bethanidine, and debrisoquin)	Decreased effect of both classes
	Adding TCA to antihypertensive	Hypertensive crisis
	Type I antiarrhythmics	Additive antiarrhythmic effect, prolonged Q-T interval, widened QRS complex, and increased risk of bundle branch block
	Directly acting sympathomimetics	Potentiation of sympathomimetic
	Disulfiram	Increased activity of both classes
	Cimetidine	Increased TCA levels
Selective serotonic uptake inhibitors	Lithium, tryptophan, buspirone, and other serotonergic drugs	Headache and serotonin syndrome
	Monoamine oxidase inhibitors	Fatal serotonin syndrome
All heterocyclic antidepressants	Neuroleptics other than fluphenthixol	Increased levels of both classes; clinically relevant for antidepressant
	Stimulants	Increased antidepressant levels
	Anticonvulsants	Decreased antidepressant levels
	Cholestyramine	Decreased antidepressant levels

Adapted from Coffey, C.E., Cummings, J.L. (Eds.) (1994). *Textbook of Geriatric Neuropsychiatry* (p. 602). Copyright 1994 by American Psychiatric Press, Inc. Reprinted with permission.

TRAZODONE

Trazodone, an atypical triazolopyridine antidepressant, has demonstrated efficacy in one acute placebo-controlled trial in late life depression.[46] It has also been studied in the treatment of behavioral complications of dementia. There is some evidence from noncontrolled studies that trazodone (150–500 mg/day) is effective for affective and behavioral disturbances in dementia.[47] The most common side effects were initial sedation, orthostatic hypotension, and excitement. Trazodone may cause ventricular arrhythmias in patients with preexisting cardiac disease. Priapism may also occur.

PSYCHOSTIMULANTS

Psychostimulants are used more frequently in the elderly and medically compromised patients than in other populations. They are effective in melancholic patients with apathy, amotivation, and abulia, either alone or as an augmentation strategy of a standard antidepressant such as a TCA.[48,49] Patients with medical illness that preclude TCAs or other antidepressants may tolerate stimulants without medical compromise.[48]

Psychostimulants have demonstrated efficacy in four placebo-controlled studies in elderly patients both with and without dementia.[49,38] Stimulants are usually used as a short-term treatment although there is some evidence for long-term treatment benefits.[49]

Methylphenidate and dextroamphetamine are the two best studied agents. More adverse effects are reported with dextroamphetamine so methylphenidate should be the first choice.[49] Potential side effects include agitation, restlessness, tremor, hyperreflexia, hallucinations, paranoia, psychosis, confusion, tachycardia, hypertension, angina, arrhythmia, circulatory collapse, and cerebral hemorrhage. Psychostimulants may aggravate psychosis and chorea and may decrease the seizure threshold. Drug interactions include increasing levels of TCAs and antipsychotics. Surprisingly, the studies of methylphenidate in the elderly report few side effects in this population.

Dosing should begin low with gradual increments (methylphenidate 2.5 mg/day every week). Typical doses of methylphenidate are 5–45 mg/day divided bid or tid for augmentation and 10–40 mg/day for primary treatment of depression.[13] Also see Chapter 4.

ELECTROCONVULSIVE THERAPY (ECT)

ECT is also an option for treating depression in demented depressed patients. Acute confusion after ECT treatments may be greater in patients with dementia, but the underlying dementia is not exacerbated.

MANIA

Mania is far less common in dementia than depression and affects about 3–17% of AD patients.[24] Mania is associated with right sided brain pathology, especially in the frontal cortex, basal ganglia, and thalamus, as well as with subcortical atrophy. There are no reported controlled prospective studies of the treatment of mania in dementia. Treatment strategies are extrapolated from studies in nondemented elderly patients. Because lithium is associated with greater toxicity in patients with underlying neurologic disease, valproate and carbamazepine, which are better tolerated, may be preferred as first-line mood stabilizers in demented patients.

CARBAMAZEPINE

Carbamazepine use has been reported in seven case reports and open pilot studies for behavioral disturbances in dementia with significant improvement in agitation with plasma levels in the subtherapeutic range. One placebo-controlled, crossover study showed no significant improvement with carbamazepine and in fact showed more cognitive deterioration with carbamazepine than placebo.[50] Another nonrandomized, placebo-controlled, crossover study with low dose carbamazepine revealed significant improvement in agitation, anxiety, aggression, and global improvement.[51]

Carbamazepine may be better tolerated than lithium in patients with brain damage.[13] Side effects were dose-related and worse with serum levels >9 mcg/ml and included sedation, confusion, ataxia, tremor, and cognitive impairment. Carbamazepine may also cause hepatitis, SIADH, lymphadenopathy, transient leukopenia, agranulocytosis, aplastic anemia, thrombocytopenia, eosinophilia, or rash. Levels must be carefully monitored, especially when used concomitantly with other hepatically metabolized agents. Medications that can increase carbamazepine levels include fluoxetine and other SSRIs, cimetidine, erythromycin, isoniazid, and valproate. Carbamazepine decreases levels of anticonvulsants, antipsychotics, benzodiazepines, and coumadin (Table 11–5).

VALPROATE

There is one open label, prospective study of valproate in nursing home patients with dementia and agitation that demonstrated decreased behavioral agitation with minimal side effects at low serum levels (13–52 mcg/ml).[52] There are no reported controlled studies of valproate in dementia. Side effects include sedation, ataxia, tremor, and cognitive impairment. Valproate may cause hepatitis, rash, alopecia, or gastrointestinal distress. Aspirin can increase valproate levels.

CALCIUM-CHANNEL ANTAGONISTS

Verapamil and nimodepine may be useful in treating mania in dementia. Dubovsky et al. report good results and minimal side effects with

TABLE 11–5. POTENTIAL INTERACTIONS OF ALTERNATIVES TO LITHIUM

Alternative	Medication	Interaction
Carbamazepine	Lithium	Neurotoxicity
	Anticonvulsants, neuroleptics, benzodiazepines, and coumadin	Decreased blood level of the other medication caused by enzyme induction
	Fluoxetine	Increased carbamazepine levels
	Neuroleptics	Neurotoxicity
	Cimetidine, erythromycin, and isoniazid	Increased carbamazepine levels
Valproic acid	Aspirin	Increased valproate levels
	Other anticonvulsants	Increased risk of hepatotoxicity, possibly caused by toxic intermediates of valproate metabolism
	Clonazepam	Absence status epilepticus
Verapamil	Carbamazepine, lithium	Increased carbamazepine and lithium levels, neurotoxicity
	Lithium, beta-blockers	Additive cardiac slowing

Adapted from Coffey, C.E., Cummings, J.L. (Eds.) (1994). *Textbook of Geriatric Neuropsychiatry* (p. 610). Copyright 1994 by American Psychiatric Press, Inc. Reprinted with permission.

verapamil 240–480 mg/day in elderly bipolar patients with dementia.[53] The use of mood stabilizers is discussed in greater detail in Chapter 5.

ANXIETY

Anxiety is a common symptom in dementia although criteria for a specific anxiety disorder may not be met. Anxiety may be related to poor sleep, memory loss, disorientation, or confusion.

BENZODIAZEPINES

The treatment of anxiety symptoms in dementia has not been well studied. Benzodiazepines are used to alleviate the anxiety, apprehension, and subjective distress that may accompany the early stages of dementia.[9] There is evidence from case reports that they may be especially helpful for hyperactivity, insomnia, intrusiveness, and impulsivity.

Benzodiazepines may cause worsening cognitive impairment in the demented elderly. Because of the risk of cognitive side effects, benzodiazepines should not be used in patients with moderate to severe dementia.[9] Side effects include sedation, ataxia, falls, delirium, and paradoxical reactions such as disinhibition and worsening behavior disturbances. Demented patients may develop benzodiazepine toxicity at relatively low doses or at previously tolerated doses. Agents with short to intermediate half-lives and no active metabolites are preferred to avoid accumulation of active metabolites and the development of toxicity. Agents such as lorazepam, oxazepam, and alprazolam are the safest benzodiazepines in the demented elderly.

Physical dependence may also develop after months of treatment, especially with shorter half-life agents. With abrupt discontinuation of benzodiazepines, patients may experience acute relapse of anxiety symptoms, rebound anxiety, or withdrawal symptoms.

Drug interactions include elevated benzodiazepine levels with cimetidine, decreased levels with anticonvulsants and corticosteroids, increased respiratory distress with opioids, and increased cognitive impairment with other central nervous system depressants.

BUSPIRONE

Buspirone is better tolerated than benzodiazepines in demented patients. It is effective for chronic anxiety in younger patients, and there is some evidence from several open studies that it may reduce agitation in dementia.[22] Buspirone also enhances dopamine neurotransmission by blocking presynaptic dopamine autoreceptors, so it may be beneficial for parkinsonian symptoms. Buspirone may cause headache, nausea, dizziness, dyskinesias, and dystonia but has no effect on cognitive function.

PSYCHOSIS

Psychotic symptoms affect 30–40% of demented patients and usually appear in the middle to late stages of the illness.[24] Hallucinations are rare in Alzheimer's disease with visual hallucinations more common than auditory. Illusions or misinterpretations of real stimuli must be ruled out. Illusions are common in patients with sensory deficits such as hearing or vision loss; sensory input is misinterpreted because of the impaired sensation. This may lead to negative or threatening interpretations of perceptions with resultant anxiety, fear, depression, or frank delusions. Hallucinations in dementia are not very responsive to medications.

Delusions may be present in the early to middle stages of dementia and tend to decrease in later stages of the illness. Paranoid delusions are the most common neuropsychiatric symptom of dementia and occur in 10–73%

of demented patients.[24] Delusions in dementia are primarily paranoid or persecutory in nature and are often attributable to memory loss. Common delusions include believing that possessions have been stolen, they are being poisoned, their spouse is not really their spouse, and their family or caregivers are impostors (Capgras syndrome).

The differential diagnosis of psychosis in dementia includes delirium and depression with psychotic features. Treatment is with antipsychotic medications. There are few good studies demonstrating efficacy of the antipsychotics for the behavioral disturbances of dementia. Schneider et al. performed a meta-analysis of the published studies.[11] The placebo response was 37.5% while the antipsychotic response was 40.5%. Eighteen percent of patients benefitted from antipsychotics over placebo. There was no significant difference between haloperidol or thioridazine and any comparison antipsychotic. Risperidone also has demonstrated efficacy in phychosis and agitation in Alzheimer's disease.[54] Antipsychotics are effective in reducing agitation, insomnia, irritability, and hostility in demented patients. However, some of the benefit may be due to the sedative effects rather than direct antipsychotic effects. No maintenance studies have been reported.

ANTIPSYCHOTICS

Choice of antipsychotic agent is based on side-effect profile because there is no evidence that any agent is more effective than another. High potency agents are more likely to cause extrapyramidal side effects while low potency agents are associated with a higher risk of anticholinergic side effects. Elderly patients with dementia are more prone to EPS, possibly from changes in the nigrostriatal pathway and higher blood levels due to increases in volume of distribution and decreased metabolism.[55] The risk of psychomotor side effects and increased confusion may not outweigh the potential benefit in some patients.

Tardive dyskinesia (TD) is more common in the elderly, especially in the first two years of treatment and occurs in 16–41% of elderly patients taking antipsychotic medications (depending on duration of exposure).[56,57] Interestingly, spontaneous dyskinesias occur in up to 5% of elderly individuals not exposed to neuroleptics. Risk factors for TD include female gender, primary affective disorder, history of acute EPS, brain damage, length of duration of neuroleptic exposure, medical illness, concurrent antiparkinsonian agents, and drug holidays. TD is less frequently reversible after withdrawal of the antipsychotic in the elderly and is irreversible in one-third to one-half of geriatric patients. Therefore, using the lowest doses possible and avoiding antiparkinsonian agents, rapid dose increases, and drug holidays are the best preventative measures. Also, the need for continued antipsychotic use should be reassessed frequently, and antipsychotic medications should be tapered or discontinued whenever possible to avoid unnecessary prolonged exposure.

The risk of neuroleptical malignant syndrome (NMS) is less in the elderly than in younger patients but increases with brain damage, neurological disease, and debilitation.[58]

While high potency antipsychotics are associated with increased risk of EPS, low potency agents are more likely to decrease the seizure threshold and exacerbate seizures in patients with an underlying seizure disorder.

Risperidone may have the advantage of being a high potency agent but less likely to cause EPS, especially at therapeutic doses. Doses in the elderly demented patients are lower than in younger patents, usually 1–2 mg/day divided bid.

Clozapine is the first-line antipsychotic agent in patients with Parkinson's disease and psychosis, because the traditional antipsychotics exacerbate the motor symptoms. It may also be useful in other types of dementia with psychosis. The risk of agranulocytosis may increase with age.[13] However, several recent reports indicate that clozapine may be used safely in elderly patients.[59,60,61,62] The most common side effects are sedation, orthostasis, hypersalivation, hyperthermia, and akathisia. There is also a risk of seizures and respiratory depression when used concomitantly with benzodiazepines.

Common drug interactions with antipsychotics are listed in Table 11–6.

Electroconvulsive therapy is an alternative to antipsychotics in dementia with psychosis or delirium.

DELIRIUM

Delirium in the context of a dementia may be difficult to differentiate from the deteriorating course of the dementia, but it is marked by a sudden change in mental status or level of functioning and implies an altered state of consciousness and arousal. Delirium can be caused by any additional insult to a brain that is already compromised. Common causes of delirium in dementia include metabolic disturbances, medications, organ failure, or an acute neurological event such as a cerebrovascular accident or subdural hemorrhage. The underlying cause or causes must be identified and treated appropriately in a timely fashion because the morbidity and mortality associated with delirium are very high.

Pharmacotherapy consists of low dose, high potency antipsychotics such as haloperidol 0.5–4 mg/day. Haloperidol may be given intravenously (IV).

TABLE 11-6. ANTIPSYCHOTIC DRUG INTERACTIONS

Medication	Interaction
Central nervous system depressants	Increased sedation, confusion, falls
Guanethidine	Decreased antihypertensive effect
Lithium	Increased extrapyramidal side effects
Anticholinergic antiparkinsonian drugs, cimetidine, and antacids	Decreased neuroleptic levels caused by inhibition of gastrointestinal absorption
Anticonvulsants	Decreased neuroleptic levels caused by increased metabolism
Tricyclic antidepressants	Increased levels of both; clinically significant only for tricyclic antidepressant
Levodopa	Decreased antiparkinsonian effect due to dopamine receptor blockade
Propranolol	Increased levels of both classes
Benzodiazepines	Physical collapse with clozapine
Carbamazepine	Increased risk of fatal bone marrow suppression with clozapine

Adapted from Coffey, C.E., Cummings, J.L. (Eds.) (1994). *Textbook of Geriatric Neuropsychiatry* (p. 617). Copyright 1994 by American Psychiatric Press, Inc. Reprinted with permission.

This route produces fewer EPS than either oral or intramuscular routes. IV haloperidol may be augmented with IV lorazepam.[63]

SLEEP DISTURBANCE

Disturbed sleep is common in dementia and delirium and may present as fragmented sleep or sleep reversal. Common causes include depression, anxiety, and grief. Benzodiazepines are good acute treatments for insomnia secondary to stress but are not effective as chronic sleeping aids. Short half-life agents do not accumulate but may wear out before the end of the night causing early morning awakening and rebound insomnia when used chronically. Long half-life agents may be accumulated and cause daytime sedation and psychomotor impairment. Zolpidem (Ambien), a new benzodiazepine type 1 selective agonist, may be safer for longer term use although this has not been clearly demonstrated.

Antihistamines such as diphenhydramine (Benadryl) are effective sedatives but may also cause daytime sedation and psychomotor impairment as well as anticholinergic side effects and cognitive impairment.

The antidepressants, amitriptyline, trazodone, and doxepin, in low doses, may be good choices for sleep.[13]

MAINTENANCE TREATMENT

While dementia is a chronic and progressive disorder, the neuro-psychiatric manifestations may fluctuate and evolve with the natural course of the underlying illness. Therefore, employing maintenance treatment as prophylaxis to prevent recurrences is not indicated. Affective and behavioral disturbances may actually decrease as dementia progresses, so pharmacotherapy should be reevaluated periodically for continued necessity. If a demented patient has a history of a chronic psychiatric illness such as recurrent major depression or chronic schizophrenia prior to the onset of the dementia, this disorder should be treated with maintenance pharmacotherapy regardless of the presence of concomitant dementia. But neuropsychiatric symptoms solely in the context of dementia should be treated acutely and possibly with continuation treatment for a period of months.

There currently is no evidence for the continued benefit of pharmacological interventions in affective or behavioral disturbances in dementia beyond acute treatment. Effective pharmacological treatments probably should be continued for six months and then reevaluated. If symptoms are still remitted and the clinical picture is stable, an attempt should then be made to taper and discontinue the medication. If symptoms return, the medication should be reinstituted and adjusted as needed to try to maintain the lowest effective dose.

REFERENCES

1. Cummings, J.L. (1992). Neuropsychiatric aspects of Alzheimer's disease and other dementing illnesses. In Yudofsky, S.C., Hales, R.E. (Eds.). *The American Psychiatric Press Textbook of Neuropsychiatry* (pp. 605–620). Washington, DC: American Psychiatric Press.
2. Skoog, I., Nilsson, L., Palmez, B., et al. (1993). A population-based study of dementia in 85-year-olds. *N Engl J Med*, 328:153–158.
3. Miller, B.L., Chang, L., Oropilla, G., Mena, I. (1994). Alzheimer's disease and frontal lobe dementias. In Coffey, C.F., Cummings, J.L. (Eds.). *Textbook of Geriatric Neuropsychiatry* (pp. 390–403). Washington, DC: American Psychiatric Press.
4. McKhann, G., Drachman, D., Folstein, M.F., et al. (1984). Clinical diagnosis of Alzheimer's disease: Report of the NINCDS-ADRDA Work Group under the auspices of the Department of Health and Human Services Task Force on Alzheimer's Disease. *Neurology*, 34:939–944.
5. Papkanm, Rubio, A., Schiffer, R.B. (1998). A review of Lewy body disease. *J Neuropsychiatry Clin Neurosci* 10:267–279.
6. Mace, N., Rabins, P. (1981). *The 36-Hour Day*. Baltimore: Johns Hopkins University Press.
7. Aronson, M. (Ed.). (1988). *Understanding Alzheimer's Disease*. New York: Charles Scribner's Sons.
8. Gruetzner, H. (1992). *Alzheimer's: A Caregiver's Guide and Sourcebook*. New York: Wiley.
9. Salzman, C. (1988). Treatment of agitation, anxiety, and depression in dementia. *Psychopharmacol Bull*, 24(1):39–42.

10. Small, G.W. (1988). Psychopharmacological treatment of elderly demented patients. *J Clin Psychiatry*, 49(Suppl 5):8–13.
11. Schneider, L.S., Pollock, V.E., Lyness, S.A. (1990). A metaanalysis of controlled trials of neuroleptic treatment in dementia. *J Am Geriatr Soc*, 38(5):553–563.
12. Rosen, J., Mulsant, B.H., Wright, B.A. (1992). Agitation in severely demented patients. *Ann Clin Psychiatry*, 4:207–215.
13. Dubovsky, S.L. (1994). Geriatric neuropsychopharmacology. In Coffey, C.F., Cummings, J.L. (Eds.). *Textbook of Geriatric Neuropsychiatry*, Washington, DC: American Psychiatric Press.
14. Zimmer, A.W., Calkins, F., Hadley E., et al. (1985). Conducting clinical research in geriatric populations. *Ann Intern Med*, 103:276–283.
15. Wagstaff, A.J., McTavish, D. (1994). Tacrine: A review of its pharmacodynamic and pharmacokinetic properties, and therapeutic efficacy in Alzheimer's disease. *Drugs and Aging*, 4(6):510–540.
16. Soares, J.C., Gershon, S. (1995). THA—Historical aspects, review of pharmacologic properties and therapeutic effects. *Dementia*, 6(4):225–234.
17. Knapp, M.J., Knopman, D.S., Soloman, P.R., et al. (1994). A 30-week randomized controlled trial of high-dose tacrine in patients with Alzheimer's disease. The Tacrine Study Group. *JAMA*, 271(13):985–991.
18. Watkins, P.B., Zimmerman, H.J., Knapp, M.J., et al. (1994). Hepatoxic effects of tacrine administration in patients with Alzheimer's disease. *JAMA*, 271(13):1023–1024.
19. Minthon, L., Nilsson, K., Edvinsson, L., et al. (1995). Long-term effects of tacrine on regional cerebral blood flow changes in Alzheimer's disease. *Dementia*, 6(5):245–251.
20. Rogers, S.L. Friedhoff, L.T. (1996). The efficacy and safety of donepezil in patients with Alzheimer's disease. Results of a U.S. multicenter, randomized, double-blind, placebo-controlled trial. The Donepezil Study Group. *Dementia*, 7(6):293–303.
21. Maletta, G.J. (1990). Pharmacologic treatment and management of the aggressive demented patient. *Psychiatric Ann*, 20(8):446–455.
22. Schneider, L.S., Sobin, P.B. (1991). Non-neuroleptic medications in the management of agitation in Alzheimer's disease and other dementias: A selective review. *Int J Geriatr Psychiatry*, 6:691–708.
23. Tariot, P.N., Schneider, L.S., Katz, L.R. (1995). Anticonvulsant and other non-neuroleptic treatment of agitation in dementia. *J Geriatr Psychiatry Neurol*, 8(Suppl 1):S28–39.
24. Wragg, R.E., Jeste, D.V. (1989). Overview of depression and psychosis in Alzheimer's disease. *Am J Psychiatry*, 146:577–587.
25. Rovner, B.W., Broadhead, J., Spencer, M., et al. (1989). Depression and Alzheimer's disease. *Am J Psychiatry*, 146(3):350–353.
26. Fedoroff, J.P., Lipsey, J.R., Starkstein, S.E., et al. (1991). Phenomenological comparisons of major depression following stroke, myocardial infarction or spinal cord lesion. *J Affect Disorders*, 22:83–89.
27. Folstein, S.E., Abbott, M.H., Chase, G.A., et al. (1983). The association of affective disorder with Huntington's disease in a case series and in families. *Psychol Med*, 13:537–542.
28. Cummings, J.L. (1992). Depression and Parkinson's disease: A review. *Am J Psychiatry*, 149:443–454.
29. Ross, E.D., Rush, A.J. (1981). Diagnosis and neuroanatomical correlates of depression in brain damaged patients. *Arch Gen Psychiatry*, 38:1344–1354.
30. McMahon, F.L., DePaulo, J.R. (1992). Clinical features of affective disorders and bereavement. *Curr Opin Psychiatry*, 5:580–584.
31. Folstein, M.F., McHugh, P.R. (1978). Dementia syndrome of depression. In Katzman, R., Terry, R.D., Bick, K.L. (Eds.). *Alzheimer's Disease: Senile Dementia and Related Disorders* (pp. 87–96). New York: Raven Press.

32. Kral, V.A. (1983). The relationship between senile dementia (Alzheimer's type) and depression. *Can J Psychiatry*, 28:304–306.
33. Reifler, B.V., Teri, L., Raskind, M., et al. (1989). Double-blind trial of imipramine in Alzheimer's disease patients with and without depression. *Am J Psychiatry*, 146:45–49.
34. Nyth, A.L., Gottfries, C.G. (1990). The clinical efficacy of citalopram in treatment of emotional disturbances in dementia disorders. A Nordic Multicentre Study. *Br J Psychiatry*, 157:894–901.
35. Reynolds, C.F., Kupfer, D.J., Hoch, C.C., et al. (1986). Two-year follow-up of elderly patients with mixed depression and dementia: Clinical and electroencephalographic sleep findings. *J Am Geriatr Soc*, 34:793–799.
36. Tollefson, G.D., Holman, S.L. (1993). Analysis of the Hamilton Depression Rating Scale factors from a double-blind, placebo-controlled trial of fluoxetine in geriatric major depression. *Int Clin Psychopharmacol*, 8:253–259.
37. Newhouse, P.A. (1996). Use of serotonin selective reuptake inhibitors in geriatric depression. *J Clin Psychiatry*, 57(Suppl 5):12–22.
38. Rockwell, E., Lam, R.W., Zisook, S. (1988). Antidepressant drug studies in the elderly. *Psychiatr Clin North Am*, 11:215–233.
39. Georgotas, A., McCue, R.E., Cooper, T.B. (1989). A placebo-controlled comparison of nortriptyline and phenelzine in maintenance therapy of elderly depressed patients. *Arch Gen Psych*, 46:783–786.
40. Reding, M.J., Young, R., DiPonte, P. (1983). Amitriptyline in Alzheimer's disease (Letter). *Neurology*, 33:522.
41. Georgotas, A., McCue, R.E., Hapworth, W., et al. (1986). Comparative efficacy and safety of MAOIs versus TCAs in treating depression in the elderly. *Biol Psychiatry*, 21:1155–1166.
42. Salzman, C. (1990). Principles of psychopharmacology. In Bienenfeld, D. (Ed.). *Verwoerdt's Clinical Geropsychiatry*, (3rd ed.) (pp. 234–249). Baltimore: Williams & Wilkins.
43. Pare, C.M.B. (1985). The present status of monoamine oxidase inhibitors. *Br J Psychiatry*, 146:576–584.
44. Tariot, P.N., Cohen, R.M., Sunderland, T., et al. (1987). L-deprenyl in Alzheimer's disease: Preliminary evidence for behavioral change with monoamine oxidase B inhibition. *Arch Gen Psychiatry*, 44:427–433.
45. Clary, C., Schweitzer, E. (1987). Treatment of MAOI hypertensive crisis with sublingual nifedepine. *J Clin Psychiatry*, 48:249–250.
46. Gerner, R., Estabrook, W., Steuer J., et al. (1980). Treatment of geriatric depression with trazodone, imipramine, and placebo: A double-blind study. *J Clin Psychiatry*, 41:216–220.
47. Houlihan, D.J., Mulsant, B.H., Sweet, R.A., et al. (1994). A naturalistic study of trazodone in the treatment of behavioral complications of dementia. *Am J Geriatr Psychiatry*, 2:78–85.
48. Katon, W., Raskind, M. (1980). Treatment of depression in the medically ill elderly with methylphenidate. *Am J Psychiatry*, 137:963–965.
49. Chiarello, R.J., Cole, J.O. (1987). The use of psychostimulants in general psychiatry: A reconsideration. *Arch Gen Psychiatry*, 44:286–295.
50. Chambers, C.A., Bain, J., Rosbottom R., et al. (1982). Carbamazepine in senile dementia and overactivity: A placebo controlled double blind trial. *IRCS Medical Science*, 10:505–506.
51. Tariot, P.N., Erb, R., Leibovici, A., et al. (1994). Carbamazepine treatment of agitation in nursing home patients with dementia: A preliminary study. *J Amer Geriatr Soc*, 42(11):1160–1166.
52. Lott, A.D., McElroy, S.L., Keys, M.A. (1995). Valproate in the treatment of behavioral agitation in elderly patients with dementia. *J Neuropsychiatry Clin Neurosci*, 7:314–319.

53. Dubovsky, S.L., Franks, R.D., Allen, S., et al. (1986). Calcium antagonists in mania: A double-blind placebo controlled study of verapamil. *Psychiatry Res*, 18:309–320.
54. Goldberg, R.J., Goldberg, J. (1997). Risperidone for dementia-related disturbed behavior in nursing home residents: A clinical experience. *Intl Psychogeriatrics*, 9(1):65–68.
55. Young, R.C., Meyers, B.S. (1991). Psychopharmacology. In Sadavoy, J., Lazarus, L.W., Jarvik, L.F. (Eds.). *Comprehensive Review of Geriatric Psychiatry* (pp. 435–467). Washington, DC: American Psychiatric Press.
56. Toerniessan, L.M., Casey, D.E., McFarland, B.H. (1984). Tardive dyskinesia in the aged. *Arch Gen Psychiatry*, 42:278–284.
57. Sweet, R.A., Mulsant, B.H., Gupta B., et al. (1995). Duration of neuroleptic treatment and prevalence of tardive dyskinesia in late life. *Arch Gen Psychiatry*, 52:478–486.
58. Mueller, P.S. (1985). Neuroleptic malignant syndrome. *Psychosomatics*, 26:654–662.
59. Oberholzer, A.F., Hendriksen, C., Monsch, A.V., et al. (1992). Safety and effectiveness of low-dose clozapine in psychogeriatric patients: A preliminary study. *Int Psychogeriatrics*, 4(2):187–195.
60. Chengappa, K.N.R., Baker, R.W., Kreinbrook, S.B., et al. (1995). Clozapine use in female geriatric patients with psychoses. *J Geriatr Psychiatry Neurol*, 8:12–15.
61. Salzman, C., Vaccaro, B., Lieff, J., et al. (1995). Clozapine in older patients with psychosis and behavioral disruption. *Am J Geriatr Psychiatry*, 3:26–33.
62. Richards, S.S., Sweet, R.A., Ganguli, R. (1996). Clozapine: Acute and maintenance treatment in late life psychoses. *Am J Gesiatr Psychiatry*, 4(4):377–378.
63. Fernandez, F., Levy, J.K., Mansell, P.W.A. (1989). Management of delirium in the terminally ill AIDS patients. *Int J Psychiatry Med*, 19:165–172.

PSYCHIATRIC SEQUELAE OF CEREBROVASCULAR ACCIDENTS

INTRODUCTION

Cerebrovascular disease (i.e., stroke) remains a leading cause of mortality and morbidity today. In addition to post-stroke medical illness, psychiatric symptomatology may arise following a stroke or a preexisting psychiatric illness may be exacerbated. These psychiatric symptoms appear to be responsive to psychopharmacologic interventions. The issue of maintenance pharmacotherapy for both post-stroke affective and psychotic illnesses is reviewed in this chapter.

REVIEW OF AFFECTIVE SYMPTOMATOLOGY POST-STROKE

Affective symptomatology has been found in 25 to 50% of patients post-stroke and has been largely untreated. Barer and Nouri[1] reported that 34 of 149 patients (23%) suffered from affective illness when examined six months post-stroke. The authors also noted that the presence of affective illness predicted a poorer functional recovery, greater degree of weakness, and a greater number of inpatient hospital days. Only 15% of the patients

337

identified by the authors with affective illness were receiving antidepressant medication. Wade et al.[2] followed up patients in a community stroke registry using a symptom inventory and found 25 to 30% of patients were depressed at each of three time points post-stroke (three weeks, six months, and one year) and that 50% of patients who were depressed acutely (at three weeks) remained depressed at one year. The authors also noted that few patients were on antidepressant medication. Robinson et al.[3] interviewed 103 stroke patients during their acute hospitalization and found that while 27% fulfilled DSM-III criteria for a major depression, an additional 50% of patients had clinically significant depressive symptoms. Finally, Wilkinson et al. reported that in 35 of 96 patients (36%) evaluated for affective symptoms at a mean of 4.9 years post-stroke were found to be depressed.[4]

Location of the stroke, left versus right, and cortical versus subcortical may contribute to the development of post-stroke depression. Robinson and Price[5] prospectively followed a series of 103 post-stroke patients for 12 months and found that strokes involving the left hemisphere were associated with more depressive symptoms than those of the right hemisphere or brain stem. The authors also noted that none of the depressed patients they identified was receiving antidepressants. Lipsey et al.[6] found in a series of 15 patients with bilateral strokes that those patients with left anterior hemispheric injury were more significantly depressed than patients with strokes in other locations. Robinson et al.[7] also found that left anterior infarcts correlated with a greater degree of depressive symptoms. In addition, right posterior infarcts were associated with greater depressive symptoms than right anterior lesions, which appeared to cause undue cheerfulness and apathy. In a series of 45 post-stroke patients, Starkstein et al.[8] found that the more proximal a left-sided infarct was to the frontal pole, the more severe the depressive symptoms. This was found in both patients with cortical and subcortical lesions. Conversely, patients with right hemisphere lesions appeared to have a higher incidence of "undue cheerfulness."

What is the relationship between post-stroke depression and overall treatment outcome? As indicated, Barer and Nouri[1] found that the presence of post-stroke affective symptoms correlated with a poorer recovery and longer hospital stay. Sinyor et al.[9] examined 64 post-stroke patients in a rehabilitation setting within several weeks of their strokes and found 47% were suffering from depression. While both depressed and nondepressed patients progressed similarly during the rehabilitation program, the depressed group appeared less motivated to the treatment staff and had a poorer functional outcome six weeks post-rehabilitation.

What is known of the outcome of post-stroke depression? Robinson et al.[10] studied post-stroke patients at one year ($n = 37$) and two years ($n = 48$) of follow-up. Acutely in hospital, 14% fulfilled DSM-III criteria for major depression and 18% for dysthymia. At two years, all the patients with major depression were improved, but 60% of the dysthymic patients had persistent symptoms. Of the remainder, i.e., those who were not depressed acutely, 34% went on to develop either a major depression or dysthymia at the two-year follow-up. The authors concluded that the time course of post-stroke depression is between one to two years and is usually self-limited, although dysthymic symptoms may persist longer.

Post-stroke mania is much less common clinically than post-stroke depression. Cummings and Mendez[11] described two patients with infarcts of the right thalamus who then developed symptoms of mania. Robinson et al.[12] examined a series of patients with secondary mania due to brain lesions (not limited to infarction) and found an association between right hemisphere lesions and mania. They also found that secondary mania was more likely to occur in patients with family histories of affective illness. Some patients with secondary mania may also experience periods of depression, resembling bipolar disorder.[13]

Post-stroke anxiety disorders and symptoms may affect both the course of recovery and the course of post-stroke depression. Schultz et al. followed a cohort of stroke patients for one year and found that the presence of anxiety symptoms at each of the evaluations (3, 6, 12, and 24 months) was associated with increased severity of depressive symptoms.[14] Aström followed a cohort of stroke patients for three years to assess the presence of generalized anxiety disorder (GAD) and its relationship to major depression. The author reported that 28% of the 80 patients followed endorsed symptoms of GAD acutely and that after one year, approximately 75% of those patients chronically endorsed GAD symptoms.[15] A lack of independence in activities of daily living and a "reduced social network" were also associated with GAD symptoms. The data suggested a high degree of comorbidity with major depression and that the prognosis of major depression plus GAD was worse than for major depression alone. The presence of anxiety in a post-stroke patient should alert the clinician to the presence of not only the possibility of an anxiety disorder, but also the possibility of an affective disorder.

PHARMACOTHERAPY OF AFFECTIVE SYMPTOMATOLOGY

Limited double-blind studies exist on the use of antidepressants for post-stroke depressive symptoms. Several such studies are reviewed below and involve nortriptyline, trazodone, citalopram, and fluoxetine.

Lipsey et al.[16] examined the effectiveness of nortriptyline in post-stroke depression in 34 patients, half of whom fulfilled DSM-III criteria for major depression in a double-blind, placebo-controlled study. Treatment duration was between four to six weeks, and all the nortriptyline patients had serum concentrations between 50–140 ng/ml at the end of the study. While at the onset of the study 50% of the drug group and 60% of the placebo group fulfilled the DSM-III criteria for major depression, 45% of the drug group and 53% of the placebo group fulfilled the criteria at the end of the study. When the two groups were examined with a series of affective symptomatology inventories, the drug group had a statistically significant improvement on each of the inventories compared with the placebo group. The side effects noted in the drug treatment group were anticholinergic in nature. The authors concluded that nortriptyline had demonstrated efficacy in the treatment of post-stroke depression.

Reding et al.[17] performed a placebo-controlled, double-blind study of trazodone in 27 post-stroke patients. Duration of treatment was approximately four weeks, and the target range of trazodone dosage was 200 mg/day. The authors noted a consistent improvement in depression scores in the trazodone group compared with the placebo group. The most common side effect in the trazodone group was sedation. The authors concluded that trazodone may have a role in the treatment of post-stroke depression.

Anderson et al.[18] treated 16 patients with "emotionalism" (i.e., crying spells without accompanying mood changes) in a double-blind, crossover fashion for three weeks of each treatment phase with either placebo or citalopram, an SSRI used clinically in treating depression outside the United States. They found that crying spells were reduced in frequency 50% during the active phase, and this effect occurred within 72 hours of initiating treatment. While none of these patients fulfilled DSM criteria for major depression, their scores on depression rating scales were noted to improve on citalopram therapy. Similar results have been reported with sertraline.[19] The other members of the SSRI class (i.e., fluoxetine, fluvoxamine) may have similar effects on emotionalism and indeed may be effective in treating post-stroke depression. In an earlier report, levodopa was used similarly with success.[20]

Stamenkovic et al.[21] performed an open study of fluoxetine in 10 post-stroke patients with DSM-III-R major depression for up to eight weeks. Of the five patients who completed the study, a marked improvement on all depression rating scales was observed at day 14 of treatment, and no one discontinued the drug because of side effects. The authors concluded that fluoxetine may be an alternative to tricyclic antidepressants in post-stroke depression.

Maintenance studies of post-stroke depression have yet to be reported, but it appears that while some cases are self-limited, a subgroup of patients have persistent chronic dysthymic symptoms. This group may require long-term pharmacotherapy.

Double-blind treatment studies of post-stroke mania have yet to be reported, due in part to the rarity of the disorder, compared with post-stroke depression. In a single patient with secondary mania, clonidine was found to diminish manic symptoms while levodopa and carbamazepine did not.[22] Anticonvulsants, antipsychotics, and lithium have also been used clinically but have yet to be formally studied. Post-stroke mania may, like primary mania, require long-term maintenance pharmacotherapy.

REVIEW OF PSYCHOTIC SYMPTOMATOLOGY POST-STROKE

Psychotic symptoms are seen much less in this population than affective symptoms and appear to be limited to patients who have infarcts of the right cerebral hemisphere. Levine and Grek[23] described the clinical characteristics of nine patients with delusions. All had infarcts of the right cerebral hemisphere. Their delusional symptoms included false identities, confabulation, unreasonable beliefs about the future, and disorientation. Preexisting brain atrophy appeared to be necessary for development of delusions post-stroke. Price and Mesulam[24] reported a series of five patients with right hemisphere infarction who developed atypical psychotic syndrome including paranoia, agitation, suspiciousness, and apathy. In some of the cases, the acute psychotic syndrome was the presenting symptom of the right cerebral infarct. The acute episodes appeared to be self-limited but were recurrent in some patients and more chronic in others.

PHARMACOTHERAPY OF PSYCHOTIC SYMPTOMATOLOGY

Pharmacological treatment of post-stroke psychosis has yet to be studied in a double-blind fashion, but reported clinical experience indicates the psychosis is difficult to treat with conventional agents.[24] Clinically, treatment with antipsychotics should be initiated at a low dose and that dose titrated upward slowly until psychotic symptoms are decreased. This patient population, largely elderly and with organic brain injury (i.e., status post-stroke),are more sensitive to psychopharmacological agent effects and side effects. The role of maintenance pharmacotherapy in this disorder remains unknown.

REFERENCES

1. Ebrahim, S., Barer, D., Nouri, F. (1987). Affective illness after stroke. *Br J Psychiatry* 151: 52–56.

2. Wade, D.T., Legh-Smith, J.E., Hewer, R.A. (1987). Depressed mood after stroke: A community study of its frequency. *Br J Psychiatry*, 151:200–205.

3. Robinson, R.G., Star, L.B., Kubos, K.L., et al. (1983). A two-year longitudinal study of post-stroke mood disorders: Findings during the initial evaluation. *Stroke*, 14:736–741.

4. Wilkinson, P.R., Wolfe, C.D., Warburton, F.G., et al. (1997). A long-term follow-up of stroke patients. *Stroke*, 28(3):507–512.

5. Robinson, R.G., Price, T.R. (1982). Post-stroke depressive disorders: A follow-up study of 103 patients. *Stroke*, 13:635–641.

6. Lipsey, J.R., Robinson, R.G., Pearlson, G.D., et al. (1983). Mood disorder following bilateral hemisphere brain injury. *Br J Psychiatry*, 143:266–273.

7. Robinson, R.G., Kubos, K.L., Starr, L.B., et al. (1984). Mood disorders in stroke patients: Importance of location of lesion. *Brain*, 107:81–93.

8. Starkstein, S.E., Robinson, R.G., Price, T.R. (1987). Comparison of cortical and subcortical lesions in the production of post-stroke mood disorders. *Brain*, 110:1045–1059.

9. Sinyor, D., Amato, P., Kaloupek, D.G., et al. (1986). Post-stroke depression: Relationship to functional impairment, coping strategies, and rehabilitation outcome. *Stroke*, 17:1102–1107.

10. Robinson, R.G., Bolduc, P.H., Price, T.R. (1987) Two-year longitudinal study of post-stroke mood disorders: Diagnosis and outcome at one and two years. *Stroke*, 18:837–843.

11. Cummings, J.L., Mendez, M.F. (1984). Secondary mania with focal cerebrovascular lesions. *Am J Psychiatry*, 141:1084–1087.

12. Robinson, R.G., Boston, J.D., Starksten, S.E. (1988). Comparison of mania with depression following brain injury causal factors. *Am J Psychiatry*, 145:172–178.

13. Starkstein, S.E., Fedoroff, P. Berthier, M.L., et al. (1991). Manic depressive and pure manic states after brain lesions. *Biol Psychiatry*, 29:149–158.

14. Schultz, S.K., Castillo, C.S., Kosier, J.T., et al. (1997). Generalized anxiety and depression. Assessment over 2 years after stroke. *Am J Geriatr Psychiatry*, 5(3):229–237.

15. Aström, M. (1996). Generalized anxiety disorder in stroke patients. A three-year longitudinal study. *Stroke*, 27(3):270–275.

16. Lipsey, J. Robinson, R.G., Pearlson, G.D., et al. (1984). Nortriptyline treatment for post-stroke depression: A double-blind study. *Lancet*, 1:297–300.

17. Reding, M.J., Orto, L.A., Winter, S.W., et al. (1986). Antidepressant therapy after stroke: A double-blind trial. *Arch Neurol*, 43:763–765.

18. Anderson, G., Vestergaard, K., Rüs, J.O. (1993). Citalopram for post-stroke pathological crying. *Lancet*, 342:837–839.

19. Mukand, J., Kaplan, M., Senno, R.G., et al. (1996). Pathological crying and laughing: Treatment with sertraline. *Arch Phys Med Rehabil*, 77(12):1309–1311.

20. Udaka, F., Yamao, S., Nagata, H., et al. (1984). Pathologic laughing and crying treated with levodopa. *Arch Neurol*, 41:1095–1096.

21. Stamenkovic, M., Schindler, S., Kasper, S. (1996). Poststroke depression and fluoxetine (letter). *Am J Psychiatry*, 153(3):446–447.

22. Bakchine, S., Lacombley, L., Benoit, N., et al. (1989). Manic-like state after orlitofrontal and right temporoparietal injury: Efficacy of clonidine. *Neurology*, 39:777–781.

23. Levine, D.N., Grek, A. (1984). The anatomic basis of delusions after right cerebral infarction. *Neurology*, 34:577–582.

24. Price, B.H., Mesulam, M. (1985). Psychiatric manifestations of right hemisphere infarctions. *J Nerv Mental Dis*, 173(10):610–613.

CHRONIC PAIN

INTRODUCTION

Chronic pain is a major cause of functional impairment and disability and is frequently associated with psychopathology. Chronic pain can adversely affect a person's psychological state, and psychopathology can influence the perception and meaning of pain. There is a complicated interaction between somatic and psychological mechanisms in chronic pain that must be sorted out and both must be addressed in treatment. Chronic pain is by definition a chronic persistent illness and requires a multidisciplinary approach to treatment. The focus of this chapter is on psychopharmacological treatment.

Pain is divided into two categories: neuropathic and nonneuropathic. Neuropathic pain results from a neural injury or neuronal dysfunction and includes post-herpetic neuralgia, nerve compression, phantom limb, painful polyneuropathies, and reflex sympathetic dystrophy. Nonneuropathic pain is nociceptive pain without evident neuronal pathology and is more frequently associated with comorbid psychopathology.

The perception of pain involves a complicated neural processing of information from the peripheral sensory cell to cerebral cortex. The pain signal can be modified at any point along this pathway. Therefore, there are many possible mechanisms leading to chronic pain that may respond to a variety of treatment modalities including psychopharmacological interventions.

PAIN PATHWAYS

The "pain pathway" begins with the primary afferent nociceptor (PAN) on the sensory ganglion cell whose cell body is in the dorsal root ganglion. The pain signal enters the spinal cord through the dorsal horn and ascends to the central nervous system via several distinct pathways that project to thalamus, midbrain, periaqueductal gray, parabrachial nucleus, hypothalamus, and amygdala. The signal is then relayed from these areas to somatosensory, orbitofrontal, and cingulate cortex. The neurotransmitters involved in the ascending pathways are substance P, excitatory amino acids (glutamate), enkephalin, GABA, and other neuropeptides. Descending tracts from cortex to brain stem back to the spinal cord are primarily noradrenergic and serotonergic and are involved in modulating and regulating the system.

PAIN PERCEPTION

The regulation and interpretation of pain perception is modulated by the cortex. The cortex modulates the descending pain pathway, attention to pain stimuli, and the interpretation of the meaning of pain. The regulation and perception of pain is a highly complex mechanism subject to wide variability between individuals and affected by psychological mechanisms.

DIAGNOSTIC CRITERIA FOR CHRONIC PAIN

The *Diagnostic and Statistical Manual of Mental Disorders*, fourth edition, provides criteria for pain disorder.[1] Pain must be present in one or more anatomical sites, warrant clinical attention, and be a focus of the clinical presentation. The pain must cause distress and functional impairment. Psychological factors play an important role in the onset, severity, exacerbation, or maintenance of the pain.

Pain is chronic if the duration is at least six months. Pain disorder may be associated with a general medical condition (this is not considered a mental disorder), associated with psychological factors, or associated with both a general medical condition and psychological factors. Patients demonstrate chronic pain through pain behavior, persistent functional impairment, and perceived disability.

EPIDEMIOLOGY

There is no definitive epidemiological data on the prevalence of chronic pain lasting greater than six months, but estimates range from 4.3 to 40% of the general population.[2]

COMORBID PSYCHOPATHOLOGY

The interaction between chronic pain, depression, other psychopathology, and disability is complex and each of these factors can exacerbate the others.

DEPRESSION

There is an association between depression and chronic pain. Patients with chronic pain have a high incidence of comorbid depression; 30–60% in most studies. Although the association between depression and chronic pain is well established, the nature of the relationship is not clear. There are several theories regarding causation:

1. The experience of chronic pain may contribute to the development of depression, and depressive symptoms may increase with the persistence of the chronic pain.
2. Preexisting psychopathology or underlying psychological mechanisms can contribute to the development of chronic pain by affecting the perception of pain and level of disability.
3. Chronic pain may be a variant of depression or "masked depression."[3]
4. There is a common neural pathway underlying both depression and chronic pain involving serotonin and enkephalin, and there is not a causal relationship between the two.[4] The only thing that is certain is that there is an association between chronic pain and depression.[5]

The presence of depression in chronic pain patients may also have relevance for level of functioning and perceived disability. There is an association between disability and depressive symptomatology in a range of medical conditions.[6,7] More severe and unremitting depressive symptomatology is associated with higher levels of disability in depressed patients who are high utilizers of health care.[8] Therefore, depression is an important contributing factor to the disability associated with chronic pain.

PREEXISTING PSYCHOPATHOLOGY

The incidence of preexisting psychopathology in chronic pain patients is higher than in the general population. Atkinson et al. found significantly higher lifetime prevalence rates of major depressive disorder and alcohol use disorder and nonsignificantly higher rates of major anxiety disorders in men with chronic low back pain than in controls.[9]

Chronic pain patients have high rates of comorbid psychopathology. Reich found Axis I diagnoses in 98% and Axis II diagnoses in 37% of chronic pain patients.[10] Depressive disorders, anxiety disorders, somatoform disorders, and personality disorders are the most common. The prevalence of other psychiatric disorders among chronic pain patients is given in Table 13–1.

TABLE 13–1. DIAGNOSES FOR PATIENTS WITH CHRONIC PAIN

Category and Diagnosis	Total ($\underline{N}$ = 283) (%)
Affective Disorders	
Major depression and bipolar disorder in remission	1.5
Current major depression single and recurrent	4.6
Dysthymic disorder	23.3
Adjustment disorder with depressed mood	28.3
Current depressive disorder (major depression and dysthymic disorder and cyclothymic disorder and adjustment disorder with depressed mood)	56.2
Somatoform Disorders	43
Anxiety Disorders	62.5
Delirium	0.4
Dementia	7.8
Substance Use Disorders	14.9
Personality Disorders	59.0
Histronic	11.7
Dependent	17.4
Passive-Aggressive	14.9
Personality Types	
Compulsive	24.5
Dependent	10.6

Adapted from Fishbain, D.A., Goldberg, M., Meagher, B.R., et al. (1986). Male and female chronic pain patients categorized by DSM-III psychiatric diagnostic criteria. *Pain*, 26:186–188. Copyright 1986. Reprinted with permission from Elsevier Science.

PAIN IN PSYCHIATRIC PATIENTS

The prevalence of chronic pain among psychiatric patients is no higher than in the general population.[11,12] Patients with a range of psychiatric disorders complain of pain, but those with chronic pain are more likely to suffer from an anxiety or dysthymic disorder than pain-free patients.[11,12] Rates of depression were no different in patients who reported pain than those who did not.[11]

NEUROPATHIC PAIN

Neuropathic pain, a result of neural injury or neuronal dysfunction, is characterized by its quality and location. The sensory quality of neuropathic pain is unique and can be distinguished from other pain the patient has experienced. Patients either experience unpleasant sensations (dysesthesia), abnormal sensations (paresthesia), or hypersensitivity to sensory, especially tactile, stimuli (allodynia). Patients describe this pain as burning, lancinating, tingling, shocking, shooting, crawling, tearing, cramping, or tightness. Hypersensitivity phenomena include allodynia, increased sensitivity to heat, and paroxysms of pain after a stimulus. Pain is located near the site of neural damage usually apparent as a sensory deficit. There is a time lapse on the order of months between the neural injury and the onset of pain.

A broad range of pathological mechanisms suggest a broad range of treatment approaches. Examples of neuropathic pain include post-herpetic neuralgia, central pain, neuroma formation, avulsion of the brachial plexus, phantom limb, lancinating neuralgias, nerve compression, painful polyneuropathies, and reflex sympathetic dystrophy (causalgia).

MECHANISMS

Different mechanisms of neuronal injury can result in different pathophysiological mechanisms for the development of chronic pain syndromes. These different syndromes require treatment approaches specifically targeted to their pathology. This topic was recently reviewed by Fields.[13]

Deafferentation, or disconnection, of the primary sensory neuron from the central nervous system due to a disruption somewhere along the "pain pathway" paradoxically can be associated with increased pain perception. Examples of this type of pain are avulsion of the brachial plexus, central pain syndrome (also called thalamic pain syndrome or post-stroke syndrome), and some polyneuropathies. Effective treatments include tricyclic antidepressants.

Nerve compression can result in damage to inhibitory myelinated primary afferents. Any damage to inhibitory neurons in the pain circuit can result in an increase of the magnitude of the pain signal that is relayed to the central nervous system.

Ectopic impulses occur when PANs fire spontaneously after damage. This is likely the mechanism for pain in post-herpetic neuralgia and painful diabetic polyneuropathy. Membrane stabilizing drugs such as anticonvulsants and antiarrythmics exert their therapeutic effect by blocking the generation of these ectopic impulses.

When stimulated, PANs release substance P, a neuropeptide that contributes to the *inflammatory response*. Substance P is a potent vasodilator, chemoattractant for white blood cells, and elicitor of histamine release from mast cells, all of which promote the inflammatory response that perpetuates or amplifies pain. Capsaicin, the active ingredient in hot chili peppers, can inactivate PANs at the right concentration, thus shutting down the inflammatory response and providing local analgesia in post-therapeutic neuralgia, post-mastectomy pain, and diabetic neuropathy.

Sympathetic activity can exacerbate pain in some patients with peripheral nerve injury. Reflex sympathetic dystrophy, or causalgia, is characterized by burning pain; a cold, swollen, and sweaty extremity; and hypersensitivity to tactile stimuli, loud noise, and cold temperature. Sympathetic blockade is an effective treatment for this type of pain.

Pain stimuli from the periphery may induce a prolonged hyperexcitable state in central neurons resulting in a *hyperpathic state*. This is analogous to a persistent memory trace for pain and can be blocked by the NMDA antagonist, ketamine.

Neuropathic pain can also result from *activation of nociceptive neurons that innervate the connective tissue sheath* around nerve trunks.

NONNEUROPATHIC PAIN

Nonneuropathic pain is nociceptive pain without evident neuronal pathology and does not include diseases with a clear neuropathic component. Examples of nonneuropathic pain include chronic low back pain, neck pain, pelvic pain, cancer pain, arthritis or rheumatologic pain, fibrositis, fibromyalgia, facial pain, tension headache, and idiopathic or psychogenic pain.

PSYCHOPHARMACOLOGICAL TREATMENT

Treatment of chronic pain is best offered in a multidisciplinary pain treatment center that can offer a broad range of treatment modalities, individually fitted to the patient's needs including surgical treatment, nerve blocks, psychopharmacology, drug detoxification, physical therapy, occupational therapy, and cognitive-behavioral pain management. This chapter focuses primarily on psychopharmacological treatment approaches that are supported by double-blind, placebo-controlled, randomized studies. For a more detailed review of the literature, we refer readers to Fields and Fishbain.[13,2]

TRICYCLIC ANTIDEPRESSANTS

Tricyclic antidepressants (TCAs) have analgesic properties in many chronic pain syndromes including both neuropathic and nonneuropathic conditions. The mechanism of action for pain control is uncertain but likely involves a combination of noradrenergic and serotonergic reuptake blockade and blockade of alpha-adrenergic, histaminergic, and muscarinic acetylcholine receptors.

Several **chronic neuropathic pain conditions** respond to TCAs. Diabetic neuropathy responds to amitriptyline,[14,15] imipramine,[16] desipramine,[15,17] and clomipramine.[16] Peripheral neuropathies respond to doxepin.[18] Postherpetic neuralgia responds to desipramine.[19] Central pain responds to clomipramine and nortriptyline.[20]

Antidepressants, particularly the TCAs, have demonstrated efficacy as "analgesics" in a variety **of chronic nonneuropathic pain conditions.** Recent meta-analyses of placebo-controlled studies of TCAs in chronic pain[21,22] demonstrate the clinically relevant antinociceptive/analgesic effect of antidepressants, despite methodological flaws of the primary studies. The test antidepressant was significantly superior to placebo in 70% of the 67 studies with significant difference in global improvement rates of 57% for the antidepressant versus 31% for placebo.[22] Onghena found the mean effect size to be 0.64, meaning that chronic pain patients taking antidepressants did better than 74% of patients taking placebo.[21] Not all antidepressants are equally effective, but these two meta-analyses came to different conclusions regarding superiority; clomipramine was found superior in the Philipp study while amitriptyline was determined superior in the Onghena study.

The analgesic/antinociceptive effect is independent of the antidepressant effect.[22,23] Decrease in pain is independent of change in depressive symptomatology, and antidepressants produce analgesia in nondepressed pain patients. However, several studies indicate a better analgesic response in depressed compared with nondepressed patients. Chronic pain responds to lower antidepressant doses than required for depression, and the onset of analgesic action is more rapid than the antidepressant response (days compared with several weeks). Although a dose-response relationship has not been clearly demonstrated, several studies suggest that higher doses and higher serum levels of TCAs correlate with improved analgesic response. Therefore, if low doses are ineffective, the dose should be increased as tolerated to antidepressant doses and therapeutic levels.[14,17]

Of the TCAs, the strongest support for efficacy is for amitriptyline, clomipramine, and doxepin, because these have been the most widely studied. TCAs have demonstrated efficacy for chronic low back pain, arthritic and rheumatic pain, muscle pain, facial pain, headache, tumor pain, fibrositis, surgical pain, and idiopathic pain.[22]

There are no controlled trials of antidepressants in neck, pelvic, or phantom pain although there is anecdotal and open study evidence for the use of TCAs in these conditions.

Antidepressants are used differently in the treatment of chronic pain than in the treatment of depression. Therapy is best started at very low doses (10–25 mg/day of a TCA given at bedtime) with small dose increments at three- to seven-day intervals. Relatively low doses (75 mg/day amitriptyline or desipramine) are required for pain control compared with much higher doses for adequate treatment of depression. There are no reports of a dose-response relationship or serum level with analgesic response, so that therapeutic drug level monitoring is not indicated. For more detail on the side effects and use of TCAs, see Chapter 4 on Depressive Disorders.

MONOAMINE OXIDASE INHIBITORS

The monoamine oxidase inhibitors (MAOIs) may have some benefit in chronic pain. There is only one well-controlled study; phenelzine produced a greater analgesic effect than amitriptyline in facial pain.[24] For guidelines on the use of MAOIs, see Chapter 4.

SELECTIVE SEROTONIN REUPTAKE INHIBITORS

Selective serotonin reuptake inhibitors (SSRIs), a newer class of antidepressants with much less noradrenergic, cholinergic, and histaminergic activity than the TCAs, have been less effective than the TCAs in the treatment of chronic pain syndromes without comorbid depression.[15,16] This suggests that the efficacy of the TCAs in pain relief is independent of the antidepressant action and involves noradrenergic, cholinergic, and/or histaminergic neurotransmitter systems. For guidelines on the use of SSRIs, see Chapter 4.

ANTIPSYCHOTICS

Antipsychotics have demonstrated efficacy in the treatment of neuropathic and nonneuropathic pain syndromes in three placebo-controlled studies; levomepromazine in a heterogenous mix of chronic pain syndromes,[25] flupenthixol in osteoarthritis,[26] and fluphenazine in tension headache.[27] Open clinical trials support the use of other antipsychotics for other neuropathic pain conditions including herpes zoster, tumor pain, and neuropathic pain. One case series suggests that antipsychotics in combination with amitriptyline can augment the analgesic effect of the TCA in postherpetic neuralgia.[28] It is unclear whether antipsychotics have a direct analgesic effect or act via another mechanism.

Antipsychotics should not be used as first-line treatments and should be reserved only for treatment refractory patients due to the side-effect profile and especially the risk of tardive dyskinesia (see Schizophrenia, Chapter 6). Patients should be informed of the risk of tardive dyskinesia with chronic use before initiating antipsychotic therapy.

ANTICONVULSANTS

Anticonvulsants are effective in the treatment of chronic neuropathic pain. The mechanism of action for analgesia is likely membrane stabilization. Carbamazepine has demonstrated efficacy in neuralgia pain, particularly trigeminal neuralgia and polyneuropathies.[22] Phenytoin, valproic acid, and clonazepam are used as second-line agents, although there have been no controlled studies of these agents. Clinically, they seem to be most effective for pain that is described as shooting, shock-like, or lancinating.[13]

There is no evidence supporting the use of anticonvulsants in nonneuropathic chronic pain syndromes. For guidelines on the use of anticonvulsants, see Chapter 5 on Bipolar Disorders.

LOCAL ANESTHETICS AND ANTIARRYTHMICS

Local anesthetics and antiarrythmics also have some membrane-stabilizing properties and can block ectopic impulses from primary afferents. Intravenous lidocaine can block pain associated with many neuropathic pain conditions including postherpetic neuralgia.[29] Mexilitene, an oral antiarrhythmic in the same class as lidocaine, is effective for diabetic neuropathy and other neuropathic pain conditions.[30,31]

ANTIHISTAMINES

Antihistamines may have some analgesic properties, but this is controversial.[32] Diphenhydramine, hydroxyzine, orphenadrine, and pyrilamine have been shown to produce analgesia. Clinically, antihistamines are used in conjunction with opioid analgesics to augment the analgesic effect of acetaminophen and aspirin.

PSYCHOSTIMULANTS

Psychostimulants may have a role in chronic cancer pain. Methylphenidate, when used adjunctively with narcotics, has analgesic properties in patients with chronic cancer pain[33] and also improves cognitive functioning.[34]

OPIOIDS

Opioids are effective in acute pain control in many neuropathic conditions. There is mixed evidence suggesting long-term benefit, but no controlled, long-term trials of opioids have been performed. The use of long-term opioids is controversial especially because of the risk of physiological dependence and addiction. Opioids seem to diminish in efficacy over time, necessitating a gradual increase in dose. If these agents are used for long-term treatment, longer acting forms are recommended, such as methadone, levorphanol, or slow-release morphine. Augmentation with other agents such as TCAs, anticonvulsants, antiarrythmics, or clonidine is also recommended prior to dose increases.[13]

BENZODIAZEPINES

The benzodiazepines diazepam and chlordiazepoxide have demonstrated efficacy in the treatment of tension and psychogenic headaches.[35,36] They have not been studied in any other chronic pain conditions. They also present problems of physiological addiction and withdrawal effects.

TREATMENT OF DEPRESSION IN CHRONIC PAIN SYNDROMES

When depressive symptoms coexist with chronic pain, an antidepressant should be the first-line agent. However, pharmacological treatment of chronic pain with antidepressants usually requires lower doses than required for the treatment of depression. Because there is a high rate of comorbid current depressive episodes in patients with chronic pain, treating the pain with low doses of antidepressants may provide analgesia but will not adequately treat the depression. Because the presence of untreated depression correlates with increased functional disability, it is imperative to adequately treat the depression for an optimal outcome. Therefore, when low doses of antidepressant do not produce an adequate analgesic response, or when there is recognized concomitant depression, doses should be raised to the antidepressant range.[37] See Chapter 4 on Depressive Disorders.

MAINTENANCE PHARMACOTHERAPY

Very few studies have been performed to assess the effects of long-term treatment. To our knowledge, there are no prospective, controlled, long-term trials of any of these agents for chronic pain treatment. Because chronic pain syndromes are by definition long-lasting, presumably long-term treatment is necessary. Continuing treatments that are efficacious acutely is the most logical recommendation, but unfortunately, there are no studies to confirm this approach.

REFERENCES

1. American Psychiatric Association. (1994). *Diagnostic and Statistical Manual of Mental Disorders*, (4th ed.), pp. 461–462.
2. Fishbain, D.A. (1996). Pain and psychopathology. *Neuropsychiatry*, 22:443–483.
3. Gupta, M.A. (1986). Is chronic pain a variant of depressive illness? A critical review. *Can J Psychiatry*, 31:241–248.
4. Gershon, S. (1986). Chronic pain: Hypothesized mechanisms and rationale for treatment. *Neuropsychobiology*, 15:22–27.
5. Romano, J.M., Turner, J.A. (1985). Chronic pain and depression: Does the evidence support a relationship? *Psychol Bull*, 97:18–34.
6. Turner, R.J., Noh, S. (1988). Physical disability and depression: A longitudinal analysis. *J Health Soc Behav*, 29:23–27.
7. Turner, R.J., Beiser, M. (1990). Major depression and depressive symptomology among the physically disabled: Assessing the role of chronic stress. *J Nerv Ment Dis*, 178:343–350.
8. Von Korff, M., Ormel, J., Katon, W., et al. (1992). Disability and depression among high utilizers of health care. A longitudinal analysis. *Arch Gen Psychiatry*, 49:91–99.
9. Atkinson, J.H., Slater, M.A., Patterson, T.L., et al. (1991). Prevalence, onset, and risk of psychiatric disorders in men with chronic low back pain: A controlled study. *Pain*, 45:111–121.
10. Reich, J., Tupen, J.P., Abramowitz, S. (1983). Psychiatric diagnosis of chronic pain patients. *Am J Psychiatry*, 140:1495–1498.
11. Chaturvedi, S.K., Michael, A. (1986). Chronic pain in a psychiatric clinic. *J Psychosom Res*, 30:347–354.
12. Chaturvedi, S.K. (1987). Prevalence of chronic pain in psychiatric patients. *Pain*, 29:231–237.
13. Fields, H.L. (1996). Evaluation and treatment of neuropathic pain. *Neuropsychiatry*, 21:433–441.
14. Max, M.B., Culhane, M., Schafer, S.C., et al. (1987). Amitriptyline relieves diabetic neuropathy pain in patients with normal or depressed mood. *Neurology*, 37:589–596.
15. Max, M.B., Lynch, S.A., Muir, J., et al. (1992). Effects of desipramine, amitriptyline, and fluoxetine on pain in diabetic neuropathy. *N Englon J Med*, 326:1250–1256.
16. Sindrup, S.H., Gram, L.F., Brosen, K., et al. (1990). The selective serotonin reuptake inhibitor paroxetine is effective in the treatment of diabetic neuropathy symptoms. *Pain*, 41:135–144.
17. Sindrup, S.H., Gram, L.F., Skjolt, T., et al. (1990). Clomipramine vs. desipramine vs. placebo in the treatment of diabetic neuropathy symptoms. A double-blind cross-over study. *Br J Clin Pharmacol*, 683–691.
18. Paladini, V.A., Battigelli, D., Antonaglia, V., et al. (1987). La doxepina nel dotore da neuropatia periferca. *Minerva Anaesthesiol*, 53:413–418.

19. Kisore-Kumar, R., Max, M.B., Schafer, S.C., et al. (1990). Desipramine relieves post-herpetic neuralgia. *Clin Pharmacol Ther*, 47:305–312.

20. Panerai, A.E., Monza, G., Movilia, P., et al. (1990). A randomized, within-patient, crossover, placebo-controlled trial on the efficacy and tolerability of the tricyclic antidepressants clomipramine and nortriptyline in central pain. *Acta Neurol Scand*, 82:34–38.

21. Onghena, P., VanHandenhove, B. (1992). Antidepressant-induced analgesia in chronic non-malignant pain: A meta-analysis of 39 placebo-controlled studies. *Pain*, 49:205–219.

22. Philipp, M., Fickinger, M. (1993). Psychotropic drugs in the management of chronic pain syndromes. *Pharmacopsychiatry*, 26:221–234.

23. Sindrup, S.H., Brosen, K., Gram, L.F. (1992). Antidepressants in pain treatment: Antidepressant or analgesic effect? *Clin Neuropharmacol*, 15(Suppl 1):636A–637A.

24. Lascelles, R.G. (1966). Atypical facial pain and depression. *Br J Psychiatry*, 112:651–659.

25. Bloomfield, S., Simard-Savoie, S., Bernier, J., et al. (1964). Comparative analgesic activity of levomepromazine and morphine in patients with chronic pain. *Can Med Assoc J*, 90:1156–1159.

26. Breivik, H., Slordahl, J. (1984). Beneficial effects of flupenthixol for osteoarthritic pain of the hip: A double-blind cross over comparison with placebo. (abstract). *Pain*, (Suppl):S 254.

27. Hakkarainen, H. (1977). Fluphenazine for tension headache; double-blind study. *Headache*, 17:216–218.

28. Taub, R. (1973). Relief of postherpetic neuralgia with psychotropic drugs. *J Neurosurg*, 39:235–239.

29. Glazer, S., Portenoy, R.K. (1991). Systemic local anesthetics in pain control. *J Pain Symp Manag*, 6:30–39.

30. Dejgard, A., Peterson, P., Kastrup, J. (1988). Mexiletine for the treatment of chronic painful diabetic neuropathy. *Lancet*, 1:9–11.

31. Chabal, C., Jacobson, L., Mariano, A., et al. (1992). The use of oral mexiletine for the treatment of pain after peripheral nerve injury. *Anesthesiology*, 76:513–517.

32. Rumore, M.M., Schlichting, D.A. (1986). Clinical efficacy of antihistamines as analgesics. *Pain*, 25:7–22.

33. Bruera, E., Chadwick, S., Brenneis, C, et al. (1987). Methylphenidate associated with narcotics for the treatment of cancer pain. *Cancer Treat Rep*, 71:67–70.

34. Bruera, E., Miller, M.J., Macmillan, K., et al. (1992). Neuropsychological effects of methylphenidate in patients receiving a continuous infusion of narcotics for cancer pain. *Pain*, 48:163–166.

35. Lance, J.W., Curran, D.A. (1964). Treatment of chronic tension headache. *Lancet II*, 1236–1239.

36. Okasha, A., Ghaleb, H.A., Sadek, A. (1973). A double-blind trial for the clinical management of psychogenic headache. *Br J Psychiatry*, 122:181–183.

37. Sullivan, M.J.L., Reesor, K., Mikail, S., et al. (1992). The treatment of depression in chronic low back pain: Review and recommendations. *Pain*, 50:5–13.

CHAPTER

14

HUMAN IMMUNODEFICIENCY VIRUS INFECTION

INTRODUCTION

The human immunodeficiency virus (HIV) emerged in the 1970s and the resulting acquired immunodeficiency syndrome (AIDS) was first recognized in 1981. Since then, a pandemic of HIV infection has spread through sexual, blood, and intrauterine transmission. An estimated 650,000–900,000 Americans were infected with HIV by 1992.[1] Each year, more than 60,000 people in the United States are diagnosed with an AIDS-defining opportunistic infection. So far, there have been more than 325,000 deaths from AIDS in the United States.[1]

HIV infection of CD4 lymphocytes impairs immune function resulting in the acquisition of opportunistic infections and certain malignancies. These eventually lead to death usually within 10 years of seroconversion and within 2 years of developing AIDS.

STAGES OF HIV DISEASE

The stages of HIV infection have been described by the Centers for Disease Control.[2] Stage I is acute infection and seroconversion and

355

may be asymptomatic or accompanied by a viral syndrome and meningoencephalitis. Stage II is the latent phase with a mean duration of nine years. During this stage, patients are asymptomatic although they are infectious. Stage III is characterized by persistent lymphadenopathy in at least two extrainguinal sites. Stage IV-A indicates the presence of constitutional symptoms such as weight loss, fever, and diarrhea. Stage IV-B marks the beginning of AIDS and indicates neuropathology including dementia, peripheral neuropathy, or myelopathy. Stage IV-C is characterized by opportunistic infections. Stage IV-D indicates HIV-related malignancies including Kaposi's sarcoma, non-Hodgkin's lymphoma, and primary central nervous system (CNS) lymphoma. Stage IV-E indicates other conditions.

PRIMARY CENTRAL NERVOUS SYSTEM PATHOLOGY

HIV is neurotropic and infects the CNS early in its course.[3] Meningoencephalitis may be the presenting condition of acute HIV infection at the time of seroconversion. CNS infection occurs before systemic involvement. Although HIV is neurotropic, it may not be virulent to the CNS until systemic immunosuppression has occurred. Histopathologic studies demonstrate that neurons and oligodendrocytes (microglia and astrocytes) are not primarily infected with HIV; it is the monocytes, macrophages, and multinucleated giant cells that are infected. HIV encephalitis involves primarily subcortical regions including central white matter, basal ganglia, thalamus, brain stem, and spinal cord. However, there may be some cortical neuronal loss. HIV leukoencephalopathy is seen histologically as myelin pallor with an inflammatory reaction involving astrocytes and multinucleated giant cells.

Primary HIV CNS infection may be manifest clinically as a variety of neuropsychiatric syndromes that may begin early in the course of illness before systemic involvement. As immunosuppression progresses, HIV replication in the CNS may also increase, possibly accounting for the emergence of more severe neuropsychiatric syndromes later in the disease. However, neurological involvement does not necessarily parallel systemic involvement.

SECONDARY CNS PATHOLOGY

In addition to primary infection of the CNS by the HIV virus, the immunosuppression caused by HIV infection leaves the CNS vulnerable to opportunistic infections. These include viral infections such as cytomegalovirus (CMV), herpes simplex virus (HSV), varicella zoster (VZ); progressive multifocal leukodystrophy (PML); fungal infections such as cryptococcus and candida; parasitic infection by toxoplasmosis; and such CNS neoplasms as primary lymphoma.[3] These conditions can cause focal neurological deficits and are also associated with neuropsychiatric syndromes and delirium.

PSYCHIATRIC DISORDERS IN HIV/AIDS

PREVALENCE OF PREMORBID PSYCHIATRIC DISORDERS IN HIV/AIDS

Many individuals at risk for HIV are also at higher risk for psychiatric disorders. For example, homosexual men have a higher prevalence of major depression than the general population.[4] Intravenous drug users have a higher incidence of depression, antisocial personality disorder, alcohol and drug dependence, and suicidality than the general population.[5]

PSYCHIATRIC DISORDER AS RISK FACTOR FOR HIV INFECTION

Some psychiatric disorders put individuals at higher risk for contracting HIV. Hypersexuality combined with poor judgment, impulsivity, and risk-taking behavior, as seen in bipolar disorder may result in an increased number of sexual partners and therefore an increased risk of contracting HIV. Schizophrenia also impairs judgment and insight, leaving patients more likely to exhibit risk-taking behavior. Alcohol- and substance-abuse disorders are associated with impulsivity and a greater number of sexual partners and therefore with increased risk of contracting HIV. Personality disorders may also increase risk factors and thus be more prevalent in HIV-positive patients. In one study, 53% of males with borderline personality disorder were homosexual, putting them at higher risk for HIV infection.[6]

NEUROPSYCHIATRIC DISORDERS ASSOCIATED WITH HIV/AIDS

SYNDROMES

There is a broad range of neuropsychiatric impairment associated with HIV infection. HIV has been called "the great imitator," like syphilis. Neuropsychiatric syndromes include cognitive impairment, dementia, delirium, affective syndromes including depression and mania, anxiety, and psychosis. Each syndrome is discussed separately with regard to presentation, epidemiology, natural history, differential diagnosis, and acute and maintenance treatment.

TIME COURSE

Mild cognitive impairment may be present during the latent phase. Affective, anxiety, or psychotic syndromes may occur at any time during the course of HIV infection. Dementia is usually a later manifestation and dementia with delirium or psychosis may herald the terminal phase of an AIDS illness.

ETIOLOGY

Neuropsychiatric impairment may be caused by a primary infection of the CNS by HIV, secondary opportunistic infections, neoplasms, or medications used to treat either the primary or secondary infections.

EVALUATION

Any change in mental status in an HIV-positive patient should be evaluated with a neurological neurodiagnostic examination and procedures as indicated clinically. Electroencephalogram (EEG) is sensitive to detect subtle early CNS involvement although it may not be very helpful in determining the etiology. Lumbar puncture and cerebrospinal fluid examination can identify an infectious process. A computed tomography should be obtained prior to lumbar puncture to rule out a mass lesion that might cause cerebral herniation. Magnetic resonance imaging (MRI) is sensitive in detecting small lesions and white matter changes.

COGNITIVE IMPAIRMENT AND DEMENTIA

The American Academy of Neurology AIDS Task Force developed diagnostic criteria for the neuropsychiatric disorders associated with HIV infection.[7] **HIV-1 associated minor cognitive/motor disorder** refers to a less severe form of neuropsychiatric impairment that may or may not progress to the more severe HIV-1 associated dementia complex. These conditions involve impairment in cognitive function, motor function, and behavior. Early cognitive changes include impaired memory, concentration, and mental slowing. Early motor symptoms include leg weakness, tremor, and ataxia. Behavioral changes include apathy, anhedonia, irritability, lability, lethargy, social withdrawal, inflexibility, emotional responsiveness, diminished spontaneity, and decreased libido. Neuroimaging studies are usually normal at this stage.

HIV-1 associated dementia complex is a severe neuropsychiatric condition and is an AIDS-defining illness. Cognitive decline begins with slowing and loss of precision in mentation and progresses to decreased verbal fluency and impaired performance on complex sequencing tasks. Higher cortical abnormalities are uncommon. Motor abnormalities include weakness, motor slowing particularly of fine and rapid alternating movements, extrapyramidal dysfunction, tremor, hyperreflexia, hypertonia, ataxia, frontal release signs, dysarthria that progresses to severe psychomotor retardation, paraparesis, myoclonus, seizures, sensory neuropathy, and bowel and bladder incontinence. Behavioral abnormalities may progress to include impaired judgment, socially inappropriate behavior, and disinhibition.

Routine bedside neuropsychological testing may not be sensitive enough to pick up subtle changes, although inattention and recent memory loss may be apparent. Neuropsychological studies should focus on attention and concentration, speed of information processing, motor functioning, abstraction and reasoning, visuospatial skills, memory, speech, and language.

The subtle early signs are not detected by routine cognitive exams such as the Mini Mental Status Exam, so formal neuropsychological testing should be performed with any neuropsychiatric presentation.

Epidemiology

HIV-1 associated dementia complex develops in the later stages of systemic infection. The incidence of dementia in HIV is 14–66%.[8] At the time of AIDS diagnosis, one-third of patients have overt symptoms of dementia and one-quarter have subclinical dementia.[9] Dementia is the presenting or only sign of AIDS in 25% of patients.[9] At autopsy, about 90% of patients have CNS involvement.[9]

Natural History

The risk of neuropsychiatric involvement increases with progression of the illness, and neuropsychiatric impairment may progress as the disease progresses. Onset of dementia is usually insidious but sometimes is abrupt or has an accelerated course in the context of a systemic illness such as pneumonia with hypoxia. The course may be variable from gradual deterioration to rapid progression to death. The mean survival time from onset of severe dementia is 1.8 months with a range of 1 to 6 months, while the total duration of dementia ranges from 1 to 9 months with a mean of 4.2 months.[9]

Differential Diagnosis

The differential diagnosis of the HIV-1 associated dementia complex includes depression with cognitive impairment, delirium (metabolic encephalopathy), and secondary opportunistic infections or neoplasms involving the CNS.

Neurodiagnostic Studies

MRI may demonstrate nonspecific white matter changes and scattered parenchymal lesions and is superior to computed tomography in this population. Electroencephalography may reveal focal or generalized dysrythmias. Examination of cerebrospinal fluid (CSF) may reveal elevated protein, mononuclear pleocytosis, or oligoclonal IgG bands. CSF cultures may be positive for opportunistic infectious organisms, particularly CMV. There are no neurodiagnostic studies that are pathognomonic for HIV-associated neuropsychiatric disorders.

Psychopharmacological Treatment

The incidence of HIV-1 associated dementia complex has declined since the regular use of antiviral agents, suggesting that these agents may slow the progression of primary CNS infection. Yarchoan reported cognitive improvement with both AZT and ddI in uncontrolled case series.[10,11] Double-blind, placebo-controlled studies demonstrated cognitive improvement in AIDS patients given a 16-week trial of AZT.[12,13]

There have been no reported longer term studies of any antiviral agents in dementia, but presumably antiviral treatment should be lifelong (as it would anyway for the systemic manifestations of HIV).

DELIRIUM

Delirium is characterized by restlessness, irritability, agitation or lethargy, depression, impaired concentration, distractibility, anxiety, and alterations in the sleep-wake cycle. Prodromal symptoms should be assessed by checking arousal, attention, short-term memory, orientation, diurnal variation, and neurologic findings such as tremor, multifocal myoclonus, and asterixis. Any of these findings should lead to a high index of suspicion for delirium and appropriate rapid intervention.

Epidemiology

Delirium is the most common neuropsychiatric manifestation in hospitalized HIV-positive patients. Up to 90% of delirious HIV patients have an organic etiology of the delirium. It has been reported in 22% of HIV patients and 57% of hospitalized AIDS patients.[14]

Natural History

HIV infection causes diffuse cerebral cellular dysfunction, leaving the brain more susceptible to additional insults including neurotoxicity with antiviral agents and antibiotics. Delirium increases the morbidity and mortality associated with any medical condition and should be treated aggressively. The onset of delirium with dementia usually heralds the terminal phase of illness.

Differential Diagnosis

The differential diagnosis of delirium includes progressive dementia or a psychotic disorder. The etiology of delirium is frequently multifactorial, and a vigorous attempt to identify and treat the underlying abnormality is imperative. Possible etiologies include metabolic abnormalities, electrolyte imbalance, hypoxia, multisystem failure, sepsis, or toxic levels of analgesics and other medications. CNS opportunistic infections (toxoplasmosis, cryptococcal meningitis, herpes encephalitis), CNS neoplasms (lymphoma), or PML are also included in the differential diagnosis. Commonly used medications in the treatment of AIDS that are associated with delirium include zidovudine, acyclovir, amphotericin B, cephalosporins, dapsone, isoniazid, 5-flucytosine, gancyclovir, metronidazole, pentamidine, trimethoprim/sulfamethoxizole, methotrexate, procarbazine hydrochloride, analgesics, anticonvulsants, corticosteroids, and psychotropic medications. Drug withdrawal, especially alcohol or benzodiazepines, may also produce delirium.

Psychopharmacological Treatment

Treatment of the underlying abnormality (or abnormalities) is imperative. For example, hypoxia should be treated with oxygen and appropriate treatment of the underlying pneumonia, electrolyte imbalances should be corrected, offending medications should be discontinued, and opportunistic infections should be appropriately treated. Nutritional status should be optimized, the sleep-wake cycle should be normalized, and patients should be kept in a quiet, consistent environment with appropriate cues, familiar objects, and frequent reorientation.

No controlled studies have been performed on the treatment of delirium in AIDS patients. An open study reported the use of a combination of intravenous (IV) haloperidol and lorazepam for acute treatment of behavioral abnormalities associated with delirium.[14] This study used relatively high doses of IV haloperidol (mean 42 mg/day) and lorazepam (mean 7.5 mg/day). Because both agents do not have active metabolites, accumulation is not a concern. While patients with AIDS are more sensitive to the extrapyramidal side effects (EPS) of antipsychotics, IV administration of haloperidol is less likely than oral administration to cause EPS, and high doses are well tolerated even in AIDS patients.

Maintenance treatment is usually not required for delirium, and there have not been any reported studies addressing maintenance treatment of delirium in AIDS patients.

DEPRESSION

Epidemiology

Depression is the most common symptom and psychiatric diagnosis in HIV-positive patients, with prevalence at least twice as high as in comparable healthy populations. In a two-year follow-up of seropositive homosexual men, 10–25% had a depressive syndrome.[15]

Natural History

Adjustment disorders and depression may be common after identification of HIV seropositive status, in the initial stage of dementia, or with secondary CNS involvement (opportunistic infection or neoplasm). Depressive disorders in HIV/AIDS patients present with a similar symptom profile as typical depressive disorders, although sleep and appetite disturbance may be more prominent in HIV-positive patients.[16] Subcortical involvement with primary HIV infection may predispose to depressive disorders.

SUICIDE

The risk of suicide is considerably higher in HIV/AIDS patients than in the general population.[17] Marzuk found the relative risk of suicide to be 36 times a comparable demographic group and 66 times the general population.[18] All suicides occurred within nine months of AIDS diagnosis. A study of an Air Force population found a 16 to 24 times increase in suicide rate among HIV-positive individuals, and half the suicide attempts were within three months of notification of seropositive status.[19] Risk factors for suicide among this group include social isolation, perceived lack of social support, HIV-related interpersonal or occupational problems, past history of depression, current adjustment disorder, personality disorder, or alcohol abuse disorder.[19]

Differential Diagnosis

Depression may be difficult to differentiate from physical illness in patients with systemic disease due to overlap between symptoms of major depression and physical symptoms of AIDS. An inclusive approach whereby all symptoms are considered even if they may be attributable to physical illness is probably the most useful. Depressive symptoms also overlap with symptoms of HIV-1 associated dementia complex and substance use or withdrawal. Delirium may also present with depressive symptoms.

An organic etiology of depression must be ruled out. Organic causes of depression in HIV disease include vitamin B_{12} deficiency, anemia, Addison's disease, other endocrinopathies, CMV, opportunistic infections, CNS malignancy, and PML. Medications that may cause depression include ketoconazole, corticosteroids, AZT, isoniazid, gancyclovir, and DDI.

A common mistake is to assume that depressive symptoms are a normal reaction to the stress of a chronic fatal illness and to not treat depression. Such cognitive symptoms as sad mood, feelings of worthlessness and guilt, suicidal thoughts, and anhedonia can help make the diagnosis of a depressive disorder and warrant treatment.

PSYCHOPHARMACOLOGICAL TREATMENT

Antidepressants that are effective in treating primary depressive disorders in healthy individuals are also effective for depression associated with HIV disease. However, response to the usual antidepressants may not be as robust as in healthy populations. In one clinic, about 85% of depressed HIV patients demonstrated some response to antidepressant pharmacotherapy, with only 50% having a complete recovery.[20]

There are few studies of antidepressants specifically in the HIV/AIDS population and there are no maintenance studies reported. Antidepressant choice is guided by side-effect profile. HIV-positive patients are more sensitive to psychotropic side effects so these agents should be used with caution, typically initiating treatment with smaller doses than usual and titrating slowly. Doses may be lower than typically used in healthy populations.

Tricyclic antidepressants (TCAs) are usually well tolerated in healthy HIV-positive patients, but the anticholinergic side effects may not be tolerated by patients with early cognitive deficits or dementia. If TCAs are used, the secondary amines, nortriptyline and desipramine, are recommended because of lower anticholinergic effects.

The selective serotonin reuptake inhibitors (SSRIs) have fewer side effects and are better tolerated in this population. Dosing may be limited by gastrointestinal side effects, which may aggravate underlying GI pathology. Drug interactions between the SSRIs and other AIDS agents that are also metabolized by the P450 IID6 should be monitored and these combinations should be avoided if possible. In particular, ketoconazole should not be coadministered with nefazodone or fluvoxamine due to inhibition at P450 3A4.

Bupropion may decrease the seizure threshold so it should be avoided in patients with a history of seizures or other CNS pathology that may predispose to seizures. Trazodone may be useful not only as an antidepressant, but also as an anxiolytic and sedative at bedtime. The most common risks with trazodone are priapism in men, orthostatic hypotension, and reflex tachycardia.

Monoamine oxidase inhibitors (MAOIs) are not recommended due to difficulty maintaining the restricted diet and potential interactions with AZT. AZT has potential catechol-O-methyltransferase inhibition and may precipitate a hypertensive crisis when coadministered with MAOIs.

Psychostimulants may be particularly useful as monotherapy or as an adjunctive agent to another antidepressant.[21,22] These agents may be especially beneficial in patients with apathy, poor nutritional status, or those who require rapid response. Psychostimulants can stimulate appetite in HIV/AIDS patients and help improve nutritional status. Stimulants may also improve psychomotor retardation and cognitive function. Methylphenidate is preferred over dextroamphetamine because it is less likely to cause motor side effects. Dextroamphetamine is more likely to unmask or aggravate abnormal involuntary movements, especially in HIV-1 associated dementia complex.[21] Methylphenidate is dosed at 5–15 mg every three to four hours, three to four times per day, with a usual dose of 30–40 mg/day, but doses up to 120 mg/day may be used. The last dose should not be given after 4 pm to avoid insomnia. Dextroamphetamine is dosed at 2.5–30 mg twice a day with a usual range of 15–60 mg/day. The most common side effects of the psychostimulants include tachycardia, hypertension, psychosis, insomnia, dyskinesias, and nausea.

The benzodiazepine alprazolam (Xanax) may be effective as an antidepressant, particularly with prominent anxiety symptoms. Doses of 0.125–0.25 mg three to four times per day up to 4 mg/day may be required. Side effects include sedation and physical dependence. Alprazolam does not have active metabolites so accumulation is not a concern.

Treatment refractory depression or life-threatening depression may be treated successfully with electroconvulsive therapy.[23] The four patients in this series did not have cognitive impairment and tolerated ECT well without cognitive changes and with resolution of their depression.

There are no reported studies of maintenance treatment for depression in HIV. We recommend maintenance treatment as outlined in Chapter 4.

MANIA

Epidemiology

Patients who develop mania early in the course of HIV are more likely to have a family history of affective disorder. Mania in patients without a personal or family history of affective disorder is associated with dementia, low CD4 cell counts, and a diagnosis of AIDS.[24] Manic syndromes are more common in AIDS than previously recognized. One series found a prevalence of mania of 8% in an infectious disease AIDS clinic.[24] Mania is primarily a late stage neuropsychiatric complication of HIV infection and is associated with cognitive impairment.

Differential Diagnosis

The differential diagnosis includes primary bipolar disorder with mania, schizophrenia, or schizoaffective disorder, primary HIV infection, or secondary causes such as medications (zidovudine, corticosteroids, gancyclovir, or antidepressants) or opportunistic infections.

Psychopharmacological Treatment

The treatment of mania in HIV is similar to treatment in HIV-negative individuals although HIV/AIDS patients are more sensitive to side effects.

Lithium may be more likely to produce toxicity in HIV-positive individuals and is usually poorly tolerated. As in other primary CNS processes, lithium may produce toxic side effects even at subtherapeutic levels. Carbamazepine and valproate, typical second-line agents, should be used with caution due to the risk of myelosupression. However, these agents may be particularly effective if there is structural brain pathology or risk of seizure disorder. Valproate coadministered with AZT may cause an increase in AZT levels. Carbamazepine coadministered with erythromycin or isoniazid may increase carbamazepine levels. High potency antipsychotics are used as first-line agents in mania.

Maintenance treatment for mania in HIV/AIDS has not been studied. We recommend maintenance treatment as outlined in Chapter 5.

ANXIETY

Epidemiology

Anxiety symptoms are common in HIV infection, and anxiety disorders may be the most common neuropsychiatric complication of HIV infection.

Differential Diagnosis

The differential diagnosis includes a psychological reaction to the illness, primary anxiety disorder, drug or alcohol intoxication or withdrawal, acute pain, or secondary causes ranging from medication side effects to CNS infections. Medications that can cause anxiety include isoniazid, acyclovir, AZT, bronchodilators, theophylline, and corticosteroids. Akathisia can mimic anxiety disorders and is caused by antipsychotics or SSRIs. Hypoxia or respiratory distress can cause anxiety.

Psychopharmacological Treatment

Benzodiazepines are the primary treatment of anxiety disorders. Preferred benzodiazepines are lorazepam and oxazepam that are both metabolized only by glucuronidation. Shorter acting agents such as alprazolam are also preferred as there is less likelihood of accumulation. Intermediate onset agents are also preferred; shorter onset agents are more likely to cause dependence. Side effects of the benzodiazepines include sedation, disinhibition, amnesia, ataxia, and motor dysfunction. Benzodiazepines should be used only for the short term.

For longer term use, buspirone is recommended because there is no risk of abuse and dependence with this agent. Buspirone, a nonbenzodiazepine anxiolytic, may be better tolerated although HIV-positive patients may be especially sensitive to the dopaminergic effects and confusion. Buspirone is best tolerated by asymptomatic patients on lower AZT doses (<300 mg/day). Patients taking high doses of AZT require higher doses of buspirone (45–60 mg/day). Buspirone may also cause dyskinesias and myoclonus.[25]

Trazodone may also be used for longer term anxiolytic use. Dosing is 25–200 mg/day and may be given in divided doses. Although trazodone is not marketed as an anxiolytic, it is effective in reducing anxiety in this patient population. Antipsychotics may be used for anxiety that is associated with psychotic symptoms such as delusions, delirium, or extreme panic. They have an immediate sedative effect, and, as with other uses of antipsychotics, EPS is a risk.

There are no maintenance studies of the treatment of anxiety in the HIV/AIDS population. We recommend buspirone or trazodone for long-term treatment rather than benzodiazepines (due to risk of dependence) or antipsychotics (due to risk of EPS, neuroleptic malignant syndrome, and tardive dyskinesia).

PSYCHOSIS

Epidemiology

Psychosis is less common in HIV/AIDS patients than other psychiatric syndromes. Only case reports exist; there are no prevalence studies of psychotic disorders in HIV patients.

Natural History

Psychosis may be an early sign of HIV disease in patients with pre-existing psychotic disorder or family history of a psychotic disorder. However, psychosis is generally a late complication of HIV infection. It may be associated with cognitive impairment of the HIV-1 associated dementia complex.

Differential Diagnosis

Psychotic symptoms may represent a brief reactive psychosis, drug intoxication, or may be directly related to CNS infection with HIV. Psychotic symptoms may be related to a primary psychotic disorder such as schizophrenia or bipolar disorder that is unrelated to HIV status or to delirium due to medication intoxication or CNS infection or malignancy. The age group at highest risk for HIV infection is also the age at which schizophrenia usually presents, so these two events may occur together by chance.[26]

Psychopharmacological Treatment

As with any psychotic disorder, the treatment of choice is antipsychotics. Several case reports suggest that HIV-positive patients are more sensitive to the extrapyramidal side effects. High-potency agents are more likely to cause EPS so midpotency agents may be better tolerated. Low-potency agents have more anticholinergic effects that can significantly impair cognitive impairment and cause delirium. The low-potency agents also lower the seizure threshold more than higher potency agents, which is a risk with intracranial mass lesions or infections that also predispose to seizures. Risperidone may be better tolerated with less EPS at therapeutic doses.

REFERENCES

1. Karon, J.M., Rosenberg, P.S., McQuillan, G., et al. (1996). Prevalence of HIV infection in the United States, 1984–1992. *JAMA*, 276(2):126–131.
2. Centers for Disease Control (1987). Revision of the CDC surveillance case definition for acquired immunodeficiency syndrome. *MMWR*, 36(Suppl 1S):1S–15S.
3. Everall, I.P., Lantos, P.L. (1991). The neuropathology of HIV: A review of the first 10 years. *Int Rev Psychiatry*, 3:307–320.
4. Perkins, D.O., Stern, R.A., Golden, R.N., et al. (1994). Mood disorders in HIV infection: Prevalence and risk factors in a nonepicenter of the AIDS epidemic. *Am J Psychiatry*, 151(2):233–236.
5. Dinwiddie, S.H., Reich, T., Cloninger, C.R. (1992). Psychiatric comorbidity and suicidality among intravenous drug users. *J Clin Psychiatry*, 53(10):364–369.

6. Zubenko, G.S., George, A.W., Soloff, P.H., et al. (1987). Sexual practices among patients with borderline personality disorder. *Am J Psychiatry*, 144(6):748–752.

7. Janssen, R.S., Cornblath, D.R., Epstein, L.G. (1991). American Academy of Neurology AIDS Task Force: Nomenclature and research case definitions for neurologic manifestations of HIV-1 infection. *Neurology*, 41:778–785.

8. Price, R.W., Brew, B., Sidtis, J., et al. (1988). The brain in AIDS: Central nervous system HIV-1 infection and AIDS dementia complex. *Science*, 239:586–591.

9. Navia, B.A., Jordan, B.D., Price, R.W. (1986). The AIDS dementia complex: I. Clinical features. *Ann Neurol*, 19:517–524.

10. Yarchoan, R., Berg, G., Browers, P., et al. (1987). Response of human-immunodeficiency-virus-associated neurological disease to 3'-azido-3'-deoxythymidine. *Lancet*, 1(8525):132–135.

11. Yarchoan R., Pluda, J.M., Thomas, R.V., et al. (1990). Long-term toxicity/activity profile of 2', 3-dideoxyinosine in AIDS or AIDS-related complex. *Lancet*, 336(8714):526–529.

12. Schmitt, F.A., Bigley, J.W., McKinnis, R., et al. (1988). Neuropsychological outcome of zidovudine (AZT) treatment of patients with AIDS and AIDS-related complex. *N Engl J Med*, 319:1573–1578.

13. Sidtis, J.J., Gatsonis, C., Price, R.W., et al. (1993). Zidovidine treatment of the AIDS dementia complex: Results of a placebo-controlled trial. AIDS Clinical Trials Group. *Ann Neurol*, 33(4):343–349.

14. Fernandez, F., Levy, J.K., Mansell, P.W.A. (1989). Management of delirium in terminally ill AIDS patients. *Int J Psychiatry Med*, 19:165–172.

15. Atkinson, J.H., Grant I. (1994). Natural history of neuropsychiatric manifestations of HIV disease. *Pscyhiatr Clin N Am*, 17:17–33.

16. Hintz S., Kuck, J., Peterkin, J.J., et al. (1990). Depression in the context of human immunodeficiency virus infection: Implications for treatment. *J Clin Psychiatry*, 51:497–501.

17. Beckett, A., Shenson, D. (1993). Suicide risk in patients with human immunodeficiency virus infection and Acquired Immunodeficiency Syndrome. *Harvard Rev Psychiatry*, 1: 27–35.

18. Marzuk, P.M., Tierney, H., Tardiff, et al. (1988). Increased risk of suicide in persons with AIDS. *JAMA*, 259:1333–1337.

19. Rundell, J.R., Kyle, K.M., Brown, G.R., et al. (1992). Risk factors for suicide attempts in a human immunodeficiency virus screening program. *Psychosomatics*, 33:24–27.

20. Treisman, G.J., Lyketsos, C.G., Fishman, M., et al. (1993). Psychiatric care for patients with HIV infection: The varying perspectives. *Psychosomatics*, 34:432–439.

21. Fernandez, F., Levy, J.K., Galizzi, H. (1988). Response of HIV-related depression to psychostimulants: Case reports. *Hosp Comm Psychiatry*, 39:628–631.

22. Holmes, V.F., Fernandez, F., Levy, J.K. (1989). Psychostimulant response in AIDS-related complex patients. *J Clin Psychiatry*, 50:5–8.

23. Schaerf, F.W., Miller, R.R., Lipsey, J.R., et al. (1989). ECT for major depression in four patients infected with human immunodeficiency virus. *Am J Psychiatry*, 146(6):782–784.

24. Lyketsos, C.G., Hanson, A.L., Fishman, M. (1993). Manic syndrome early and late in course of HIV. *Am J Psychiatry*, 150:326–327.

25. Fernandez, F. (1989). Anxiety and the neuropsychiatry of AIDS. *J Clin Psychiatry*, 50(11): 9–14.

26. Vogel-Scibilia, J.E., Mulsant, B.H., Keshavan, M.S. (1988). HIV infection presenting as psychosis: A critique. *Acta Psychiatr Scand*, 78:652–656.

15

TRAUMATIC BRAIN INJURY AND POST-CONCUSSIVE SYNDROME

INTRODUCTION

Head trauma is a common cause of morbidity and mortality. Approximately 2 million head injuries occur per year in the United States, and 25% of them require inpatient hospital treatment. A concussion is a head injury associated with a transient loss of consciousness. The neuropathological correlate of a concussion is diffuse axonal injury, i.e., a shearing force injury to longer axons of the cortex and subcortex of the brain. In other words, imagine a bowl of jello (i.e., the brain and skull) struck from the side—the jello will be subject to a variety of shock waves with different vectors changing its internal structure. This correlates with the effects of diffuse axonal injury in the brain. Approximately 50% of mild head injuries with or without loss of consciousness progress to the post-concussive syndrome.[1]

This chapter deals with the pharmacological treatments for a well-defined clinical entity, post-concussive syndrome, following mild head injury, which is a head injury with a loss of consciousness of 30 minutes or less, an initial high Glasgow Coma Scale that does not deteriorate, no skull fracture or intracerebral blood on computerized tomographic (CT) scan, and a nonfocal neurological exam.[2]

TABLE 15–1. POST-CONCUSSIVE SYMPTOM
FREQUENCY

Study/Follow-up/Symptoms	n	Percent
Jakobsen et al. 1987 (N=55)		
At 1 month, at 3 months		
Headache	16	29.15
Fatigue	16	29.5
Impaired concentration	9	16.9
Vertigo	6	11.5
Irritability	5	9.2
Rutherford et al. 1979 (N=131)		
At 1 year		
Headache	11	8.4
Irritability	7	5.3
Anxiety	5	3.8
Depression	2	1.5
Insomnia	3	2.3
Fatigue	3	2.3
Loss of concentration	4	3.1
Loss of memory	5	3.8
Amnesia	2	1.5
Diplopia	1	0.8
Visual defect	3	2.3
Hearing defect	2	1.5
Dizziness	6	4.6
Epilepsy	0	0
Sensitivity to alcohol	0	0
Others	1	0.8
Middelboe et al. 1992 (N=28)		
At 1 year		
Headache	9	32
Dizziness	7	25
Memory deficit	7	25
Concentration deficit	7	25
Fatigue	6	21
Irritability	6	21
Anxiety	5	18
Sleep disturbance	5	18
Sight disturbance	5	18
Alcohol intolerance	3	11
Gastrointestinal symptoms	3	11
Hearing disturbance	2	7
Disturbance in smell	1	3
Tactile disturbance	1	3
		(*Contd.*)

TABLE 15–1. (Continued)

Study/Follow-up/Symptoms	n	Percent
Edna et al. 1987 (N=485)		
At 3–5 years		
Headache	113	23
Impaired memory	90	20
Dizziness	90	19
Fatigue	89	18
Irritability (noise and light)	88	18
Impaired concentration	68	14
Insomnia	65	13
Tinnitus	61	13
Hearing defect	51	11
Depression	45	9
Anxiety	37	8
Double vision	12	2

From Brown, S.J., Fann, J.R., Grant, I. (1994). Post-concussional disorder: Time to acknowledge a common source of neurobehavioral morbidity. *J Neuropsychiatry Clin Neurosci*, 6:18. Copyright 1994 by American Psychiatric Press, Inc. Reprinted with permission.

POST-CONCUSSIVE SYNDROME

Post-concussive syndrome is characterized by both neurological and psychiatric signs and symptoms. Headache, dizziness, tinnitus, and vertigo are the most common neurological sequelae, while irritability, fatigue, insomnia, anxiety, depression, and impairment of concentration and memory are the common psychiatric sequelae.

While post-concussive syndrome may be transient in many patients, resolving within three months, a more chronic course may develop: 15–33% of patients are symptomatic at one year, 15% at three years.[3,4] More recently, Brown et al. summarized the results of four previous studies of sequelae of mild head injury demonstrating the chronicity of post-concussive syndrome.[5] Their results are shown in Table 15–1.

The treatment of post-concussive syndrome requires a team approach, including the disciplines of psychiatry, rehabilitation medicine, social work, and psychology. Individual symptoms may be amenable to psychopharmacological intervention and are discussed below.

Before proceeding to individual, symptom-based treatment strategies, a few general principles are mentioned regarding psychopharmacological treatment of this population. Head injury patients, in general, are more sensitive to psychopharmacological drugs, particularly to their side effects.

Anticholinergic side effects (e.g., sedation and delirium) may be seen at much lower dosages in this population than in the nonbrain injured. Mild head injury patients may develop post-traumatic seizures, and psychopharmacological agents are known to decrease seizure threshold (increase the potential to have a seizure). Particular agents of concern are clomipramine, chlorpromazine, clozapine, and buproprion, although other agents may be implicated. As a result, treatment should be initiated in consultation with a physician experienced in treating brain injuries and at a low initial dose with slow dose increases under close supervision.

IRRITABILITY

Irritability—being quick to anger—is a persistent symptom after mild head injury. Edna et al. reported an 18% prevalence three to five years after head injury.[6] Brooks et al. noted that 64% of head injury patients were irritable as reported by family members.[7] Data on treatment of irritability are limited but clinical experience has demonstrated effectiveness of the SSRIs, particularly sertraline, in reducing irritability. Duration of such treatment also remains unstudied, but given the chronic course of irritability in a subset of these patients, the treatment may be lifelong, especially if the patient fails an attempt to wean off the medication. Use and side effects of the SSRIs are discussed in Chapter 4 on depression.

Irritability and mild aggression lie on a continuum of behavior. The treatment of milder forms of aggression after mild head injury remains unstudied. Clinically, however, if a patient fails to respond to treatment with an SSRI, one may attempt a trial of buspirone, increasing it first to dosages of 30 mg/day, the recommended dosage for treatment of generalized anxiety disorder, but it may be necessary to increase the dose higher.

INSOMNIA

Sleep disturbance is a common chronic sequelae of mild head injury. Insomnia is the most common form of sleep disturbance, although excessive somnolence is seen rarely.[8] The authors also noted that approximately 20 months post-injury, 52% of patients endorsed sleep disturbance. Edna et al. reported a 13% prevalence of insomnia in their patients at three to five years.[6]

Data on the pharmacological treatment of insomnia following mild head injury does not exist currently. Clinically, one would need to determine if the sleep disturbance was present alone or was part of a depressive syndrome. If the condition is part of a depressive illness, treatment with an antidepressant (i.e., an SSRI as a first-line agent) may resolve the insomnia. If the insomnia appears the sole complaint, a trial of trazodone may be warranted. As the symptom appears to be chronic, the benzodiazepines, zolpidem, or benadryl would not be favored choices due to their side-effect profiles and tolerance to their sedative effects with continued use, which may be required in this patient population. Use of trazodone is discussed more fully in Chapter 4 on depression. However, trazodone is generally well tolerated for long-term use, and tolerance to its sedative effects does not appear to develop.

ANXIETY

Anxiety is seen chronically in post-concussive syndrome, from approximately 4–18% at one year to 8% at three to five years.[3,9,6] It is characterized by a chronic, low-to-moderate level of anxiety that may resemble generalized anxiety disorder.

Clinical experience has demonstrated a possible role for buspirone as treatment for post-head injury anxiety symptoms. Well-controlled studies have not been reported. The clinician may start with a low dose (5 mg/day) and increase slowly (one 5 mg tablet every three days) until a dose of 20–30 mg/day is reached. Although 30 mg/day is the initial target dose in generalized anxiety disorder, this population may respond to a slightly lower dosage or may have greater difficulty with dizziness, its major side effect. Therefore, the dictum of "starting low and going slow" is best followed. Further details on buspirone are discussed in Chapter 7 on anxiety disorders.

DEPRESSION

The prevalence of depression post-mild head injury has been reported as 1.5% at one year to 9% at three to five years.[3,6] Mild head injury appears to induce depressive symptoms, as demonstrated in a case-control study.[10] Experimental data on antidepressant treatments are lacking; however, clinical experience has demonstrated the effectiveness of antidepressant therapy in this population. The SSRIs appear to be the best tolerated given their side-effect profile, but low starting doses should be used, and the dose titrated upward slowly until the desired clinical effect is obtained. If sleep disturbance is a prominent part of the depressive syndrome, a tricyclic antidepressant (nortriptyline) in low doses may be tried as monotherapy or, alternatively, trazodone may be combined with an SSRI. Data do not exist on the optimum duration of treatment, but given the chronicity of symptoms in a subset of these patients, failure at drug weaning may indicate the need for long-term pharmacotherapy.

REFERENCES

1. Mardel, S. (1989). Minor head injury may not be "minor." *Postgrad Med*, 85(6):213–225.
2. Evans, R.W. (1992). The postconcussion syndrome and the sequelae of minor head injury. *Neurologic Clinics*, 10(4):815–847.
3. Rutherford, W.H., Merrett, J.D., McDonald, J.R. (1979). Symptoms at one year following concussion from minor head injuries. *Injury*, 10:225–230.
4. Denker, P.G. (1944). The postconcussion syndrome: Prognosis and evaluation of the organic factors. *NY State J Med*, 44:379–384.
5. Brown, S.J., Fann, J.R., Grant, I. (1994). Postconcussional disorder: Time to acknowledge a common source of neurobehavioral morbidity. *J Neuropsychiatry Clin Neurosci*, 6:15–22.
6. Edna, T.H. (1987). Disability 3-5 years after minor head injury. *J Oslo City Hospital*, 37:41–48.
7. Brooks, N., Campsie, L., Symington, C., et al. (1986). The five year outcome of severe blunt head injury: A relative's view. *J Neurol Neurosurg Psychiatry*, 49:764–770.
8. Cohen, M., Oksenberg, A., Snir, D., et al. (1992). Temporally related changes of sleep complaints in traumatic brain injured patients. *J Neurol Neurosurg Psychiatry*, 55:313–315.
9. Middelboe, T., Birket-Smith, M., Andersen, H.S., et al. (1992). Personality traits in patients with postconcussional sequelae. *J Personality Disorders*, 6:246–255.
10. Schoenhuber, R., Gentilini, M. (1988). Anxiety and depression after mild head injury: A case control study. *J Neurol Neurosurg Psych*, 51:722–724.
11. Jakobsen, J., Baasdsgaard, S.E., Thomsen, S., et al. (1987). Prediction of post-concussional sequelae by reaction time test. *Acta Neurol Scand*, 75:341–345.

INDEX